Clinical Risks and Perinatal Outcomes in Pregnancy and Childbirth

Clinical Risks and Perinatal Outcomes in Pregnancy and Childbirth

Guest Editors

Apostolos Mamopoulos
Ioannis Tsakiridis

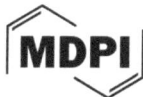

Basel • Beijing • Wuhan • Barcelona • Belgrade • Novi Sad • Cluj • Manchester

Guest Editors

Apostolos Mamopoulos
Third Department of
Obstetrics and Gynaecology
School of Medicine
Faculty of Health Sciences
Aristotle University of
Thessaloniki
Thessaloniki
Greece

Ioannis Tsakiridis
Third Department of
Obstetrics and Gynecology
School of Medicine
Faculty of Health Sciences
Aristotle University of
Thessaloniki
Thessaloniki
Greece

Editorial Office
MDPI AG
Grosspeteranlage 5
4052 Basel, Switzerland

This is a reprint of the Special Issue, published open access by the journal *Journal of Clinical Medicine* (ISSN 2077-0383), freely accessible at: https://www.mdpi.com/journal/jcm/special_issues/F72RCZF0A6.

For citation purposes, cite each article independently as indicated on the article page online and as indicated below:

Lastname, A.A.; Lastname, B.B. Article Title. *Journal Name* **Year**, *Volume Number*, Page Range.

ISBN 978-3-7258-3651-2 (Hbk)
ISBN 978-3-7258-3652-9 (PDF)
https://doi.org/10.3390/books978-3-7258-3652-9

© 2025 by the authors. Articles in this book are Open Access and distributed under the Creative Commons Attribution (CC BY) license. The book as a whole is distributed by MDPI under the terms and conditions of the Creative Commons Attribution-NonCommercial-NoDerivs (CC BY-NC-ND) license (https://creativecommons.org/licenses/by-nc-nd/4.0/).

Contents

Sien Lenie, Laure Sillis, Karel Allegaert, Annick Bogaerts, Anne Smits,
Kristel Van Calsteren, et al.
Alcohol, Tobacco and Illicit Drug Use During Pregnancy in the Longitudinal BELpREG Cohort
in Belgium Between 2022 and 2024
Reprinted from: *J. Clin. Med.* 2025, 14, 613, https://doi.org/10.3390/jcm14020613 1

Maria Tzitiridou-Chatzopoulou, Georgia Zournatzidou, Eirini Orovou, Lazaros Lavasidis,
Arsenios Tsiotsias, Panagiotis Eskitzis and Dimitrios Papoutsis
Intermittent Preventive Treatment of Malaria in Pregnancy and the Impact on Neonates in
African Countries as Assessed by Entropy Weight and TOPSIS Methods
Reprinted from: *J. Clin. Med.* 2024, 13, 6231, https://doi.org/10.3390/jcm13206231 20

Maria Tzitiridou-Chatzopoulou and Georgia Zournatzidou
Bibliometric Analysis on of the Impact of Screening to Minimize Maternal Mental Health on
Neonatal Outcomes: A Systematic Review
Reprinted from: *J. Clin. Med.* 2024, 13, 6013, https://doi.org/10.3390/jcm13196013 32

Antonios Siargkas, Ioannis Tsakiridis, Athanasios Gatsis, Catalina De Paco Matallana,
Maria Mar Gil, Petya Chaveeva and Themistoklis Dagklis
Risk Factors of Velamentous Cord Insertion in Singleton Pregnancies—A Systematic Review
and Meta-Analysis
Reprinted from: *J. Clin. Med.* 2024, 13, 5551, https://doi.org/10.3390/jcm13185551 50

Yuichiro Narita, Hiroyuki Tsuda, Eri Tsugeno, Yumi Nakamura, Miho Suzuki,
Yumiko Ito, et al.
Association between Subclinical Hypothyroidism and Adverse Pregnancy Outcomes in
Assisted Reproduction Technology Singleton Pregnancies: A Retrospective Study
Reprinted from: *J. Clin. Med.* 2024, 13, 5137, https://doi.org/10.3390/jcm13175137 69

Virginia A. Aparicio, Nuria Marín-Jiménez, Jose Castro-Piñero, Marta Flor-Alemany,
Irene Coll-Risco and Laura Baena-García
Association between Flexibility, Measured with the Back-Scratch Test, and the Odds of Oxytocin
Administration during Labour and Caesarean Section
Reprinted from: *J. Clin. Med.* 2024, 13, 5245, https://doi.org/10.3390/jcm13175245 78

Kirstin Tindal, Fiona L. Cousins, Stacey J. Ellery, Kirsten R. Palmer, Adrienne Gordon,
Caitlin E. Filby, et al.
Investigating Menstruation and Adverse Pregnancy Outcomes: Oxymoron or New Frontier?
A Narrative Review
Reprinted from: *J. Clin. Med.* 2024, 13, 4430, https://doi.org/10.3390/jcm13154430 89

Claire de Moreuil, Brigitte Pan-Petesch, Dino Mehic, Daniel Kraemmer, Theresa Schramm,
Casilda Albert, et al.
Predelivery Haemostatic Biomarkers in Women with Non-Severe Postpartum Haemorrhage
Reprinted from: *J. Clin. Med.* 2024, 13, 4231, https://doi.org/10.3390/jcm13144231 105

Elena Mellado-García, Lourdes Díaz-Rodríguez, Jonathan Cortés-Martín,
Juan Carlos Sánchez-García, Beatriz Piqueras-Sola, Juan Carlos Higuero Macías, et al.
Comparative Analysis of Therapeutic Showers and Bathtubs for Pain Management and Labor
Outcomes—A Retrospective Cohort Study
Reprinted from: *J. Clin. Med.* 2024, 13, 3517, https://doi.org/10.3390/jcm13123517 117

Elena Mellado-García, Lourdes Díaz-Rodríguez, Jonathan Cortés-Martín,
Juan Carlos Sánchez-García, Beatriz Piqueras-Sola, María Montserrat Prieto Franganillo
and Raquel Rodríguez-Blanque
Hydrotherapy in Pain Management in Pregnant Women: A Meta-Analysis of Randomized Clinical Trials
Reprinted from: *J. Clin. Med.* **2024**, *13*, 3260, https://doi.org/10.3390/jcm13113260 128

Carlos H. Becerra-Mojica, Miguel A. Parra-Saavedra, Ruth A. Martínez-Vega,
Luis A. Díaz-Martínez, Raigam J. Martínez-Portilla, Johnatan Torres-Torres and
Bladimiro Rincon-Orozco
Performance of the First-Trimester Cervical Consistency Index to Predict Preterm Birth
Reprinted from: *J. Clin. Med.* **2024**, *13*, 3906, https://doi.org/10.3390/jcm13133906 138

Kyriaki Mitta, Ioannis Tsakiridis, Evaggelia Giougi, Apostolos Mamopoulos,
Ioannis Kalogiannidis, Themistoklis Dagklis and Apostolos Athanasiadis
Comparison of Fetal Crown-Rump Length Measurements between Thawed and Fresh Embryo Transfer
Reprinted from: *J. Clin. Med.* **2024**, *13*, 2575, https://doi.org/10.3390/jcm13092575 149

Zivile Sabonyte-Balsaitiene, Tomas Poskus, Eugenijus Jasiunas, Diana Ramasauskaite
and Grazina Drasutiene
Incidence and Risk Factors of Perianal Pathology during Pregnancy and Postpartum Period: A Prospective Cohort Study
Reprinted from: *J. Clin. Med.* **2024**, *13*, 2371, https://doi.org/10.3390/jcm13082371 158

Maciej Ziętek, Małgorzata Szczuko and Tomasz Machałowski
Gastrointestinal Disorders and Atopic Dermatitis in Infants in the First Year of Life According to ROME IV Criteria—A Possible Association with the Mode of Delivery and Early Life Nutrition
Reprinted from: *J. Clin. Med.* **2024**, *13*, 927, https://doi.org/10.3390/jcm13040927 174

Kyriaki Mitta, Ioannis Tsakiridis, Themistoklis Dagklis, Ioannis Kalogiannidis,
Apostolos Mamopoulos, Georgios Michos, et al.
Ultrasonographic Evaluation of the Second Stage of Labor according to the Mode of Delivery: A Prospective Study in Greece
Reprinted from: *J. Clin. Med.* **2024**, *13*, 1068, https://doi.org/10.3390/jcm13041068 185

Sophia Tsokkou, Dimitrios Kavvadas, Maria-Nefeli Georgaki, Kyriaki Papadopoulou,
Theodora Papamitsou and Sofia Karachrysafi
Genetic and Epigenetic Factors Associated with Postpartum Psychosis: A 5-Year Systematic Review
Reprinted from: *J. Clin. Med.* **2024**, *13*, 964, https://doi.org/10.3390/jcm13040964 196

Johann Hêches, Sandra Marcadent, Anna Fernandez, Stephen Adjahou, Jean-Yves Meuwly,
Jean-Philippe Thiran, et al.
Accuracy and Reliability of Pelvimetry Measures Obtained by Manual or Automatic Labeling of Three-Dimensional Pelvic Models
Reprinted from: *J. Clin. Med.* **2024**, *13*, 689, https://doi.org/10.3390/jcm13030689 209

Rosalia Pascal, Irene Casas, Mariona Genero, Ayako Nakaki, Lina Youssef,
Marta Larroya, et al.
Maternal Stress, Anxiety, Well-Being, and Sleep Quality in Pregnant Women throughout Gestation
Reprinted from: *J. Clin. Med.* **2023**, *12*, 7333, https://doi.org/10.3390/jcm12237333 221

**Renata Saucedo, María Isabel Peña-Cano, Mary Flor Díaz-Velázquez,
Aldo Ferreira-Hermosillo, Juan Mario Solis-Paredes, Ignacio Camacho-Arroyo
and Jorge Valencia-Ortega**
Gestational Weight Gain Is Associated with the Expression of Genes Involved in Inflammation in Maternal Visceral Adipose Tissue and Offspring Anthropometric Measures
Reprinted from: *J. Clin. Med.* **2023**, *12*, 6766, https://doi.org/10.3390/jcm12216766 . . . . **237**

Piotr Gibała, Anna Jarosz-Lesz, Zuzanna Sołtysiak-Gibała, Jakub Staniczek and Rafał Stojko
Multifactorial Colonization of the Pregnant Woman's Reproductive Tract: Implications for Early Postnatal Adaptation in Full-Term Newborns
Reprinted from: *J. Clin. Med.* **2023**, *12*, 6852, https://doi.org/10.3390/jcm12216852 . . . . **246**

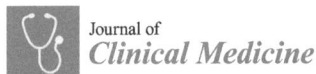

Article

Alcohol, Tobacco and Illicit Drug Use During Pregnancy in the Longitudinal BELpREG Cohort in Belgium Between 2022 and 2024

Sien Lenie [1,†], Laure Sillis [1,2,3,†], Karel Allegaert [1,3,4,5], Annick Bogaerts [3,4,6], Anne Smits [3,4,7], Kristel Van Calsteren [4,8], Jan Y. Verbakel [9,10], Veerle Foulon [1,3] and Michael Ceulemans [1,2,3,*]

1. Clinical Pharmacology and Pharmacotherapy, Department of Pharmaceutical and Pharmacological Sciences, KU Leuven, 3000 Leuven, Belgium; sien.lenie@kuleuven.be (S.L.); laure.sillis@kuleuven.be (L.S.); karel.allegaert@kuleuven.be (K.A.); veerle.foulon@kuleuven.be (V.F.)
2. Research Foundation Flanders, 1000 Brussels, Belgium
3. L-C&Y, Child and Youth Institute KU Leuven, 3000 Leuven, Belgium; annick.bogaerts@kuleuven.be (A.B.); anne.smits@uzleuven.be (A.S.)
4. Department of Development and Regeneration, KU Leuven, 3000 Leuven, Belgium; kristel.vancalsteren@uzleuven.be
5. Department of Hospital Pharmacy, Erasmus MC, 3015 GD Rotterdam, The Netherlands
6. Faculty of Health, University of Plymouth, Devon PL4 8AA, UK
7. Neonatal Intensive Care Unit, University Hospitals Leuven, 3000 Leuven, Belgium
8. Department of Obstetrics and Gynaecology, University Hospitals Leuven, 3000 Leuven, Belgium
9. Department of Public Health and Primary Care, KU Leuven, 3000 Leuven, Belgium; jan.verbakel@kuleuven.be
10. Nuffield Department of Primary Care Health Sciences, University of Oxford, Oxford OX2 6GG, UK
* Correspondence: michael.ceulemans@kuleuven.be
† These authors contributed equally to this work.

Abstract: Background/Objectives: Substance use during pregnancy is associated with adverse outcomes for both mother and child. This study aimed to determine the prevalence and determinants of alcohol, tobacco and illicit drug use before and during pregnancy in Belgium. **Methods:** An observational study was conducted using data from the longitudinal BELpREG registry. The study included women aged 18 years or older who completed at least one questionnaire on substance use during pregnancy between 2022 and 2024. Data were analyzed using descriptive statistics and logistic regressions. **Results:** In total, 1441 women were included. Preconception prevalences of alcohol, tobacco and illicit drug use were 82.2%, 10.0% and 4.2%. These self-reported prevalences dropped in the first trimester to 12.9%, 4.1% and 0.6%, respectively. Considering the rates of substance use in pregnancy but before pregnancy awareness, the overall prevalence of alcohol, tobacco and illicit drug use in the first trimester was 41.0%, 6.6% and 1.2%, respectively. Women with a higher education (aOR (adjusted odds ratio), 2.12; 95% CI (confidence interval): 1.14–3.96), unplanned pregnancies (aOR, 2.88; 95% CI: 1.77–4.67), spontaneous pregnancies (aOR, 2.94; 95% CI: 1.51–5.75), cohabitants drinking alcohol daily (aOR, 2.01; 95% CI: 1.09–3.70), and those using tobacco in the first trimester (aOR, 5.37; 95% CI: 2.70–10.66) were more likely to report alcohol use. In addition, women with a lower education (aOR, 7.67; 95% CI: 3.76–15.67), unplanned pregnancies (aOR, 3.31; 95% CI: 1.53–7.15), cohabitants using tobacco (aOR, 9.11; 95% CI: 4.48–18.52), and those who used alcohol (aOR, 6.67; 95% CI: 3.07–14.64) or illicit drugs (aOR, 39.03; 95% CI: 3.72–409.83) in the first trimester were more likely to report tobacco use. **Conclusions:** Despite a significant reduction in substance use in pregnancy compared to before pregnancy, a relevant portion of women continue to use substances, particularly in the early stages before pregnancy awareness. Targeted public health interventions and (more) awareness among caregivers are needed to further promote substance use cessation before conception.

Keywords: pregnancy; substance use; preconception care; observational research; Belgium

1. Introduction

Substance use during pregnancy, including alcohol, tobacco and illicit drug use, is a significant public health concern due to its association with adverse maternal (miscarriage, preterm birth, or placental abruption) [1–6] and neonatal outcomes (small for gestational age (SGA), prematurity, or fetal alcohol syndrome (FAS)) [1–8]. Likewise, maternal complications such as maternal anemia and postpartum depression have been associated with perinatal substance use [4,6,9–11]. Substance use in pregnancy, even in small amounts, has also been linked to teratogenic effects, including craniofacial abnormalities, organ malformations and neurodevelopmental impairment such as lower IQ or behavioral problems [2,3,7,8,12]. Additionally, substance use prior to conception, which may be linked to poorer maternal preconception health, has been associated with adverse pregnancy and neonatal outcomes [13–15]. These findings emphasize the importance of avoiding substance use before and in pregnancy to ensure optimal maternal and infant health.

Although adverse effects following substance use during pregnancy have been extensively described, pregnant women may be somewhat unaware of the potential impact of the associated risks or will not value the risk as important. In 2016, only 48% of the pregnant women (in their 20th week of pregnancy) who received care in a public university hospital in Spain knew that the teratogenic effects of prenatal alcohol exposure are lifelong and 27.1% could not specify any risks when asked [16]. Furthermore, a low perception of risks was correlated with more frequent alcohol use [16]. As a safe lower limit for alcohol has not been defined, health authorities worldwide, including the World Health Organization [17], recommend complete abstinence from alcohol use during pregnancy. Similarly, abstinence from tobacco and illicit drug use is also strongly advised.

Despite the recommendations of avoiding any substance use during pregnancy, the most recent data from Belgium collected in 2016 showed that substance use in a highly educated cohort of pregnant women visiting a tertiary obstetrics clinic was prevalent, with about 6% reporting alcohol or tobacco use during the previous week (almost equally divided over the gestational trimesters) [18]. Given the outdated nature of these findings and the well-known adverse effects of substance use in pregnancy, updated and more comprehensive data were urgently needed to reflect current prevalences and identify determinants of such use in Belgium. In fact, insights into substance use in pregnancy are vital to assess the need for public health interventions, while identifying specific subgroups which should be primarily targeted.

Therefore, this study aimed to determine the current prevalence of alcohol, tobacco and illicit drug use before and during pregnancy in Belgium, as well as the characteristics associated with alcohol and tobacco use during pregnancy.

2. Materials and Methods

2.1. Study Design and Population

An observational study was performed using data collected in the BELpREG pregnancy registry (see www.belpreg.be/en, accessed on 3 December 2024). The BELpREG registry is the only ongoing, prospective, longitudinal, perinatal cohort in Belgium using digital self-reported questionnaires to collect real-world data on periconceptional exposures and mother–infant outcomes. BELpREG aims to gain more knowledge on the utilization and safety of exposure to medications, vaccines, health products and other substances around pregnancy [19]. BELpREG was established in November 2022. All pregnant persons

18 years or older and receiving healthcare in Belgium are considered eligible to participate in the BELpREG cohort. Upon enrolment, participants complete the first ("enrolment") questionnaire, followed by subsequent ("follow-up") questionnaires every four weeks during pregnancy until eight weeks postpartum. Additionally, participants receive two questionnaires on child health and development at 6 and 12 months after birth. The BELpREG questionnaires were developed using the core data elements compiled within the IMI ConcePTION project [20] and supplemented with variables defined by the European Medicines Agency and existing, similar registration systems [21]. Individuals can enroll in BELpREG at any time during pregnancy, although enrolment as early on as possible in pregnancy is preferred. BELpREG recruits pregnant women through various channels, including social media (advertising), healthcare professional referrals and via printed and digital posters and flyers. BELpREG questionnaires are available in Dutch, French and English (with the French and English translations added in January 2024). More details on the development and design of the BELpREG pregnancy registry have previously been described elsewhere [19,22].

Data extraction for this study took place on 13 August 2024. All BELpREG participants who had completed at least one questionnaire on substance use during pregnancy by the time of data extraction were included in this study. The number of questionnaires completed by each participant varied between one and eleven, as enrolment could occur at any time during pregnancy. Further, participants were not required to already have delivered. Participants who had not completed the substance use questions at enrolment, or missed a follow-up questionnaire in pregnancy, could still complete questions related to substance use in a later follow-up questionnaire and hence, were included in this study.

Ethics approval was obtained from EC Research UZ/KU Leuven (S66464); all participants provided an electronic informed consent prior to study enrolment. The study is reported using the STROBE checklist (see Supplementary Material S1) [23].

2.2. Study Outcomes

Participants were asked about their exposure to alcohol, tobacco (i.e., defined as cigarettes or vaping, the latter defined as e-cigarettes containing nicotine) and illicit drug use in the preconception period (i.e., defined as the year before conception), during the 1st trimester (i.e., gestational week 1–12), 2nd trimester (i.e., week 13–26) and 3rd trimester (i.e., week 27 until the last follow-up questionnaire before delivery).

Preconception use of alcohol, tobacco and illicit drug use was assessed at the enrolment questionnaire by asking questions on any exposures in the year before pregnancy (yes/no).

Alcohol, tobacco and illicit drug use *during* pregnancy were queried in the enrolment and four-weekly follow-up questionnaires in pregnancy (yes/no). Participants who reported not using any substances during pregnancy at the enrolment questionnaire were asked about the timing of alcohol, tobacco and illicit drug use cessation (i.e., in the year before pregnancy, since trying to get pregnant, since I knew I was pregnant). Additional questions focused on the amount of alcohol and tobacco use during pregnancy. More specifically, with respect to alcohol, the amount of alcohol use was asked based on the following three questions: (1) the frequency of drinking alcohol during pregnancy (i.e., monthly or less, 2–4 times a month, 2–3 times a week, 4 or more times a week), (2) the number of standard glasses of alcohol (i.e., defined as the amount of a drink that is usually served in a pub or at a restaurant, e.g., 25cl beer or 10cl wine) used per occasion (i.e., <1, 1 or 2, 3 or 4, 5 or 6, 7 or 9, 10 or more) and (3) binge drinking during pregnancy, which was defined as the consumption of six or more standard glasses of alcohol on one occasion (i.e., never, less than monthly, monthly, weekly, daily or almost daily). With respect to tobacco use, the amount of tobacco used was assessed based on the mean daily number of cigarettes between two consecutive BELpREG questionnaires. The categories 1–10 cigarettes/day, 11–20 cigarettes/day, 21–30 cigarettes/day, >30 cigarettes/day were used until July 2024, after which the following modified categories were used to obtain more detailed data: <1 cigarette/day, 1–5 cigarettes/day, 6–10 cigarettes/day, 11–20 cigarettes/day and >20 cigarettes/day. Lastly, the type of illicit drugs used in pregnancy was questioned (i.e., cannabis, XTC, amphetamines, hallucinogens, cocaine, ketamine, heroine, GHB, or other).

The questionnaires on substance use were based on established European standards (e.g., with respect to binge drinking), and were further refined with the input from expert centers in our country (i.e., Flemish Expertise Centre for Alcohol and Other Drugs and the Flemish Institute for Healthy Living) [19]. A detailed overview of the substance use-related questions is provided in Supplementary Material S2.

2.3. Covariates

The following covariates, for which an association with either alcohol or tobacco use during pregnancy has previously been reported, were available in and extracted from the enrolment questionnaire: maternal age [24–34], maternal ethnical background [26,28,31,32,34–36], marital status [29,30,37,38], maternal education [25,26,29,30,34,36–41], paternal education [31], maternal employment in the past year [30,31,40,41], household annual gross income [25,37], preconception body mass index (BMI) [26,28,36], chronic condition prior to pregnancy [26], (un)planned pregnancy [27,29,31], method of conception [28], gravidity [25,26,28,29,31,40], previous planned termination of pregnancy [32], intention to breastfeed [31] and substance use among cohabitants [31,41]. A detailed overview of the questions related to these covariates is provided in Supplementary Material S2.

2.4. Data Handling and Analysis

Descriptive statistics were used to determine the characteristics of the total study population and the participants who had reported any substance use in the first trimester.

Descriptive statistics were also used to report the prevalence of alcohol, tobacco and illicit drug use in the preconception period, in each trimester and during pregnancy. To calculate the timing of substance use during pregnancy, gestational age was defined based on the expected delivery date, which was determined by ultrasound (as the preferred option), the start date of the last menstrual period, or the moment of conception in case of assisted reproductive technology (ART), along with the date of survey completion. The prevalence for each trimester was calculated based on the gestational age at the moment of survey completion. The prevalence for each trimester was determined using data of the enrolment and/or follow-up questionnaires of participants who had fully completed that trimester and who had provided data on substance use during that specific trimester. For the calculation of the prevalence of the entire pregnancy, only participants who had given birth by the time of data extraction were considered by combining all registrations of substance use obtained during pregnancy. With respect to binge drinking, this variable was dichotomized (yes/no) and also used for the calculations per trimester or total pregnancy.

The amount of alcohol and tobacco use during pregnancy was analyzed as follows. First, the total number of standard glasses of alcohol was calculated considering the frequency of alcohol use and the number of glasses of alcohol used per occasion. The latter two questions were combined to the number of standard glasses of alcohol per day. Taking into account the number of days between two consecutive questionnaires, the total number of standard glasses over this period was calculated. Second, the mean number of cigarettes per day was calculated based on the mean daily number of cigarettes reported across the various questionnaires/periods. Therefore, the mean number of cigarettes per day was recoded from never used tobacco, <1, 1–5, 1–10, 6–10, 11–20, 21–30, >20 and >30 cigarettes per day into 0, 0.5, 2.5, 5, 7.5, 15, 25, 25 and 35 cigarettes per day choosing the midpoint, to be able to pool data from the initial and modified response categories [42,43]. The time period for alcohol and tobacco use was determined in the same way as for the calculation of the prevalence of alcohol, tobacco and illicit drug use.

In addition to descriptive statistics, backward multivariable logistic regressions were applied to determine characteristics associated with alcohol and tobacco use in the first pregnancy trimester. Only participants who reported any alcohol or tobacco use during pregnancy and who were beyond the first trimester by the time of data extraction were considered for the regression analysis (i.e., dependent variable). Regressions were only performed if numbers allowed, which was the case for alcohol and tobacco but not for illicit drug use. The following independent variables were used in the models: maternal age, maternal ethnical background, marital status, maternal education, preconception BMI, chronic condition before pregnancy, (un)planned pregnancy, method of conception, gravidity, previous planned termination of pregnancy, daily alcohol drinking cohabitant, a tobacco-using cohabitant, an illicit drug-using cohabitant, preconception alcohol use, preconception tobacco use, alcohol use during the 1st trimester, tobacco use during the 1st trimester and illicit drug use in the 1st trimester. Non-significant covariates ($p > 0.05$) were removed from the model one-by-one until only significant covariates remained. Collinearity among the covariates was checked using Pearson correlation coefficients, with a cut-off value of 0.90. The results are shown as adjusted odds ratios (aORs) with 95% confidence intervals (95% CI). A sensitivity analysis was conducted to identify determinants of alcohol and tobacco use in the first trimester, utilizing univariable and multivariable logistic regressions with a stepwise approach. Covariates with a p-value < 0.10 in the univariable analyses were included in the multivariable models. Statistical analyses were conducted using IBM SPSS Statistics version 29.

3. Results

3.1. Characteristics of the Study Population

In total, 1651 pregnant women had been enrolled in the BELpREG cohort by 13 August 2024. Out of these, 1441 women had completed at least one questionnaire on substance use and were included for this study. Figure 1 provides an overview of the study sample, highlighting the number of participants used for the calculation of the prevalence of substance use prior to and during pregnancy (first, second, and third trimesters and entire pregnancy).

Table 1 presents the characteristics of the study population in general and according to alcohol and tobacco use in the first trimester. About half of the participants were aged between 30 and 34 years (50.9%). Most participants identified as Caucasian (96.9%) and had a partner (95.4%). Further, 85.2% had a high education level. Among participants with a partner, 68.3% of their partners were also highly educated. The employment rate in the past year among participants was 95.2%.

With respect to maternal health, 57.2% had a preconception BMI between 18.5 and 25 kg/m^2. A chronic condition prior to pregnancy was reported by 38.2% of the participants. Among those participants suffering from chronic conditions, the most common conditions were allergic rhinitis (due to pollen) (15.5%), asthma (11.3%), migraine (11.1%), allergic or hypersensitivity conditions (8.0%) and hypothyroidism (7.1%).

Moreover, most of the pregnancies were planned (89.9%), 52.7% of the participants were multigravidae and 17.8% cited undergoing assisted reproductive technology (ART) prior to the index pregnancy. A previous planned termination of pregnancy was reported by 12.4% of multigravida participants. Lastly, the intention to breastfeed at the time of enrolment in the BELpREG registry was high (83.2%).

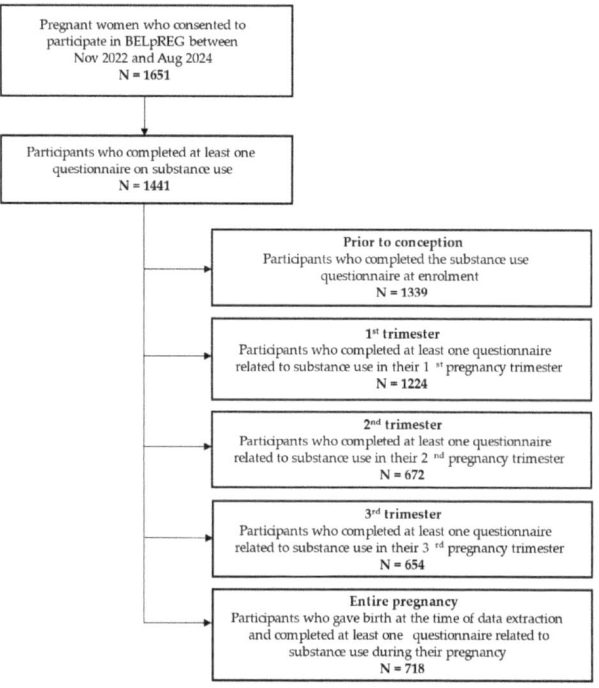

Figure 1. Overview of the study sample, highlighting the five different groups used for the calculation of the prevalence of substance use prior to and during pregnancy (i.e., 1st, 2nd and 3rd trimesters and entire pregnancy).

Table 1. Characteristics of the study population in general and after stratification according to self-reported alcohol and tobacco use in the first pregnancy trimester.

Characteristics	All Pregnant Women (N = 1441)		Pregnant Women Who Used Alcohol in the 1st Trimester [1] (N = 158)		Pregnant Women Who Used Tobacco in the 1st Trimester [1] (N = 50)	
	N	%	N	%	N	%
Sociodemographic variables						
Maternal age (in years)						
18–24	27	1.9	4	2.5	3	6.0
25–29	449	31.2	50	31.6	15	36.0
30–34	733	50.9	82	51.9	20	40.0
35–39	176	12.2	21	13.3	11	22.0
≥40	21	1.5	1	0.6	1	2.0
Missing	35	2.4	-	-	-	-
Maternal ethnical background						
Caucasian	1397	96.9	157	99.4	48	96.0
Non-Caucasian or I do not know	19	1.4	1	0.6	2	4.0
Missing	25	1.7	-	-	-	-

Table 1. Cont.

Characteristics	All Pregnant Women (N = 1441)		Pregnant Women Who Used Alcohol in the 1st Trimester [1] (N = 158)		Pregnant Women Who Used Tobacco in the 1st Trimester [1] (N = 50)	
	N	%	N	%	N	%
Marital status						
Partner	1375	95.4	157	99.4	47	94.0
No partner	41	2.8	1	0.6	3	6.0
Missing	25	1.7	-	-	-	-
Maternal education [2]						
Low/medium	188	13.1	20	12.7	29	58.0
High	1228	85.2	138	87.3	21	42.0
Missing	25	1.7	-	-	-	-
Paternal education [2]						
Low/medium	429	31.2	41	26.1	30	65.2
High	939	68.3	116	73.9	16	34.8
Missing	7	0.5	-	-	-	-
Maternal employment status in the past year						
Employed	1372	95.2	156	98.7	50	100.0
Not employed	44	3.1	2	1.3	0	0.0
Missing	25	1.7	-	-	-	-
Annual household gross income						
EUR < 45,000	171	11.9	19	12.0	11	22.0
EUR 45,000–65,000	342	23.7	30	19.0	17	34.0
EUR > 65,000	562	39.0	76	48.1	7	14.0
I do not know/I would rather not tell	341	23.7	33	20.9	15	30.0
Missing	25	1.7	-	-	-	-
Maternal preconception BMI (kg/m^2)						
<18.5	48	3.3	4	2.5	1	2.0
18.5–25	824	57.2	101	63.9	27	54.0
25–30	342	23.7	37	23.4	14	28.0
>30	201	13.9	16	10.1	8	16.0
Missing	26	1.8	-	-	-	-
Chronic medical condition prior to pregnancy [3]						
Yes	550	38.2	51	32.3	20	40.0
No	866	60.1	107	67.7	30	60.0
Missing	25	1.7	-	-	-	-
Pregnancy-related variables						
Planned pregnancy						
Yes	1295	89.9	125	79.1	33	66.0
No	121	8.4	25	20.9	17	34.0
Missing	25	1.7	-	-	-	-

Table 1. Cont.

Characteristics	All Pregnant Women (N = 1441)		Pregnant Women Who Used Alcohol in the 1st Trimester [1] (N = 158)		Pregnant Women Who Used Tobacco in the 1st Trimester [1] (N = 50)	
	N	%	N	%	N	%
Method of conception						
Spontaneous	1159	80.4	148	93.7	47	94.0
ART [4]	257	17.8	10	6.3	3	6.0
Missing	25	1.7	-	-	-	-
Gravidity						
Primigravida	657	45.6	76	48.1	18	36.0
Multigravida	759	52.7	82	51.9	32	64.0
Missing	25	1.7	-	-	-	-
Previous planned termination of pregnancy						
Yes	94	12.4	13	15.9	9	28.1
No	663	87.4	69	84.1	23	71.9
Missing	2	0.2	-	-	-	-
Intention to breastfeed						
Yes	1199	83.2	128	81.0	41	82.0
No or I do not know yet	217	15.1	30	19.0	9	18.0
Missing	25	1.7	-	-	-	-
Environmental variables at the time of enrolment						
Cohabitant who was drinking alcohol daily						
Yes	74	5.1	16	10.1	6	12.0
No	1265	87.8	142	89.9	44	88.0
Missing	102	7.1	-	-	-	-
Cohabitant who was using tobacco						
Yes	173	12.0	22	13.9	30	60.0
No	1166	80.9	136	86.1	20	40.0
Missing	102	7.1	-	-	-	-
Cohabitant who was using illicit drugs						
Yes	34	2.4	6	3.8	5	10.0
No	1305	90.6	152	96.2	45	90.0
Missing	102	7.1	-	-	-	-

[1] Considering pregnant women who reported alcohol and/or tobacco use during the first trimester. [2] High education is defined as any formal degree obtained in higher education or university. [3] A chronic condition prior to pregnancy was defined as any diagnosed chronic condition before the start of the index pregnancy. [4] ART is defined as assisted reproductive technology.

Upon enrolment in the BELpREG registry, 5.1% indicated having a cohabitant who was drinking alcohol daily (i.e., at the time the pregnant woman enrolled in the pregnancy registry), 12.0% reported having a cohabitant using tobacco and 2.4% answered having a cohabitant who was using illicit drugs. The median gestational age at enrolment in the BELpREG registry, at the time of data extraction, was 16 weeks (IQR (interquartile range): 10–25 weeks).

3.2. Prevalences of Alcohol, Tobacco and Illicit Drug Use

Table 2 shows the prevalence of alcohol, tobacco and illicit drug use before and during pregnancy. Regarding exposure *prior to conception*, 82.2% reported alcohol use, 10.0% tobacco use and 4.2% illicit drug use.

Table 2. Prevalences and the amount of self-reported alcohol, tobacco and illicit drug use before and during pregnancy.

	Preconception [1] N = 1339	Trimester 1 [2] N = 1224	Trimester 2 [2] N = 972	Trimester 3 [3] N = 654	Total Pregnancy [4] N = 718
Alcohol use					
Prevalence	1100 (82.2%)	158 (12.9%)	35 (3.6%)	31 (4.7%)	105 (14.6%)
Total number of standard glasses					
<1		40 (25.3%)	2 (5.7%)	5 (16.1%)	22 (21.0%)
1–5		76 (48.1%)	16 (45.7%)	11 (35.5%)	51 (48.6%)
5–10		18 (11.4%)	11 (31.4%)	12 (38.7%)	17 (16.2%)
10–20		10 (6.3%)	1 (2.9%)	1 (3.2%)	9 (8.6%)
20–40		10 (6.3%)	5 (14.3%)	2 (6.5%)	4 (3.8%)
>40		4 (2.5%)	0 (0.0%)	0 (0.0%)	2 (1.9%)
Binge drinking [5]		50 (4.1%)	7 (0.7%)	5 (0.8%)	33 (4.6%)
Tobacco use					
Prevalence	134 (10.0%)	50 (4.1%)	19 (2.0%)	14 (2.1%)	29 (4.0%)
Mean number of cigarettes per day					
<1		0 (0.0%)	1 (5.3%)	1 (7.1%)	13 (44.8%)
1–5		45 (90.0%)	17 (89.5%)	11 (78.6%)	15 (51.7%)
5–10		5 (10.0%)	1 (5.3%)	2 (14.3%)	1 (3.4%)
Illicit drug use					
Prevalence	56 (4.2%)	7 (0.6%)	6 (0.6%)	1 (0.2%)	3 (0.4%)

[1] Preconception was defined as the year prior to conception; for this variable, all women who completed the enroll questionnaire on substance use were considered. [2] Per trimester: considering all women who were beyond the first or second trimester at the time of data extraction and provided data on substance use during the respective trimester. [3] Third trimester: considering all women who had already given birth at the time of data extraction and provided data on substance use during the third trimester. [4] Total pregnancy: considering all women who had already given birth at the time of data extraction. [5] Binge drinking was defined as the consumption of ≥6 standard glasses of alcohol on one occasion.

During the first trimester, the self-reported prevalence of alcohol, tobacco and illicit drug use was 12.9%, 4.1% and 0.6%, respectively. *During the second trimester*, alcohol use was reported by 3.6%, tobacco use by 2.0% and illicit drug use by 0.6%. Prevalences for the *third trimester* were 4.7% for alcohol use, 2.1% for tobacco use and 0.2% for illicit drug use. Considering the entire pregnancy (i.e., including only women who had already delivered by the time of data extraction), 14.6% of the participants reported alcohol use, 4.0% tobacco use and 0.4% illicit drug use during pregnancy. Notably, pregnant women who reported substance use cessation only after becoming aware of their pregnancy were excluded from these prevalence calculations.

Further, binge drinking was reported by 10.0% of the women prior to conception, 4.1% in the first trimester, 2.0% in the second trimester, 2.1% in the third trimester and 4.6% over the entire pregnancy.

Finally, the few women who reported the use of illicit drugs during pregnancy (n = 7) had used cannabis (n = 5), cocaine (n = 3) and ketamine (n = 1). Among these women, two used more than one illicit drug during pregnancy.

3.3. Quantity of Alcohol and Tobacco Use During Pregnancy

Table 2 illustrates the amount of self-reported alcohol and tobacco used in pregnancy. Nearly half of the participants who had delivered by the time of data extraction (48.6%) reported having drunk 1–5 standard glasses of alcohol *throughout the entire pregnancy*, 21.0% less than 1 glass and 16.2% 5–10 glasses. With regard to the first trimester, 25.3% consumed less than 1 glass, 48.1% 1–5 glasses and about 1/4 more than 5 standard glasses.

For tobacco use, the mean number of cigarettes used per day *in the first trimester* for most women using tobacco (90.0%) was 1–5 cigarettes. Similar results were found for the second and third trimester. With regard to the entire pregnancy, about half of the women using tobacco consumed on average less than 1 cigarette a day or 1–5 cigarettes a day. However, when the maximum reported mean number of cigarettes per day was considered, much higher amounts were observed. More specifically, some women reported having used up to 10–20 cigarettes per day, corresponding to 14.0% in the first trimester, 16.7% in the second trimester, 21.4% in the third trimester and 20.7% over the entire pregnancy.

3.4. Prevalences of Early Pregnancy Exposures Before Pregnancy Awareness

Participants who reported substance use prior to but not in pregnancy were asked when they stopped using the substance(s). Overall, 32.3% (n = 344) of participants who indicated that they had not consumed alcohol during pregnancy reported that they ceased alcohol use only after being aware of their pregnancy. Adding this early-pregnancy exposure to the reported exposures during pregnancy (as detailed in Table 2), the total prevalence of any alcohol use in the first trimester was 41.0% (n = 344). Similarly, for tobacco and illicit drug use, 2.6% (n = 31) and 0.7% (n = 8) of participants, respectively, who reported no use in pregnancy admitted to quitting only after becoming aware of their pregnancy. This led to a first-trimester prevalence of any tobacco or illicit drug use of 6.6% (n = 81) and 1.2% (n = 15), respectively. In this cohort, the median gestational age at the time of pregnancy awareness was 4 weeks (IQR: 4–5 weeks).

3.5. Determinants of Alcohol Use in the First Pregnancy Trimester

Table 3 presents the associations between maternal characteristics and alcohol use in the first trimester. Tobacco use in the first trimester, (un)planned pregnancy, daily alcohol use by cohabitant(s), maternal education and the method of conception were found to be associated with alcohol use in the first trimester.

Table 3. Associations between maternal characteristics and alcohol use during the first trimester.

	Alcohol Use in the 1st Trimester	
	aOR [1]	95% CI
Tobacco use in 1st trimester		
Yes	5.37	2.70–10.66
Method of conception		
Spontaneous	2.94	1.51–5.75
Planned pregnancy		
No	2.88	1.77–4.67
Maternal education		
High	2.12	1.14–3.96
Cohabitant who was drinking alcohol daily		
Yes	2.01	1.09–3.70

[1] aOR = adjusted odds ratios, adjusted for maternal education, planned pregnancy, method of conception, cohabitant who was drinking alcohol daily, or tobacco use during the 1st trimester. The results were derived by conducting a backward multivariable logistic regression where non-significant covariates ($p > 0.05$) were removed from the model one-by-one.

An increased likelihood of alcohol use in the first trimester was found for the following covariates: tobacco use in the first trimester, spontaneous pregnancy, unplanned pregnancy, high education level and alcohol use by cohabitant(s). First, tobacco use in the first trimester strongly increased the odds of alcohol use in the first trimester (aOR, 5.37; 95% CI: 2.70–10.66). Second, women who conceived spontaneously were more likely to drink alcohol in the first trimester (aOR, 2.94; 95% CI: 1.51–5.75). Further, an unplanned pregnancy was associated with a nearly threefold increase in the likelihood of alcohol use (aOR, 2.88; 95% CI: 1.77–4.67), while pregnant participants with a high level of education were also more likely to drink alcohol in the first trimester (aOR, 2.12; 95% CI: 1.14–3.96). Finally, having a cohabitant who was drinking alcohol daily doubled the odds of alcohol use by the pregnant woman herself (aOR, 2.01; 95% CI: 1.09–3.70).

All participants who had reported alcohol use in the first trimester also cited alcohol use in the year prior to conception. Hence, preconception alcohol use is an important determinant but could not be included in the regression analysis due to statistical limitations.

3.6. Determinants of Tobacco Use in the First Pregnancy Trimester

Table 4 presents the associations between maternal characteristics and tobacco use in the first trimester. Tobacco use by a cohabitant, alcohol use in the first trimester, maternal education, (un)planned pregnancy and illicit drug use in the first trimester were found to be associated with tobacco use in the first trimester.

Table 4. Associations between maternal characteristics and tobacco use during the first trimester.

	Tobacco Use During the 1st Trimester	
	aOR [1]	95% CI
Cohabitant who was a tobacco user		
Yes	9.11	4.48–18.52
Maternal education		
Low/medium	7.67	3.76–15.67
Alcohol use in 1st trimester		
Yes	6.67	3.07–14.64
Planned pregnancy		
No	3.31	1.53–7.15
Illicit drug use in 1st trimester		
Yes	39.03	3.72–409.83

[1] aOR = adjusted odds ratios, adjusted for maternal education, (un)planned pregnancy, cohabitant who was a tobacco user, alcohol use in the 1st trimester, or illicit drug use in the 1st trimester. The results were derived by conducting a backward multivariable logistic regression where non-significant covariates ($p > 0.05$) were removed from the model one-by-one.

First, a tobacco-using cohabitant strongly increased the odds of tobacco use in the first trimester (aOR, 9.11; 95% CI: 4.48–18.52). Second, alcohol use in the first trimester was strongly associated with tobacco use in the same period (aOR, 6.67; 95% CI: 3.07–14.64). Third, pregnant participants with a low or medium level of education were more likely to use tobacco in the first trimester (aOR, 7.67; 95% CI: 3.76–15.67). Moreover, an unplanned pregnancy was associated with a threefold increase in the likelihood of tobacco use in the first trimester (aOR, 3.31; 95% CI: 1.53–7.15). Finally, although the number of illicit drug users in the first trimester was very limited in our cohort, significantly increased odds of tobacco use in the first trimester were observed among such drug users, despite a very wide confidence interval (aOR, 39.03; 95% CI: 3.72–409.83).

Similar to alcohol use in the first trimester, all participants who reported tobacco use in the first trimester also indicated tobacco use in the year prior to conception. As a result, preconception tobacco use is an important determinant but could not be included in the regressions due to statistical limitations.

A sensitivity analysis was conducted to identify determinants of alcohol and tobacco use in the first trimester using multivariable logistic regressions with a *stepwise approach*. This stepwise method identified the same determinants as presented for both alcohol use (Table S3 in the Supplementary Material S3) and tobacco use during the first trimester (Table S4 in the Supplementary Material S3), except for maternal education level, which was no longer observed as a determinant for alcohol use during the first trimester.

4. Discussion

4.1. Main Findings

This study aimed to provide evidence on the prevalence of alcohol, tobacco and illicit drug use before and during pregnancy in Belgium and determinants of alcohol and tobacco use during pregnancy. The data used in this study had recently been collected by the BELpREG pregnancy registry in Belgium and therefore provide an up-to-date and comprehensive view on this relevant topic in a Western European country.

First, the study found that 82.2% of the pregnant women reported alcohol use, 10.0% tobacco use and 4.2% illicit drug use in the year prior to conception. In our study, alcohol use in the year before pregnancy (82.2%) was somewhat higher compared to the general population of women in Belgium (70.1%) [44], illustrating that alcohol use seems to be the norm in Belgium and is socially accepted. Tobacco use rates (10.0%), in the year prior to conception, were slightly lower compared to the general population (14.6%) [45].

In the first trimester, the self-reported prevalence of alcohol, tobacco and illicit drug use dropped to 12.9%, 4.1% and 0.6%, respectively. Overall, the prevalence of alcohol use was in line with previous studies [18,40,46,47]. Similar prevalences on binge drinking, as observed in our study, have also previously been reported [46]. Moreover, tobacco use in pregnancy was found to be on the lower side of the range of previously found prevalence estimates [28,29,31–34,38,41,48]. In contrast, illicit drug use in pregnancy was found to be ten times lower in our study cohort compared to previous studies from other countries [47,49]. The trend of a lower exposure to illicit drugs was, in our cohort, also reflected by the numbers prior to conception and might be explained by the highly educated sample and different drug regulations across countries affecting the (reporting of) use [47,49,50].

Nevertheless, it is clear that a significant proportion of pregnant women continue to use substances until pregnancy identification. Specifically, 32.3% of women ceased alcohol use only after learning about their pregnancy in the first trimester. The prevalences for tobacco use (2.6%) and use of illicit drugs (0.7%) until pregnancy awareness were much lower. This resulted in a composite, total prevalence of alcohol use in the first trimester of 41.0%, for tobacco use of 6.6% and for illicit drug use of 1.2%. Although previous studies reported even higher prevalences of alcohol use in pregnancy before pregnancy awareness [27,51], our observed numbers are alarming as they show that early pregnancy exposures to substances in the first and most vulnerable weeks of pregnancy still very often occur in our pregnant population. This underscores the need for more emphasis and dissemination to the public on the importance of preconception care, including the recommendations of total abstinence from alcohol, tobacco and illicit drug use [27,51].

When looking at the quantities of alcohol and tobacco use in pregnancy, however, the used amount was generally rather limited. About 21.0% cited drinking less than one standard glass of alcohol in the entire pregnancy and about half of the participants reported drinking one to five standard glasses in total. Some pregnant women described alcohol use as "having a sip of an alcoholic beverage" or "accidently receiving an alcoholic drink instead of a non-alcoholic version." Similarly, 44.8% of participants who reported tobacco use indicated an average consumption of less than one cigarette per day throughout their pregnancy. In contrast, 51.7% of smokers indicated an average use of one to five cigarettes per day over the course of their pregnancy.

With respect to potential determinants, women with a high education level, an unplanned pregnancy, a spontaneous pregnancy, a daily alcohol drinking cohabitant and tobacco use in the first trimester were more likely to drink alcohol in the first trimester. Similar findings were previously reported for education level [37,39,40], pregnancy planning [27] and tobacco use in pregnancy [24,26,35]. Similar trends have also previously been observed in the general population in Belgium and elsewhere, where individuals with higher education levels tend to have higher alcohol consumption rates [44,52]. This has been argued to be a result of greater gender equality in highly developed countries [52]. Further, women with a low/medium education level, an unplanned pregnancy, a tobacco-using cohabitant and using alcohol or illicit drugs in the first trimester were more likely to use tobacco in the first trimester. Many similarities can be drawn with previous studies showing that women with low/medium levels of education [29–32,34,38,41], those who had an unplanned pregnancy [29,31], those with a tobacco-using cohabitant [41] and those using alcohol or illicit drugs in the first trimester [29,31] were more likely to use tobacco in the first trimester. Finally, all participants with self-reported alcohol or tobacco use in the first trimester already used these substances in the year prior to conception.

4.2. Methodological Considerations

This study has some strengths. First, we used a large, longitudinal cohort, enhancing the trustworthiness of the findings. Second, the use of anonymous data reported to the BELpREG registry likely reduced information or social desirability bias, leading to more accurate and reliable data. Moreover, BELpREG questionnaires are sent out every four weeks in pregnancy, minimizing the risk of recall bias. Participants are also required to complete the substance use-related questions in the BELpREG questionnaires, limiting the possibility of missing values. Next, when designing the BELpREG questionnaires related to alcohol, tobacco and illicit drug use, input was sought from the respective centers of expertise in our country on these matters (i.e., Flemish Expertise Centre for Alcohol and Other Drugs and the Flemish Institute for Healthy Living), with the aim of collecting comprehensive and reliable self-reported data on substance use [19]. Further, our study not only provides up-to-date evidence on the extent of the use of various substances during the entire pregnancy but also about substance use before pregnancy awareness, which may not be perceived by women as substance use in pregnancy or after conception. Lastly, a sensitivity analysis was conducted using a different statistical approach for the multivariable logistic regressions, enhancing the robustness and reliability of the findings.

Some limitations should be addressed. First, self-reported data may entail the risk of reporting bias. Currently, no objective measurements or comparisons are in place to verify the self-reported data on substance use in BELpREG. Second, selection bias occurred given the higher education level and employment rates in our sample, limiting the generalizability of the findings. When interpreting the findings from the BELpREG cohort, demographics of participants should be considered related to population statistics. The BELpREG cohort has a higher proportion of mothers aged 30–34 years, while mothers aged 18–24 years are less represented [53]. The BELpREG cohort also contains more highly educated individuals with higher household income levels, has higher employment rates and more women with a Caucasian ethnicity [54–56]. Finally, in BELpREG, 17.8% of the pregnancies did not occur spontaneously, which is nearly double the population statistic of 9.6% [53]. It cannot be excluded that these differences affected the prevalence of substance use in pregnancy.

For example, while the overrepresentation of highly educated women may have led to an overestimation of the prevalence of alcohol consumption, the underrepresentation of both spontaneous and unplanned pregnancies and of women with lower education levels may have led to an underestimation of the actual numbers of alcohol consumption and smoking in the perinatal population, respectively. In addition, the BELpREG registry only became accessible to French-speaking individuals from January 2024 onwards, resulting in an underrepresentation of French-speaking individuals (10.6%) and challenging the generalizability of the results for the entire country. For instance, regarding the general population in Belgium, alcohol use is higher in Flanders, while smoking rates are higher in Wallonia [44,45]. Due to the low number of illicit drug users, an exploration of determinants was not possible. Additionally, individual substance use trajectories in pregnancy were not studied. Given the overall low numbers of substance-exposed women in pregnancy, especially after pregnancy awareness and throughout pregnancy, the interpretation of individual trajectories in this cohort might be, for the time being, challenging. A backward regression approach also comes with some limitations, such as the risk of overfitting, the loss of important variables and ignoring interaction terms and the likelihood that variables with a strong univariate link are predominantly retained. Moreover, no questions were included on the amount of vaping and illicit drug use. Data on any substance use between the last questionnaire in pregnancy and delivery were also lacking. Consequently, prevalence estimates of substance use in the third trimester and over the entire pregnancy might be an underestimation. Yet, this is considered rather unlikely, as de novo substance use initiated in the weeks between the last questionnaire in pregnancy and the delivery is improbable. Lastly, no data were available on the amount of alcohol or tobacco use in pregnancy among women who reported substance use cessation since pregnancy awareness, so no conclusions can be drawn about the extent of alcohol and tobacco use by these women in early pregnancy, requiring further investigation.

Interestingly, Table S5 (see Supplementary Material S4) provides a comparison of the characteristics between participants who had delivered and those who had not yet delivered or were lost to follow-up by the time of data extraction. Overall, no significant differences were observed between the two groups. Given the lack of differences and the larger sample size of first-trimester pregnant women, the latter group was chosen to find determinants associated with substance use, thereby improving statistical power and precision. Moreover, most exposures to substances occurred in the first trimester and data completeness was higher for this period compared to the entire pregnancy.

Finally, the relationship between substance use before or in pregnancy and the occurrence of adverse pregnancy or neonatal outcomes was beyond the scope of this study.

4.3. Future Perspectives

The findings underscore the need for targeted interventions to improve public health. All pregnant women who reported alcohol or tobacco use in the first trimester also indicated alcohol or tobacco use in the year prior to conception. Additionally, most exposures to substances occurred prior to conception or in early pregnancy before pregnancy awareness. These findings underscore the need for robust preconception interventions aimed at promoting healthy lifestyle (changes) before conception [57,58]. Interestingly, unplanned pregnancy was identified as a determinant of both alcohol and tobacco use in pregnancy, prompting the need to optimize the use of effective (hormonal) contraception in the population and to consider interventions to prevent unplanned pregnancies. Future research should explore which tailored interventions can be designed to address pregnancy planning and preconception health and to minimize unplanned pregnancies [57,58].

As polysubstance use in the first trimester occurred, interventions should specifically target pregnant women using various substances simultaneously. Early identification and support for these women can help mitigate the risks. Tailored programs addressing the specific needs and challenges faced by these individuals could be more effective in promoting positive lifestyle changes [59]. Interventions should also focus on the social environment of pregnant women, as alcohol or tobacco use by cohabitants relates to maternal tobacco and alcohol use in pregnancy. Therefore, multicomponent family-based interventions are needed. Recently, the Born in Belgium Professionals tool was designed to help healthcare professionals in Belgium detect antenatal psychosocial vulnerabilities during pregnancy [60,61]. This tool also includes a comprehensive screening for substance use and has the potential to direct pregnant women to personalized professional care.

In future studies, when our BELpREG cohort has grown further, we aim to include a broad range of mental health disorders and related covariates for regression analyses, as these conditions might influence substance use. Likewise, individual substance use trajectories could also be further studied.

5. Conclusions

This study highlighted the prevalence and determinants of alcohol, tobacco and illicit drug use before and during pregnancy in Belgium. Despite a significant reduction in substance use in pregnancy, a notable portion of women continue to use substances until they become aware of their pregnancy. Determinants associated with substance use in the first gestational trimester include substance use by cohabitants, maternal education level, (un)planned pregnancies and method of conception. The results underscore the need for policy makers to enable targeted public health interventions to further enhance substance use cessation before conception. Healthcare providers should be aware of these findings and proactively address substance use during counseling sessions, both before and in the early stages of pregnancy.

Supplementary Materials: The following supporting information can be downloaded at: https://www.mdpi.com/article/10.3390/jcm14020613/s1, Table S1: STROBE checklist; Table S2: Overview questions; Tables S3 and S4: Sensitivity analysis; Table S5: Sample comparison.

Author Contributions: Conceptualization, L.S., K.A., A.B., A.S., J.Y.V., V.F., K.V.C. and M.C.; methodology, S.L., L.S. and M.C.; software, S.L., L.S. and M.C.; validation, S.L., L.S., V.F. and M.C.; formal analysis, S.L and L.S.; investigation, L.S. and M.C.; resources, L.S., V.F. and M.C.; data curation, S.L. and L.S.; writing—original draft preparation, S.L., L.S. and M.C.; writing—review and editing, K.A., A.B., A.S., J.Y.V., K.V.C. and V.F.; visualization, S.L. and L.S.; supervision, M.C. and V.F.; project administration, S.L., L.S. and M.C.; funding acquisition, M.C. and V.F. All authors have read and agreed to the published version of the manuscript.

Funding: The BELpREG registry was established with financial support from the Internal Funds KU Leuven and received independent research grants from P&G Health, Tilman, UCB, Almirall, KelaPharma, Sanofi, and Johnson & Johnson. The research activities of Laure Sillis are supported by a Strategic Basic PhD Fellowship of the Research Foundation Flanders (FWO, 1S62625N). The research activities of Michael Ceulemans are supported by a fundamental research Senior Postdoctoral Fellowship of the Research Foundation Flanders (FWO, 1246425N). The research activities of Anne Smits are supported by a Senior Clinical Investigatorship of the Research Foundation Flanders (FWO) (18E2H24N).

Institutional Review Board Statement: The study was conducted in accordance with the Declaration of Helsinki and approved by the Ethics Committee Research of UZ/KU Leuven (S66464; 25 May 2022).

Informed Consent Statement: Informed consent was obtained from all subjects involved in the study.

Data Availability Statement: The data presented in this manuscript are available on request from the corresponding author due to ethical and privacy reasons.

Acknowledgments: The authors are thankful to all BELpREG participants and to all healthcare professionals who motivated pregnant women to enroll in the BELpREG registry. The authors would like to thank Digile for their technical support to the BELpREG registry and Medipim for their support in upgrading the BELpREG questionnaires.

Conflicts of Interest: The authors declare no conflicts of interest. The companies providing research grants for the BELpREG initiative had no role in the design of the study; in the collection, analysis, or interpretation of data; in the writing of the manuscript; or in the decision to publish the results.

References

1. Avsar, T.S.; McLeod, H.; Jackson, L. Health outcomes of smoking during pregnancy and the postpartum period: An umbrella review. *BMC Pregnancy Childbirth* **2021**, *21*, 254. [CrossRef] [PubMed]
2. Mamluk, L.; Edwards, H.B.; Savovic, J.; Leach, V.; Jones, T.; Moore, T.H.M.; Ijaz, S.; Lewis, S.J.; Donovan, J.L.; Lawlor, D.; et al. Low alcohol consumption and pregnancy and childhood outcomes: Time to change guidelines indicating apparently 'safe' levels of alcohol during pregnancy? A systematic review and meta-analyses. *BMJ Open* **2017**, *7*, e015410. [CrossRef] [PubMed]
3. Volkow, N.D.; Compton, W.M.; Wargo, E.M. The Risks of Marijuana Use During Pregnancy. *JAMA* **2017**, *317*, 129–130. [CrossRef] [PubMed]
4. Corsi, D.J.; Walsh, L.; Weiss, D.; Hsu, H.; El-Chaar, D.; Hawken, S.; Fell, D.B.; Walker, M. Association Between Self-reported Prenatal Cannabis Use and Maternal, Perinatal, and Neonatal Outcomes. *JAMA* **2019**, *322*, 145–152. [CrossRef] [PubMed]
5. Gabrhelik, R.; Mahic, M.; Lund, I.O.; Bramness, J.; Selmer, R.; Skovlund, E.; Handal, M.; Skurtveit, S. Cannabis Use during Pregnancy and Risk of Adverse Birth Outcomes: A Longitudinal Cohort Study. *Eur. Addict. Res.* **2021**, *27*, 131–141. [CrossRef] [PubMed]
6. Gunn, J.K.; Rosales, C.B.; Center, K.E.; Nunez, A.; Gibson, S.J.; Christ, C.; Ehiri, J.E. Prenatal exposure to cannabis and maternal and child health outcomes: A systematic review and meta-analysis. *BMJ Open* **2016**, *6*, e009986. [CrossRef] [PubMed]
7. O'Leary, C.M. Fetal alcohol syndrome: Diagnosis, epidemiology, and developmental outcomes. *J. Paediatr. Child Health* **2004**, *40*, 2–7. [CrossRef] [PubMed]
8. Feldman, H.S.; Jones, K.L.; Lindsay, S.; Slymen, D.; Klonoff-Cohen, H.; Kao, K.; Rao, S.; Chambers, C. Prenatal alcohol exposure patterns and alcohol-related birth defects and growth deficiencies: A prospective study. *Alcohol. Clin. Exp. Res.* **2012**, *36*, 670–676. [CrossRef] [PubMed]
9. Pacho, M.; Aymerich, C.; Pedruzo, B.; Salazar de Pablo, G.; Sesma, E.; Bordenave, M.; Dieguez, R.; Lopez-Zorroza, I.; Herrero, J.; Laborda, M.; et al. Substance use during pregnancy and risk of postpartum depression: A systematic review and meta-analysis. *Front. Psychiatry* **2023**, *14*, 1264998. [CrossRef] [PubMed]
10. Pentecost, R.; Latendresse, G.; Smid, M. Scoping Review of the Associations Between Perinatal Substance Use and Perinatal Depression and Anxiety. *J. Obs. Gynecol. Neonatal. Nurs.* **2021**, *50*, 382–391. [CrossRef]
11. Grzywacz, E.; Brzuchalski, B.; Smiarowska, M.; Malinowski, D.; Machoy-Mokrzynska, A.; Bialecka, M.A. Significance of Selected Environmental and Biological Factors on the Risk of FASD in Women Who Drink Alcohol during Pregnancy. *J. Clin. Med.* **2023**, *12*, 6185. [CrossRef]
12. Muggli, E.; Matthews, H.; Penington, A.; Claes, P.; O'Leary, C.; Forster, D.; Donath, S.; Anderson, P.J.; Lewis, S.; Nagle, C.; et al. Association Between Prenatal Alcohol Exposure and Craniofacial Shape of Children at 12 Months of Age. *JAMA Pediatr.* **2017**, *171*, 771–780. [CrossRef] [PubMed]
13. Pielage, M.; El Marroun, H.; Odendaal, H.J.; Willemsen, S.P.; Hillegers, M.H.J.; Steegers, E.A.P.; Rousian, M. Alcohol exposure before and during pregnancy is associated with reduced fetal growth: The Safe Passage Study. *BMC Med.* **2023**, *21*, 318. [CrossRef] [PubMed]
14. Lassi, Z.S.; Imam, A.M.; Dean, S.V.; Bhutta, Z.A. Preconception care: Caffeine, smoking, alcohol, drugs and other environmental chemical/radiation exposure. *Reprod Health* **2014**, *11* (Suppl. 3), S6. [CrossRef]
15. Zhou, Q.; Song, L.; Chen, J.; Wang, Q.; Shen, H.; Zhang, S.; Li, X. Association of Preconception Paternal Alcohol Consumption With Increased Fetal Birth Defect Risk. *JAMA Pediatr.* **2021**, *175*, 742–743. [CrossRef] [PubMed]
16. Corrales-Gutierrez, I.; Mendoza, R.; Gomez-Baya, D.; Leon-Larios, F. Pregnant Women's Risk Perception of the Teratogenic Effects of Alcohol Consumption in Pregnancy. *J. Clin. Med.* **2019**, *8*, 907. [CrossRef] [PubMed]

17. World Health Organization. *Guidelines for the Identification and Management of Substance Use Disorders in Pregnancy*; World Health Organization: Geneva, Switzerland, 2014.
18. Ceulemans, M.; Van Calsteren, K.; Allegaert, K.; Foulon, V. Health products' and substance use among pregnant women visiting a tertiary hospital in Belgium: A cross-sectional study. *Pharmacoepidemiol. Drug Saf.* **2019**, *28*, 1231–1238. [CrossRef]
19. Sillis, L.; Foulon, V.; Allegaert, K.; Bogaerts, A.; De Vos, M.; Hompes, T.; Smits, A.; Van Calsteren, K.; Verbakel, J.Y.; Ceulemans, M. Development and design of the BELpREG registration system for the collection of real-world data on medication use in pregnancy and mother-infant outcomes. *Front. Drug. Saf. Regul.* **2023**, *3*, 1166963. [CrossRef]
20. Richardson, J.L.; Moore, A.; Bromley, R.L.; Stellfeld, M.; Geissbuhler, Y.; Bluett-Duncan, M.; Winterfeld, U.; Favre, G.; Alexe, A.; Oliver, A.M.; et al. Core Data Elements for Pregnancy Pharmacovigilance Studies Using Primary Source Data Collection Methods: Recommendations from the IMI ConcePTION Project. *Drug. Saf.* **2023**, *46*, 479–491. [CrossRef]
21. European Medicines Agency. *Guideline on Good Pharmacovigilance Practices (GVP) Product- or Population-Specific Considerations III: Pregnant and Breastfeeding Women*; EMA/653036/2019—Draft for Public Consultation; European Medicine Agency: Amsterdam, The Netherlands, 2019.
22. Ceulemans, M.; Sillis, L.; Allegaert, K.; Bogaerts, A.; De Vos, M.; Hompes, T.; Smits, A.; Van Calsteren, K.; Verbakel, J.Y.; Foulon, V. Letter to the Editor re Davis et al., 2023: BELpREG, the first of its kind real-world data source on medication use in pregnancy in Belgium. *Pharmacoepidemiol. Drug Saf.* **2024**, *33*, e5751. [CrossRef]
23. von Elm, E.; Altman, D.G.; Egger, M.; Pocock, S.J.; Gotzsche, P.C.; Vandenbroucke, J.P.; Initiative, S. The Strengthening the Reporting of Observational Studies in Epidemiology (STROBE) statement: Guidelines for reporting observational studies. *J. Clin. Epidemiol.* **2008**, *61*, 344–349. [CrossRef] [PubMed]
24. Skagerstrom, J.; Alehagen, S.; Haggstrom-Nordin, E.; Arestedt, K.; Nilsen, P. Prevalence of alcohol use before and during pregnancy and predictors of drinking during pregnancy: A cross sectional study in Sweden. *BMC Public Health* **2013**, *13*, 780. [CrossRef] [PubMed]
25. Skagerstrom, J.; Chang, G.; Nilsen, P. Predictors of drinking during pregnancy: A systematic review. *J. Womens Health (Larchmt)* **2011**, *20*, 901–913. [CrossRef] [PubMed]
26. Kitsantas, P.; Gaffney, K.F.; Wu, H.; Kastello, J.C. Determinants of alcohol cessation, reduction and no reduction during pregnancy. *Arch. Gynecol. Obs.* **2014**, *289*, 771–779. [CrossRef] [PubMed]
27. McCormack, C.; Hutchinson, D.; Burns, L.; Wilson, J.; Elliott, E.; Allsop, S.; Najman, J.; Jacobs, S.; Rossen, L.; Olsson, C.; et al. Prenatal Alcohol Consumption Between Conception and Recognition of Pregnancy. *Alcohol. Clin. Exp. Res.* **2017**, *41*, 369–378. [CrossRef] [PubMed]
28. Tsakiridis, I.; Mamopoulos, A.; Papazisis, G.; Petousis, S.; Liozidou, A.; Athanasiadis, A.; Dagklis, T. Prevalence of smoking during pregnancy and associated risk factors: A cross-sectional study in Northern Greece. *Eur. J. Public Health* **2018**, *28*, 321–325. [CrossRef]
29. Smedberg, J.; Lupattelli, A.; Mardby, A.C.; Nordeng, H. Characteristics of women who continue smoking during pregnancy: A cross-sectional study of pregnant women and new mothers in 15 European countries. *BMC Pregnancy Childbirth* **2014**, *14*, 213. [CrossRef]
30. de Wolff, M.G.; Backhausen, M.G.; Iversen, M.L.; Bendix, J.M.; Rom, A.L.; Hegaard, H.K. Prevalence and predictors of maternal smoking prior to and during pregnancy in a regional Danish population: A cross-sectional study. *Reprod Health* **2019**, *16*, 82. [CrossRef] [PubMed]
31. Riaz, M.; Lewis, S.; Naughton, F.; Ussher, M. Predictors of smoking cessation during pregnancy: A systematic review and meta-analysis. *Addiction* **2018**, *113*, 610–622. [CrossRef]
32. Sequi-Canet, J.M.; Sequi-Sabater, J.M.; Marco-Sabater, A.; Corpas-Burgos, F.; Collar Del Castillo, J.I.; Orta-Sibu, N. Maternal factors associated with smoking during gestation and consequences in newborns: Results of an 18-year study. *J. Clin. Transl. Res.* **2022**, *8*, 6–19.
33. Rumrich, I.K.; Vahakangas, K.; Viluksela, M.; Gissler, M.; Surcel, H.M.; Korhonen, A.; De Ruyter, H.; Hanninen, O. Smoking during pregnancy in Finland—Trends in the MATEX cohort. *Scand. J. Public Health* **2019**, *47*, 890–898. [CrossRef] [PubMed]
34. Kondracki, A.J. Prevalence and patterns of cigarette smoking before and during early and late pregnancy according to maternal characteristics: The first national data based on the 2003 birth certificate revision, United States, 2016. *Reprod Health* **2019**, *16*, 142. [CrossRef] [PubMed]
35. O'Keeffe, L.M.; Kearney, P.M.; McCarthy, F.P.; Khashan, A.S.; Greene, R.A.; North, R.A.; Poston, L.; McCowan, L.M.; Baker, P.N.; Dekker, G.A.; et al. Prevalence and predictors of alcohol use during pregnancy: Findings from international multicentre cohort studies. *BMJ Open* **2015**, *5*, e006323. [CrossRef] [PubMed]
36. Kitsantas, P.; Gaffney, K.F.; Wu, H. Identifying high-risk subgroups for alcohol consumption among younger and older pregnant women. *J. Perinat. Med.* **2015**, *43*, 43–52. [CrossRef]

37. Shmulewitz, D.; Hasin, D.S. Risk factors for alcohol use among pregnant women, ages 15-44, in the United States, 2002 to 2017. *Prev. Med.* **2019**, *124*, 75–83. [CrossRef]
38. Houston-Ludlam, A.N.; Bucholz, K.K.; Grant, J.D.; Waldron, M.; Madden, P.A.F.; Heath, A.C. The interaction of sociodemographic risk factors and measures of nicotine dependence in predicting maternal smoking during pregnancy. *Drug Alcohol Depend.* **2019**, *198*, 168–175. [CrossRef] [PubMed]
39. Mardby, A.C.; Lupattelli, A.; Hensing, G.; Nordeng, H. Consumption of alcohol during pregnancy-A multinational European study. *Women Birth* **2017**, *30*, e207–e213. [CrossRef] [PubMed]
40. Corrales-Gutierrez, I.; Mendoza, R.; Gomez-Baya, D.; Leon-Larios, F. Understanding the Relationship between Predictors of Alcohol Consumption in Pregnancy: Towards Effective Prevention of FASD. *Int. J. Environ. Res. Public Health* **2020**, *17*, 1388. [CrossRef]
41. Hamadneh, S.; Hamadneh, J.; Alhenawi, E.; Khurma, R.A.; Hussien, A.G. Predictive factors and adverse perinatal outcomes associated with maternal smoking status. *Sci. Rep.* **2024**, *14*, 3436. [CrossRef]
42. Azagba, S.; Ebling, T.; Korkmaz, A. The Changing Faces of Smoking: Sociodemographic Trends in Cigarette Use in the U.S., 1992–2019. *Int. J. Ment. Health Addict.* **2024**. [CrossRef]
43. Bover Manderski, M.T.; Steinberg, M.B.; Wackowski, O.A.; Singh, B.; Young, W.J.; Delnevo, C.D. Persistent Misperceptions about Nicotine among US Physicians: Results from a Randomized Survey Experiment. *Int. J. Environ. Res. Public Health* **2021**, *18*, 7713. [CrossRef] [PubMed]
44. Gisle, L.; Demararest, S.; Drieskens, S. *Health Interview Survey 2018: Alcohol Use*; D/2019/14.440/56; Sciensano: Brussels, Belgium, 2018.
45. Gisle, L.; Demararest, S.; Drieskens, S. *Health Interview Survey 2018: Smoking*; D/2019/14.440/57; Sciensano: Brussels, Belgium, 2018.
46. Denny, C.H.; Acero, C.S.; Naimi, T.S.; Kim, S.Y. Consumption of Alcohol Beverages and Binge Drinking Among Pregnant Women Aged 18–44 Years—United States, 2015–2017. *Morb. Mortal. Wkly. Rep.* **2019**, *68*, 365–368. [CrossRef] [PubMed]
47. Harrison, P.A.; Sidebottom, A.C. Alcohol and drug use before and during pregnancy: An examination of use patterns and predictors of cessation. *Matern. Child Health J.* **2009**, *13*, 386–394. [CrossRef] [PubMed]
48. Liao, S.; Luo, B.; Feng, X.; Yin, Y.; Yang, Y.; Jing, W. Substance use and self-medication during pregnancy and associations with socio-demographic data: A cross-sectional survey. *Int. J. Nurs. Sci.* **2015**, *2*, 28–33. [CrossRef]
49. Haight, S.C.; King, B.A.; Bombard, J.M.; Coy, K.C.; Ferre, C.D.; Grant, A.M.; Ko, J.Y. Frequency of cannabis use during pregnancy and adverse infant outcomes, by cigarette smoking status—8 PRAMS states, 2017. *Drug Alcohol Depend.* **2021**, *220*, 108507. [CrossRef] [PubMed]
50. Cerda, M.; Wall, M.; Keyes, K.M.; Galea, S.; Hasin, D. Medical marijuana laws in 50 states: Investigating the relationship between state legalization of medical marijuana and marijuana use, abuse and dependence. *Drug Alcohol Depend.* **2012**, *120*, 22–27. [CrossRef]
51. Ishitsuka, K.; Hanada-Yamamoto, K.; Mezawa, H.; Saito-Abe, M.; Konishi, M.; Ohya, Y.; Japan, E.; Children's Study, G. Determinants of Alcohol Consumption in Women Before and After Awareness of Conception. *Matern. Child Health J.* **2020**, *24*, 165–176. [CrossRef] [PubMed]
52. Grittner, U.; Kuntsche, S.; Gmel, G.; Bloomfield, K. Alcohol consumption and social inequality at the individual and country levels--results from an international study. *Eur. J. Public Health* **2013**, *23*, 332–339. [CrossRef] [PubMed]
53. Goemaes, R.; Fomenko, E.; Laubach, M.; De Coen, K.; Roelens, K.; Bogaerts, A. *Perinatal Health in Flenders—Year 2023*; Study Center for Perinatal Epidemiology: Brussels, Belgium, 2024.
54. Statistics Flanders. Population and Society. Available online: https://www.vlaanderen.be/statistiek-vlaanderen/bevolking-en-samenleving (accessed on 13 November 2024).
55. Growing Up; Child and Youth Govermental Agency. Numerical Report Household Income and Poverty. Available online: https://www.opgroeien.be/kennis/cijfers-en-onderzoek/gezinsinkomen-en-kansarmoede (accessed on 13 November 2024).
56. Statbel. Employment and Unemployment. Available online: https://statbel.fgov.be/en/themes/work-training/labour-market/employment-and-unemployment (accessed on 13 November 2024).
57. Backhausen, M.G.; Ekstrand, M.; Tyden, T.; Magnussen, B.K.; Shawe, J.; Stern, J.; Hegaard, H.K. Pregnancy planning and lifestyle prior to conception and during early pregnancy among Danish women. *Eur. J. Contracept. Reprod Health Care* **2014**, *19*, 57–65. [CrossRef] [PubMed]
58. Goossens, J.; Beeckman, D.; Van Hecke, A.; Delbaere, I.; Verhaeghe, S. Preconception lifestyle changes in women with planned pregnancies. *Midwifery* **2018**, *56*, 112–120. [CrossRef]
59. Goossens, J.; Delbaere, I.; Dhaenens, C.; Willems, L.; Van Hecke, A.; Verhaeghe, S.; Beeckman, D. Preconception-related needs of reproductive-aged women. *Midwifery* **2016**, *33*, 64–72. [CrossRef] [PubMed]

60. Amuli, K.; Decabooter, K.; Talrich, F.; Renders, A.; Beeckman, K. Born in Brussels screening tool: The development of a screening tool measuring antenatal psychosocial vulnerability. *BMC Public Health* **2021**, *21*, 1522. [CrossRef] [PubMed]
61. Born in Belgium Professionals. Born in Belgium Professionals. Available online: https://borninbelgiumpro.be/ (accessed on 29 November 2024).

Disclaimer/Publisher's Note: The statements, opinions and data contained in all publications are solely those of the individual author(s) and contributor(s) and not of MDPI and/or the editor(s). MDPI and/or the editor(s) disclaim responsibility for any injury to people or property resulting from any ideas, methods, instructions or products referred to in the content.

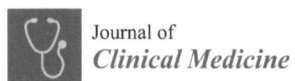 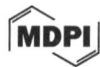

Article

Intermittent Preventive Treatment of Malaria in Pregnancy and the Impact on Neonates in African Countries as Assessed by Entropy Weight and TOPSIS Methods

Maria Tzitiridou-Chatzopoulou [1], Georgia Zournatzidou [2,*], Eirini Orovou [1], Lazaros Lavasidis [1], Arsenios Tsiotsias [1], Panagiotis Eskitzis [1] and Dimitrios Papoutsis [1]

[1] Department of Midwifery, School of Healthcare Sciences, University of Western Macedonia, Keptse, 50200 Ptolemaida, Greece; mtzitiridou@uowm.gr (M.T.-C.); eorovou@uowm.gr (E.O.); lavasidis@yahoo.gr (L.L.); atsiotsias@uowm.gr (A.T.); peskitzis@uowm.gr (P.E.); dpapoutsis@uowm.gr (D.P.)
[2] Department of Business Administration, University of Western Macedonia, 51100 Grevena, Greece
* Correspondence: gzournatzidou@uowm.gr

Abstract: **Background/Objectives**: In regions of Africa with a high prevalence of malaria, pregnant women in their first or second trimester should be administered intermittent preventive treatment in pregnancy (IPTp). However, infants may contract malaria despite the IPTp therapy that their mothers have received. The objective of the present investigation was to assess the symptoms and various treatments for neonatal malaria. **Methods**: Entropy weight and TOPSIS were used to achieve the study goal. The TOPSIS multi-attribute decision-making system was used to assess newborn malaria symptoms and select the optimal treatment, even for mothers receiving IPTp medication during pregnancy. The entropy weight approach calculated TOPSIS attribute weights. The present research used UNICEF data for 14 African nations in 2023. **Results**: The results indicated that neonates whose mothers received IPTp therapy ultimately contracted malaria, with diarrhea being the primary symptom. It is important to note that health providers administer a combination of zinc and oral rehydration solution (ORS) to infants as the most effective treatment for malaria symptoms, thereby abandoning the first-line treatment for malaria, artemisinin-based combination therapy (ACT). **Conclusions**: The most effective treatment for neonatal malaria is a combination of zinc and ORS, although less than half of children in Africa have access to ORS. Therefore, the findings of this study may encourage African countries to prioritize co-pack therapy in their procurement and supply, healthcare provider training, and expenditures. This therapy will also help alleviate the symptoms of malaria in neonates.

Keywords: Intermittent preventive treatment; pregnancy; neonatal outcome; Africa; zinc; ORS

Citation: Tzitiridou-Chatzopoulou, M.; Zournatzidou, G.; Orovou, E.; Lavasidis, L.; Tsiotsias, A.; Eskitzis, P.; Papoutsis, D. Intermittent Preventive Treatment of Malaria in Pregnancy and the Impact on Neonates in African Countries as Assessed by Entropy Weight and TOPSIS Methods. *J. Clin. Med.* **2024**, *13*, 6231. https://doi.org/10.3390/jcm13206231

Academic Editors: Ioannis Tsakiridis and Apostolos Mamopoulos

Received: 18 September 2024
Revised: 15 October 2024
Accepted: 16 October 2024
Published: 18 October 2024

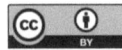

Copyright: © 2024 by the authors. Licensee MDPI, Basel, Switzerland. This article is an open access article distributed under the terms and conditions of the Creative Commons Attribution (CC BY) license (https://creativecommons.org/licenses/by/4.0/).

1. Introduction

Malaria during pregnancy is a significant global health issue that has major impacts on the well-being of both mothers and babies. In 2021, the African region under the jurisdiction of the World Health Organization (WHO) saw a substantial impact of malaria infection, which affected about 13.3 million pregnancies. Therefore, the region experienced a 11% mortality rate among newborns and a 20% mortality rate among fetuses. The World Health Organization (WHO) recommends that women who live in areas with moderate to high malaria transmission rates receive at least three doses of sulfadoxine-pyrimethamine as an intermittent preventive treatment for malaria in pregnancy (IPTp) [1,2]. It is necessary to provide this drug after every routine appointment at a prenatal care clinic, starting in the second trimester of pregnancy. Research has shown that the administration of IPTp decreases the prevalence of low birthweight infants by 29%, acute maternal anemia by 38%, and neonatal mortality by 31%. IPTp is among the few healthcare interventions that have shown an effective reduction in perinatal mortality. Although it is very cost-effective, the extent of coverage it offers remains inadequate [3].

Only a minority of pregnant women living in areas with regular malaria transmission contract symptomatic malaria infections [4,5]. However, these infections are linked to maternal morbidity, which encompasses illnesses like anemia, as well as harmful effects on the child, such as spontaneous abortion, low birth weight, and infant mortality. In areas with low malaria transmission rates, where women of reproductive age lack immunity to the disease, malaria infection in pregnant women can result in anemia, increase the risk of severe malaria, and potentially result in spontaneous abortion, infant mortality, and low birth weight. In areas with high malaria transmission rates, the prevalence of malaria is higher in locations with a significant population of primigravidae [4,6,7]. As the number of pregnancies rises, the incidence of malaria and the parasite load in the blood decrease. Parasite infection is diagnosed using microscopic examination, polymerase chain reaction (PCR) to identify specific nucleic acids, and rapid diagnostic testing utilizing specialist kits to detect plasmodium antigens. Moreover, the WHO strongly supports the use of IPTp with sulfadoxine-pyrimethamine (SP) as a treatment for uncomplicated malaria in pregnant women and children under the age of 5 in the current malaria-endemic areas of Africa, while it recommends the administration of at least three doses of IPTp for malaria to all pregnant women, irrespective of their plasmodial infection status. This is because IPTp has shown efficacy in avoiding maternal anemia and mitigating the likelihood of low birth weight in neonates [8].

Newborns may be more susceptible to malaria because of IPTp, as indicated by observational studies. By fortifying the neonatal immune system to resist the blood-stage of *P. falciparum*, exposure to *P. falciparum* during pregnancy increases the likelihood of *P. falciparum* infection in early life [9,10]. Nevertheless, the possibility of this phenomenon having clinical significance has not been adequately defined. There is a lack of capacity in observational studies on infant malaria and prenatal malaria exposure to incorporate common risk factors that are shared by the mother and neonate, such as postnatal environmental variables or a shared genetic predisposition to higher sensitivity. Therefore, the results of this investigation are restricted. Therefore, it is conceivable that the link between malaria during pregnancy and the risk to infants is due to postnatal exposure to malaria, rather than direct exposure to malaria parasites during gestation. IPTp in pregnancy clinical research offers a distinctive opportunity to investigate whether maternal malaria exposure influences the susceptibility of neonates to malarias. By employing a randomized regimen, this is feasible, as it guarantees that the exposure levels are comparable among all participants [11–13].

Thus, the current study aims to evaluate the symptoms and treatment of malaria in infants in fourteen African countries, which are among those with the highest proportion of pregnant women who have received the IPTp therapy, although their infants have contracted malaria and received specific treatment based on the symptoms they have. To approach the research objective of the current study, the two methods of entropy weight and TOPSIS have been used. For the purposes of the study, six criteria have been used that are related to the different symptoms of infants regarding malaria and the treatment they receive from health providers based on these symptoms. The analysis indicates that infants whose mothers received three doses of IPTp therapy during pregnancy contracted malaria, and the symptom that they mostly experienced was diarrhea, which is treated with ORS and zinc therapy. Additionally, one more novel aspect of the current research is that it indicates that febrile infants receiving artemisinin-based combination therapy (ACT) is not a usual case in the countries under investigation. Despite ACT now being generally accepted as the best treatment for uncomplicated falciparum malaria and one of the most effective treatments for infants with malaria, the current study highlights that this is not a panacea.

The structure of the paper is as follows: Section 2 presents the key points of the related literature review in the field under investigation, Section 3 describes the materials and methods used for the analysis, Section 4 presents the results of both entropy weight and TOPSIS analysis, Section 5 discusses the results, implications and limitations of the study, and Section 6 concludes the paper.

2. Literature Review

Malaria infection during pregnancy is a significant public health concern. Pregnancy impairs a woman's immune system, increasing the likelihood of illness, anemia, severe disease, and mortality, and rendering expecting women more susceptible to malaria. The developing child is at increased risk of spontaneous abortion, stillbirth, premature delivery, and low birth weight because of maternal malaria. Infant mortality is substantially affected by low birth weight [14–16].

To prevent and manage malaria in expecting women, the World Health Organization (WHO) suggests the implementation of a comprehensive array of interventions. In areas where P. falciparum transmission is moderate to high, individuals are encouraged to utilize insecticide-treated nets, cases are promptly and effectively treated, and intermittent preventive treatment with sulfadoxine-pyrimethamine (IPTp-SP) is implemented. IPTp-SP is linked to a decrease in maternal parasitemia, a decrease in the incidence of low-birth-weight neonates, and an increase in the mean birth weight, according to data from countries with high malaria prevalence [17].

Nevertheless, IPTp therapy administered to expecting women does not ensure that their infants will be completely protected from contracting malaria. Infants born to mothers who underwent IPTp treatment are susceptible to malaria and may display a variety of symptoms. To be more specific, the primary symptoms of this condition may be diverse and frequently resemble other common neonate illnesses, such as pneumonia, meningitis/encephalitis, or gastroenteritis [4,18,19]. The sole symptoms that may be present are fever and headache, or there may be a predominance of gastrointestinal symptoms, such as diarrhea. The primary symptom is fever, but the distinct regular tertian and quartan patterns are observed in less than 25% of children. Nevertheless, children are more susceptible to experiencing elevated fevers, which can lead to febrile convulsions if they exceed 40 °C.

Furthermore, oral anti-malaria medications may be rendered ineffective by the frequent occurrence of nausea and vomiting. The most prevalent comorbidities associated with malaria are acute diarrhea and pneumonia, which are significant predictors of mortality. A concomitant bacterial or viral respiratory disease, such as pneumonia, may be diagnosed in a neonate with malaria. Additionally, a child who is experiencing respiratory distress due to malaria may be diagnosed with pneumonia. In the same vein, the presence of severe diarrhea may suggest clinical malaria or be the result of a concurrent infection with a diarrheal pathogen [20,21].

Artemisinin-based combination therapy (ACT) is employed to treat malaria in infants. Infants experience elevated rates of malaria morbidity and mortality in regions with an endemic malaria problem [22,23]. Consequently, the WHO advises the use of ACT for the treatment of uncomplicated malaria. To facilitate the treatment of minors, pediatric formulations of ACT have been created. The primary objective of pediatric malaria treatment is to administer the first-line formula of ACT, which is comprised of artemether + lumefantrine, artesunate + amodiaquine, artesunate + mefloquine, artesunate + sulfadoxine-pyrimethamine, and dihydroartemisinin + piperaquine. However, the treatment described in the formula is not the sole effective method. Another formula is the combination of oral rehydration solution (ORS). The global standard for diarrhea treatment is ORS. In its most basic form, ORS is a combination of sodium, sugar, and water that can expedite the body's fluid replacement process [24]. ORS is administered to neonates who are experiencing diarrhea, which is one of the most prevalent symptoms of malaria in infants. Lastly, there are a limited number of studies that have assessed the influence of treatments on malaria in infants. Consequently, the current study is unique in that it evaluates the influence of the most prevalent symptoms and their respective remedies on malaria in neonates born to mothers who received three or more dosages of IPTp therapy [7,25].

3. Materials and Methods
3.1. Data

To evaluate the symptoms of malaria in infants, despite their mothers having received three doses of IPT therapy, as well as the treatment that the healthcare provider gave them, we have considered six criteria (Table 1).

Table 1. Dependent variables and criteria with their computation units.

	Indicator ID	Indicator Description	Data Source
	IPTP	Pregnant women (15–49) who received three or more doses of intermittent preventive therapy during their previous prenatal care visits	Household surveys including MICS, DHS and other national surveys
C1	DIARCARE	Care-seeking for diarrhea for infants with malaria symptoms	Household surveys including MICS, DHS and other national surveys
C2	ORS	Treatment of gastroenteritis in neonates who were administered oral rehydration salts (ORS sachets or pre-packaged ORS fluids)	Household surveys including MICS, DHS and other national surveys
C3	ORTCF	Treatment for diarrhea in infants who have received oral rehydration therapy (oral rehydration salts, recommended homemade fluids, or increased fluids) and have continued to feed	Household surveys including MICS, DHS and other national surveys
C4	ORSZINC	Treatment of diarrhea in neonates who were administered ORS and zinc	Household surveys including MICS, DHS and other national surveys
C5	ZINC	Zinc treatment for diarrhea in neonates who have received zinc supplements	Household surveys including MICS, DHS and other national surveys
C6	MLRACT	First-line treatment for febrile infants who have previously received ACT (first-line antimalarial drug) for malaria	Household surveys including MICS, DHS and other national surveys

Also, the selected variables and data were retrieved from the database of UNICEF. The data referred to fourteen African countries (Figure 1) for the year 2023. Among those, Mali, Mozambique, and Benin are the countries with the highest rate of pregnant women who have received IPTp therapy and whose infants contracted malaria.

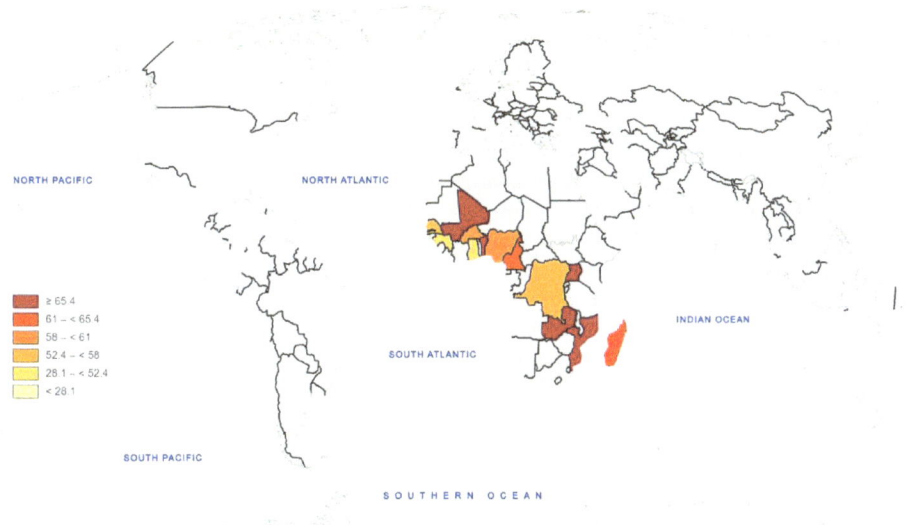

Figure 1. IPTp for pregnant women (aged 14–49) who received three or more doses for the year 2023.

3.2. Entropy Weight Method

The TOPSIS method is currently being implemented in the current research as a multicriteria decision-making approach. This approach entails the evaluation of multiple elements within a well-defined framework in relation to the data analysis method. Entropy weighing is the process of assigning weights to a diverse array of variables or factors according to the degree of uncertainty or unpredictability, as determined by entropy. Moreover, the TOPSIS model, a composite methodology that integrates entropy and TOPSIS approaches, was introduced by Kaur et al. (2023) [26]. The entropy weight approach is the primary objective of this system, which is to assess the significance of each assessment indicator. It then utilizes the method of selecting the most optimal solution to rank assessment items.

According to Dwivedi et al. (2023), the basic concept of the entropy weight the TOPSIS technique aims to identify the ideal solution by comparing the attribute values of several alternatives and selecting the one that has either the greatest or lowest value for each characteristic [27]. An evaluation object's optimality is evaluated by analyzing its relative closeness to the best and worst options. Assessment items are deemed ideal when they are positioned near the most efficient solution and furthest away from the least desirable choice. On the other hand, it is deemed less than ideal if it does not match these characteristics. Entropy plays a crucial part in the TOPSIS approach by incorporating information from the original data without placing any limitations on the sample size. It offers a wide range of functions and has minimum loss of information.

The initial presumption that there are available approaches is made prior to the presentation of n alternatives $A = \{A_1, A_2, A_3, \ldots, A_n\}$ and m criteria $M = \{M_1, M_2, M_3, \ldots, M_m\}$, where $i \in A$, $j \in M$, $i = \{1, 2, 3, \ldots, n\}$, $j = \{1, 2, 3, \ldots, m\}$. The matrix $X' = (x''_{ij})$ in Equation (1) is a decision matrix of $n \times m$. The relative importance of the criterion A weight vector can be used to represent M as follows: $W = \{w_1, w_2, w_3, \ldots, w_m\}$, which satisfies $\sum_{j=1}^{m} w_j = 1$.

$$X' = \begin{bmatrix} x'_{11} & x'_{12} & x'_{1m} \\ x'_{21} & \ldots & x'_{2m} \\ x'_{n1} & x'_{n2} & x'_{nm} \end{bmatrix} \qquad (1)$$

The weight is determined by assessing the degree of data dispersion in the Shannon entropy weighting approach. Initially, we employ the min–max method to standardize the n original options. The subsequent step involves adjusting the standardized equation to the right by 0.001 units to facilitate future logarithmic calculations.

$$x_{ij} = \frac{x'_{ij} - \min(x'_j)}{\max(x'_j) - \min(x'_j)} + 0.001, \text{ where } i = 1, 2, 3, \ldots, n, \text{ and } j = 1, 2, 3, \ldots, m. \qquad (2)$$

Equation (4) was used to calculate the entropy value, represented as e_j. Entropy is a measure of the extent to which data are distributed. The entropy value drops as the data exhibit more fluctuation, indicating a higher level of information in the data. As the data become more concentrated, the entropy value rises, which suggests a reduction in the amount of information present in the data.

$$r_{ij} = \frac{x_{ij}}{\sum_{i=1}^{n} x_{ij}}, i = 1, 2, 3, \ldots, n, \text{ and } j = 1, 2, 3, \ldots, m. \qquad (3)$$

$$e_j = -\frac{1}{\ln n} \sum_{i=1}^{n} r_{ij}, i = 1, 2, 3, \ldots, n \text{ and } j = 1, 2, 3, \ldots, m. \qquad (4)$$

The weight w_j is determined by Equation (5).

$$w_j = \frac{1 - e_j}{\sum_{j=1}^{m}(1 - e_j)} \qquad (5)$$

3.3. TOPSIS Method

In 1981, Hwang and Yoon devised the TOPSIS methodology, which quantifies the alternatives' proximity to the optimal solutions. To ascertain the degree of proximity, we compute the Euclidean distance between each potential option and both the optimal and suboptimal alternatives. The most advantageous value for each evaluation criterion is chosen to determine the optimal solution, while the least beneficial value for each assessment criterion is used to characterize the suboptimal solution. Finally, we select the most advantageous alternative, which closely resembles the ideal resolution and significantly deviates from the unfavorable option, as the preferred decision. At the outset, we implemented individual standardization of the positive and negative attributes of the choice matrix in Equation (1) to reduce any disparities in dimensions among the various criteria. In numerous domains, we underscored the necessity of attaining uniformity through application of the min–max methodology. When determining the entropy weight, this method facilitates the process of assessing the advantages and disadvantages. A technique for order preference by similarity to the ideal solution is denoted by the acronym TOPSIS.

$$positive : x_{ij}^+ = \frac{x'_{ij} - \min(x'_j)}{\max(x'_j) - \min(x'_j)}$$

$$negative : x_{ij}^- = \frac{\max(x'_j) - x'_{ij}}{\max(x'_j) - \min in(x'_j)} \quad (6)$$

$$\min(x'_j) = \{\min_i x'_{ij} | 1 < i < n, 1 < j < m\}$$

$$\max(x'_j) = \{\max_i x'_{ij} | 1 < i < n, 1 < j < m\}$$

As illustrated in Equation (7), the dimensionless normalized decision matrix x_{ij} is generated by normalizing the positive and negative criteria to generate the initial choice matrix in Equation (6).

$$X' = \begin{bmatrix} x_{11} & x_{12} & \cdots & x_{1m} \\ x_{21} & \cdots & \cdots & x_{2m} \\ \vdots & \cdots & \cdots & \vdots \\ x_{n1} & x_{n2} & \cdots & x_{nm} \end{bmatrix}, \text{ where } i = 1, 2, 3, \ldots, n \text{ and } j = 1, 2, 3, \ldots, m. \quad (7)$$

Moreover, the decision matrix in Equation (8) is obtained by multiplying each individual element $v_{ij} = w_j \times x_{ij}$, where $w_j = (w_1, w_2, w_3, \ldots, w_m)$ is obtained from Equation (5) and meets the condition $\sum_{j=1}^m w_j = 1$ and x_{ij}, as generated using Equation (7).

$$V = \begin{bmatrix} v_{11} & v_{12} & \cdots & v_{1m} \\ v_{21} & \cdots & \cdots & v_{2m} \\ \vdots & \cdots & \cdots & \vdots \\ v_{n1} & v_{n2} & \cdots & v_{nm} \end{bmatrix} = \begin{bmatrix} w_1 x_{11} & w_2 x_{12} & \cdots & w_m x_{1m} \\ w_1 x_{21} & w_2 x_{22} & \cdots & w_m x_{2m} \\ \vdots & \cdots & \cdots & \vdots \\ w_1 x_{n1} & w_2 x_{n2} & \cdots & w_m x_{nm} \end{bmatrix} \quad (8)$$

The positive ideal solution (PIS) is the highest value, and the negative ideal solution (NIS) is the lowest value for each criterion, as defined by Equation (9). The distance of each option from the PIS and NIS is determined using Equations (10) and (11).

$$PIS : P^+ = \{v_1^+, v_2^+, v_3^+, \ldots, v_m^+\} = \{(\max_i v_{ij} | j \in M)\}$$
$$NIS : P^- = \{v_1^-, v_2^-, v_3^-, \ldots, v_m^-\} = \{(\min_i v_{ij} | j \in M)\} \quad (9)$$

$$d_i^+ = \sqrt{\sum_{j=1}^{m}(v_{ij} - v_j^+)^2}, \, i = 1, 2, 3, \ldots, n, \text{ and } j = 1, 2, 3, \ldots, m. \tag{10}$$

$$d_i^- = \sqrt{\sum_{j=1}^{m}(v_{ij} - v_j^-)^2}, \, i = 1, 2, 3, \ldots, n, \text{ and } j = 1, 2, 3, \ldots, m. \tag{11}$$

Below is the computation for the coefficient of relative proximity (RC).

$$RC_i = \frac{d_i^-}{d_i^- + d_i^+}, \, i = 1, 2, 3, \ldots, n \tag{12}$$

4. Results

The research analysis was performed using the predefined choice matrix, which was divided into three major areas. The ensuing sections provide an overview of the stages of various times. The data in the decision matrix were first normalized using the N1 method. The aim of this strategy was to homogenize the data to simplify comparisons. After completing Step 1, we created a normalized matrix for each Ni. The normalized matrices may be found in Table A1 in Appendix A. In addition, the next step of the analysis included assigning weights to each criterion and creating a weighted normalized matrix using the methods described in Section 3.1 of the present research. This experiment used the entropy-weighted TOPSIS approach. Table 2 provides a comprehensive examination of the weights applied to each chosen criterion.

Table 2. Entropy-weight TOPSIS approach to determining criteria weight.

Criterion	C1	C2	C3	C4	C5	C6
e_j	0.991	0.971	0.987	0.404	0.562	1.122
$D = 1 - e_j$	0.009	0.029	0.013	0.596	0.438	−0.122
W_j	0.009	0.030	0.014	0.619	0.455	−0.127

C4 > C5 > C2 > C3 > C1 > C6. Determination of the weights of the selected criteria used.

Subsequently, the Euclidean distance between the positive ideal solution (PIS) and the negative ideal solution (NIS) was computed. Equations (10) and (11) yielded the normalized Euclidean distance for both positive and negative solutions for each option. Table 3 presents the results.

Table 3. Calculation of the Euclidean distance between PIS and NIS.

S_i+	S_{i-}	Si+ Si−	Si−/(Si+ Si−)
0.082385	0.095601	0.177985	0.537126
0.145773	0.0307	0.176473	0.173966
0.134343	0.040964	0.175308	0.233672
0.0309	0.168381	0.199282	0.844941
0.135921	0.053811	0.189732	0.283618
0.129315	0.047055	0.176369	0.266796
0.151772	0.028847	0.180619	0.159712
0.168552	0.023639	0.192191	0.122997
0.156242	0.025005	0.181247	0.137963
0.066952	0.108894	0.175846	0.619257
0.095928	0.077601	0.173529	0.447192
0.119909	0.055778	0.175686	0.317484
0.161518	0.023051	0.184568	0.12489
0.131546	0.048147	0.179692	0.26794

The Euclidean distances of each alternative from the PIS and NIS.

By employing the entropy-weight TOPSIS method, it was demonstrated that criterion four (C4: infants with diarrhea and treatment with ORS and zinc) and criterion five (C5: infants with diarrhea and treatment with zinc supplements) are of the most significant importance to mothers who have received IPTp therapy to prevent malaria. The results above indicate that, even though mothers in the selected African countries had received IPTp therapy, their neonates appear to be suffering from malaria. Health providers have decided to administer a treatment that consists of a combination of ORS and zinc. Zinc supplementation has been demonstrated to decrease morbidity from infectious diseases in these populations, particularly through morbidity reductions from respiratory infections and diarrhea. In addition, the combination of zinc and ORS can be beneficial in fortifying the immune system of neonates with malaria. This therapy may prevent diarrhea episodes for a period of up to three months and expedite the recovery process. However, ORS is accessible to fewer than half of children in Africa. Consequently, the World Health Organization must incorporate co-packaged ORS and zinc into its Essential Medicines List. This will encourage African countries to prioritize the co-pack in their procurement and supply, healthcare provider training, and expenditures. Additionally, this therapy will alleviate the symptoms of malaria in neonates. Additionally, our analysis showed that one of the most common therapies for malaria in infants (C6: malaria first-line treatment for febrile infants receiving ACT) was not widespread in the selected African countries assessed in the current study.

5. Discussion

Neonatal malaria refers to the diagnosis of malaria in infants within the first 28 days of life. In a recent meta-analysis by Danwang et al., it was shown that the overall prevalence of clinical newborn malaria among the 28,083 neonates included was 12.0% between the 7th and 28th days of life, despite the presence of substantial heterogeneity [28]. Congenital malaria is caused by passage of malaria parasites through the placenta before birth. Neonatal parasitemia is often characterized by the presence of asexual parasites in the cord blood or peripheral blood of newborns during the first week of life. Light microscopy has proven the occurrence of clinical congenital malaria; however, the reported incidence varies significantly depending on factors such as the characteristics of the research population, the seasonal patterns of malaria prevalence, and the study technique [25,29]. The frequency of congenital malaria transmission in African nations with significant is 46.7%.

Furthermore, infants are relatively protected from malaria during their first months of life; however, infection can occur at any age and can progress to febrile illness and anemia. Infants over the age of six months are at an increased risk since they have not yet developed partial immunity, as well as the fact that their maternal antibodies and embryonic hemoglobin are diminishing [30]. Consequently, it is essential that infants receive sufficient antimalarial treatment. Additionally, IPTp therapy offers an additional layer of protection by administering antimalarial medication to expecting women at predetermined intervals, regardless of their malaria infection status. The goal is to reduce the negative consequences of a malaria infection on the mother and her embryo during pregnancy, and on the neonate. The disparities in ANC access are the subject of a new recommendation in the updated WHO guidance on IPTp. Access to IPTp can be influenced by sociodemographic factors, including age, marital status, religion, and urban/rural domicile. The adoption of IPTp is significantly influenced by socioeconomic factors, such as education, employment, and wealth index, as well as health system barriers [31,32].

The objective of the present investigation was to evaluate the most prevalent symptoms of neonatal malaria in fourteen African countries where mothers receive IPTp therapy during pregnancy. The most effective therapies for infants with malaria are also identified in this research, in addition to concentrating on symptoms. Fever is the most prevalent clinical symptom of malaria in neonates, as indicated by the existing literature (88–100%). Respiratory distress (20–57%), pallor and anemia (38% each), hepatomegaly (31–80%), refusal to feed (40–70%), jaundice, and diarrhea (25% each) are additional manifestations.

Nevertheless, the present investigation indicates that diarrhea is the most prevalent symptom in neonates whose mothers have received IPTp treatment, rendering them susceptible to malaria [33]. Additionally, the combination of zinc and ORS therapy reduces the duration and severity of neonatal diarrhea, as well as its frequency over the subsequent 2–3 months. Although it is possible to describe access to treatment for neonatal diarrheal disease caused by malaria among infants as unequal, the reason for this unequal access is linked to age group, area of residence, and wealth index quintiles, particularly in countries such as those included in the current analysis. Additionally, the study's results have the potential to disrupt the cycle of unsuccessful first-line malaria treatment. Throughout the recent past, malaria medicines have been repeatedly compromised by antimicrobial resistance (AMR). In the past two decades, we have made substantial strides in the prevention and treatment of malaria by enhancing the implementation of a variety of control measures, such as diagnostics, insecticide-treated bed nets, and artemisinin-based medications [34,35]. However, antimalarial remedies become less effective as malaria parasites develop the ability to elude their effects over time. Antimalarial drugs may require additional time to eliminate parasites when this occurs, a phenomenon referred to as partial antimalarial resistance.

Although zinc is crucial for cellular growth, differentiation, and metabolism, zinc deficiency is associated with a reduction in infection resistance and a decline in juvenile growth. Mild to moderate zinc deficiency may be prevalent worldwide, despite the rarity of severe zinc deficiency in humans. Zinc supplementation has been shown to reduce the duration and severity of diarrhea and prevent subsequent episodes, even though the mechanisms by which it exerts its anti-diarrheal effect are still unclear. Nevertheless, the management of malaria-induced pediatric diarrhea should be improved by incorporating zinc supplements, rehydration therapy with ORS, and counseling for ongoing nutrition and prevention. Lastly, policymakers should prioritize the enhancement of first-line treatment for neonatal malaria. For decades, artemisinin-based combination therapy (ACT) has been the primary treatment for malaria. Healthcare providers are no longer prioritizing it as their primary treatment option, according to the research. It is possible that this is due to the existence of potential resistance. A search for potential alternatives to ACT has been initiated in response to the emerging prospect of resistance. Therefore, future research should focus on improvement of primary treatments for neonatal malaria and integration of this therapy with zinc and ORS combination therapy.

6. Conclusions

Health systems in sub-Saharan Africa (SSA) have consistently acknowledged malaria as a critical public health issue, and it continues to be a primary contributor to maternal and neonatal morbidity and mortality in the region. In most sub-Saharan African countries, the utilization of insecticide-treated nets (ITNs) and antimalarial intermittent preventive therapy in pregnancy (IPTp) has experienced a substantial increase. Strategic initiatives and robust political commitments by national and international organizations have led to this result. Consequently, the incidence of malaria has decreased. Malaria in pregnancy (MiP) remains a significant preventable factor in maternal and neonatal morbidity and mortality, with an estimated 75,000 to 200,000 neonates dying in endemic regions. An expanding body of evidence supports this assertion.

Even though women receive IPTp treatment during pregnancy, the objective of this investigation was to evaluate the most prevalent symptoms of malaria in infants in fourteen African countries. The study's results indicate that diarrhea is the most prevalent symptom in infants whose mothers have undergone IPTp therapy, rendering them susceptible to malaria. The combination of zinc and ORS treatment reduces the duration, intensity, and frequency of neonatal gastroenteritis during the subsequent 2–3 months. Infants suffering from malaria-induced diarrhea face unequal access to treatment, primarily due to factors related to age group, geographic location, and wealth index quintiles, especially in the countries under review.

Moreover, the findings of this research may call into question the effectiveness of first-line malaria treatment. Antimicrobial resistance (AMR) has increasingly undermined malaria therapies in recent decades. Over the last two decades, the improved use of several control measures such as diagnostics, insecticide-treated bed nets, and artemisinin-based medicines has achieved significant progress in the prevention and treatment of malaria. The effectiveness of antimalarial therapies diminishes when malaria parasites acquire the capacity to circumvent their effects over time. Partial antimalarial resistance may necessitate a longer duration of antimalarial drugs to eradicate the parasites. Future research proposals must target the improvement of first-line therapy for newborn malaria and advance clinical treatment. Considering the possibility of resistance, we have started research to investigate possible alternatives to ACT. Consequently, future research should concentrate on enhancing primary therapy for malaria in newborns and integrating it with a combination of zinc and oral rehydration solution (ORS).

Author Contributions: Conceptualization, G.Z.; Methodology, M.T.-C., E.O., A.T. and P.E.; Software, E.O. and A.T.; Validation, G.Z., E.O., P.E. and D.P.; Formal analysis, M.T.-C., G.Z. and D.P.; Investigation, L.L., A.T. and P.E.; Resources, M.T.-C., L.L. and D.P.; Data curation, G.Z. and L.L.; Writing—original draft, M.T.-C., G.Z., E.O., L.L., A.T., P.E. and D.P.; Supervision, P.E.; Project administration, G.Z. and L.L. All authors have read and agreed to the published version of the manuscript.

Funding: This research received no external funding.

Institutional Review Board Statement: Not applicable.

Informed Consent Statement: Not applicable.

Data Availability Statement: Dataset available on request from the authors.

Conflicts of Interest: The authors declare no conflicts of interest.

Appendix A

Table A1. Normalized matrix.

C1	C2	C3	C4	C5	C6
0.0869	0.0673	0.0732	0.0318	0.0552	0.0937
0.0922	0.0581	0.0792	0.0112	0.0225	0.0899
0.0615	0.0374	0.0423	0.0158	0.0257	0.0801
0.0542	0.1404	0.0930	0.0649	0.0761	0.1109
0.0744	0.0302	0.0575	0.0116	0.0311	0.0413
0.0408	0.0406	0.0465	0.0160	0.0329	0.1032
0.0837	0.0939	0.0880	0.0124	0.0133	0.0724
0.0669	0.0949	0.0899	0.0059	0.0072	0.0717
0.0786	0.0758	0.0822	0.0080	0.0164	0.0797
0.0522	0.0715	0.0622	0.0410	0.0560	0.1035
0.0974	0.0806	0.1071	0.0327	0.0392	0.1099
0.0754	0.0925	0.0549	0.0216	0.0349	0.1228
0.0695	0.0740	0.0527	0.0078	0.0112	0.0747
0.0663	0.0428	0.0714	0.0137	0.0329	0.0797

Explaining the procedure of considering the determinants of the matrix and dividing each element by the determinants of the matrix. This approach outlines the development of the normalized matrix.

References

1. Van Eijk, A.M.; Hill, J.; Alegana, V.A.; Kirui, V.; Gething, P.W.; ter Kuile, F.O.; Snow, R.W. Coverage of malaria protection in pregnant women in sub-Saharan Africa: A synthesis and analysis of national survey data. *Lancet Infect. Dis.* **2011**, *11*, 190–207. [CrossRef] [PubMed]
2. van Eijk, A.M.; Larsen, D.A.; Kayentao, K.; Koshy, G.; Slaughter, D.E.C.; Roper, C.; Okell, L.C.; Desai, M.; Gutman, J.; Khairallah, C.; et al. Effect of Plasmodium falciparum sulfadoxine-pyrimethamine resistance on the effectiveness of intermittent preventive therapy for malaria in pregnancy in Africa: A systematic review and meta-analysis. *Lancet Infect. Dis.* **2019**, *19*, 546–556. [CrossRef] [PubMed]

3. Ndyomugyenyi, R.; Tukesiga, E.; Katamanywa, J. Intermittent preventive treatment of malaria in pregnancy (IPTp): Participation of community-directed distributors of ivermectin for onchocerciasis improves IPTp access in Ugandan rural communities. *Trans. R. Soc. Trop. Med. Hyg.* **2009**, *103*, 1221–1228. [CrossRef] [PubMed]
4. Venkatesan, M.; Alifrangis, M.; Roper, C.; Plowe, C.V. Monitoring antifolate resistance in intermittent preventive therapy for malaria. *Trends Parasitol.* **2013**, *29*, 497–504. [CrossRef]
5. Obaideen, K.; Abu Shihab, K.H.; Madkour, M.I.; Faris, M.A.I.E. Seven decades of Ramadan intermittent fasting research: Bibliometrics analysis, global trends, and future directions. *Diabetes Metab. Syndr. Clin. Res. Rev.* **2022**, *16*, 102566. [CrossRef]
6. Zhao, H.; Jiang, C.; Zhao, M.; Ye, Y.; Yu, L.; Li, Y.; Luan, H.; Zhang, S.; Xu, P.; Chen, X.; et al. Comparisons of Accelerated Continuous and Intermittent Theta Burst Stimulation for Treatment-Resistant Depression and Suicidal Ideation. *Biol. Psychiatry* **2023**, *96*, 26–33. [CrossRef]
7. Mbonye, A.K.; Hansen, K.S.; Bygbjerg, I.C.; Magnussen, P. Intermittent preventive treatment of malaria in pregnancy: The incremental cost-effectiveness of a new delivery system in Uganda. *Trans. R. Soc. Trop. Med. Hyg.* **2008**, *102*, 685–693. [CrossRef]
8. Ndyomugyenyi, R.; Katamanywa, J. Intermittent preventive treatment of malaria in pregnancy (IPTp): Do frequent antenatal care visits ensure access and compliance to IPTp in Ugandan rural communities? *Trans. R. Soc. Trop. Med. Hyg.* **2010**, *104*, 536–540. [CrossRef]
9. Tijani, M.K.; Persson, K.E.M. Malaria, Immunity, and Immunopathology. In *Reference Module in Life Sciences*; Elsevier: Amsterdam, The Netherlands, 2024. [CrossRef]
10. Adhikary, K.; Chatterjee, A.; Chakraborty, S.; Bhattacherjee, A.; Banerjee, P. Malaria: Epidemiology, pathogenesis, and therapeutics. In *Viral, Parasitic, Bacterial, and Fungal Infections: Antimicrobial, Host Defense, and Therapeutic Strategies*; Academic Press: Cambridge, MA, USA, 2022; pp. 341–363. [CrossRef]
11. Michaels, M.G.; Sánchez, P.J.; Lin, P.L. Congenital Toxoplasmosis, Syphilis, Malaria, and Tuberculosis. In *Avery's Diseases of the Newborn*; Elsevier: Amsterdam, The Netherlands, 2023; pp. 487–511.e7. [CrossRef]
12. Tzitiridou-Chatzopoulou, M.; Orovou, E.; Zournatzidou, G. Digital Training for Nurses and Midwives to Improve Treatment for Women with Postpartum Depression and Protect Neonates: A Dynamic Bibliometric Review Analysis. *Healthcare* **2024**, *12*, 1015. [CrossRef]
13. Tzitiridou-Chatzopoulou, M.; Kountouras, J.; Zournatzidou, G. The Potential Impact of the Gut Microbiota on Neonatal Brain Development and Adverse Health Outcomes. *Children* **2024**, *11*, 552. [CrossRef]
14. Long, B.; MacDonald, A.; Liang, S.Y.; Brady, W.J.; Koyfman, A.; Gottlieb, M.; Chavez, S. Malaria: A focused review for the emergency medicine clinician. *Am. J. Emerg. Med.* **2024**, *77*, 7–16. [CrossRef] [PubMed]
15. Ampofo, G.D.; Tagbor, H. Community delivery of malaria chemoprevention in pregnancy. *Lancet Glob. Health* **2023**, *11*, e487–e488. [CrossRef] [PubMed]
16. Anstey, N.M.; Tham, W.H.; Shanks, G.D.; Poespoprodjo, J.R.; Russell, B.M.; Kho, S. The biology and pathogenesis of vivax malaria. *Trends Parasitol.* **2024**, *40*, 573–590. [CrossRef] [PubMed]
17. Uyaiabasi, G.N.; Olaleye, A.; Elikwu, C.J.; Funwei, R.I.; Okangba, C.; Adepoju, A.; Akinyede, A.; Adeyemi, O.O.; Walker, O. The question of the early diagnosis of asymptomatic and subpatent malaria in pregnancy: Implications for diagnostic tools in a malaria endemic area. *Eur. J. Obstet. Gynecol. Reprod. Biol. X* **2023**, *19*, 100233. [CrossRef] [PubMed]
18. Mbonye, A.K.; Schultz Hansen, K.; Bygbjerg, I.C.; Magnussen, P. Effect of a community-based delivery of intermittent preventive treatment of malaria in pregnancy on treatment seeking for malaria at health units in Uganda. *Public Health* **2008**, *122*, 516–525. [CrossRef]
19. Slutsker, L.; Leke, R.G.F. First-trimester use of ACTs for malaria treatment in pregnancy. *Lancet* **2022**, *401*, 81–83. [CrossRef]
20. O'Mahony, E.; Ryan, F.; Hemandas, H.; Al-Sabbagh, A.; Cunnington, A.; Fitzgerald, F. Cryptic Congenital Malaria Infection Causing Fever of Unknown Origin in an Infant. *J. Pediatr.* **2024**, *275*, 114237. [CrossRef]
21. Figueroa-Romero, A.; Saura-Lázaro, A.; Fernández-Luis, S.; González, R. Uncovering HIV and malaria interactions: The latest evidence and knowledge gaps. *Lancet HIV* **2024**, *11*, e255–e267. [CrossRef]
22. Vásquez-Echeverri, E.; Yamazaki-Nakashimada, M.A.; Venegas Montoya, E.; Scheffler Mendoza, S.C.; Castano-Jaramillo, L.M.; Medina-Torres, E.A.; González-Serrano, M.E.; Espinosa-Navarro, M.; Bustamante Ogando, J.C.; González-Villarreal, M.G.; et al. Is Your Kid Actin Out? A Series of Six Patients With Inherited Actin-Related Protein 2/3 Complex Subunit 1B Deficiency and Review of the Literature. *J. Allergy Clin. Immunol. Pract.* **2023**, *11*, 1261–1280.e8. [CrossRef]
23. Custy, C.; Mitchell, M.; Dunne, T.; McCaffrey, A.; Neylon, O.; O'Gorman, C.; Cremona, A. A thematic analysis of barriers and facilitators of physical activity, and strategies for management of blood glucose levels around physical activity for adolescents with type 1 diabetes. *Clin. Nutr. Open Sci.* **2024**, *56*, 265–286. [CrossRef]
24. Elwyn, R.; Mitchell, J.; Kohn, M.R.; Driver, C.; Hay, P.; Lagopoulos, J.; Hermens, D.F. Novel ketamine and zinc treatment for anorexia nervosa and the potential beneficial interactions with the gut microbiome. *Neurosci. Biobehav. Rev.* **2023**, *148*, 105122. [CrossRef] [PubMed]
25. Adebusuyi, S.A.; Olorunfemi, A.B.; Fagbemi, K.A.; Nderu, D.; Amoo AO, J.; Thomas, B.N.; Velavan, T.P.; Ojurongbe, O. Performance of rapid diagnostic test, light microscopy, and polymerase chain reaction in pregnant women with asymptomatic malaria in Nigeria. *IJID Reg.* **2024**, *12*, 100416. [CrossRef] [PubMed]
26. Kaur, H.; Gupta, S.; Dhingra, A. Selection of solar panel using entropy TOPSIS technique. *Mater. Today Proc.* **2023**; *in press*. [CrossRef]

27. Dwivedi, P.P.; Sharma, D.K. Evaluation and ranking of battery electric vehicles by Shannon's entropy and TOPSIS methods. *Math. Comput. Simul.* **2023**, *212*, 457–474. [CrossRef]
28. Danwang, C.; Kirakoya-Samadoulougou, F.; Samadoulougou, S. Assessing field performance of ultrasensitive rapid diagnostic tests for malaria: A systematic review and meta-analysis. *Malar. J.* **2021**, *20*, 245. [CrossRef]
29. Kassie, G.A.; Azeze, G.A.; Gebrekidan, A.Y.; Lombebo, A.A.; Adella, G.A.; Haile, K.E.; Welda, G.D.; Efa, A.G.; Asgedom, Y.S. Asymptomatic malaria infection and its associated factors among pregnant women in Ethiopia; a systematic review and meta-analysis. *Parasite Epidemiol. Control* **2024**, *24*, e00339. [CrossRef]
30. Ogbuanu, I.U.; Otieno, K.; Varo, R.; Sow, S.O.; Ojulong, J.; Duduyemi, B.; Kowuor, D.; Cain, C.J.; Rogena, E.A.; Onyango, D.; et al. Burden of child mortality from malaria in high endemic areas: Results from the CHAMPS network using minimally invasive tissue sampling. *J. Infect.* **2024**, *88*, 106107. [CrossRef]
31. Barrett, J.R.; Pipini, D.; Wright, N.D.; Cooper, A.J.; Gorini, G.; Quinkert, D.; Lias, A.M.; Davies, H.; Rigby, C.A.; Aleshnick, M.; et al. Analysis of the diverse antigenic landscape of the malaria protein RH5 identifies a potent vaccine-induced human public antibody clonotype. *Cell* **2024**, *187*, 4964–4980.e21. [CrossRef]
32. Matambisso, G.; Brokhattingen, N.; Maculuve, S.; Cístero, P.; Mbeve, H.; Escoda, A.; Bambo, G.; Cuna, B.; Melembe, C.; Ndimande, N.; et al. Sustained clinical benefit of malaria chemoprevention with sulfadoxine-pyrimethamine (SP) in pregnant women in a region with high SP resistance markers. *J. Infect.* **2024**, *88*, 106144. [CrossRef]
33. Peterkin, T.; Eke, E.; Don-Aki, J.; Jaiyeola, O.; Suhowatsky, S.; Noguchi, L. Increased Uptake of Intermittent Preventive Treatment for Prevention of Malaria in Pregnancy and Scale-Up of Group Antenatal Care in Nasarawa State, Nigeria. *Am. J. Obstet. Gynecol.* **2024**, *230*, S627. [CrossRef]
34. Fernandes, S.; Were, V.; Gutman, J.; Dorsey, G.; Kakuru, A.; Desai, M.; Kariuki, S.; Kamya, M.R.; ter Kuile, F.O.; Hanson, K. Cost-effectiveness of intermittent preventive treatment with dihydroartemisinin–piperaquine for malaria during pregnancy: An analysis using efficacy results from Uganda and Kenya, and pooled data. *Lancet Glob. Health* **2020**, *8*, e1512–e1523. [CrossRef]
35. Adeyemo, M.O.A.; Adeniran, G.O.; Adeniyi, V.A.; Olabisi, E.O.; Oyekale, R.A.; Akinwale, O.; Adejare, S.F.; Olaleye, O.J.; Fafowora, R.O.; Akinbowale, B.T. Assessment of uptake of intermittent preventive treatment of malaria among pregnant women attending antenatal clinic in public health facilities in Osogbo metropolis, Osun state, Nigeria. *Int. J. Afr. Nurs. Sci.* **2024**, *20*, 100742. [CrossRef]

Disclaimer/Publisher's Note: The statements, opinions and data contained in all publications are solely those of the individual author(s) and contributor(s) and not of MDPI and/or the editor(s). MDPI and/or the editor(s) disclaim responsibility for any injury to people or property resulting from any ideas, methods, instructions or products referred to in the content.

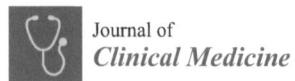

Systematic Review

Bibliometric Analysis on of the Impact of Screening to Minimize Maternal Mental Health on Neonatal Outcomes: A Systematic Review

Maria Tzitiridou-Chatzopoulou [1] and Georgia Zournatzidou [2,*]

1   Midwifery Department, School of Healthcare Sciences, University of Western Macedonia, GR50 100 Kozani, Greece; mtzitiridou@uowm.gr
2   Department of Business Administration, University of Western Macedonia, GR511 00 Grevena, Greece
*   Correspondence: gzournatzidou@uowm.gr

Abstract: (1) **Background**: Prenatal depression, maternal anxiety, puerperal psychosis, and suicidal thoughts affect child welfare and development and maternal health and mortality. Women in low-income countries suffer maternal mental health issues in 25% of cases during pregnancy and 20% of cases thereafter. However, MMH screening, diagnosis, and reporting are lacking. The primary goals of the present study are twofold, as follows: firstly, to evaluate the importance of screening maternal mental health to alleviate perinatal depression and maternal anxiety, and, secondly, to analyze research patterns and propose novel approaches and procedures to bridge the current research gap and aid practitioners in enhancing the quality of care offered to women exhibiting symptoms of perinatal depression. (2) **Methods**: We conducted a bibliometric analysis to analyze the research topic, using the bibliometric tools Biblioshiny and VOSviewer, as well as the R statistical programming language. To accomplish our goal, we obtained a total of 243 documents from the Scopus and PubMed databases and conducted an analysis utilizing network, co-occurrence, and multiple correlation approaches. (3) **Results**: Most of the publications in the field were published between the years 2021 and 2024. The results of this study highlight the significance of shifting from conventional screening methods to digital ones for healthcare professionals to effectively manage the symptoms of maternal mental health associated with postpartum depression. Furthermore, the results of the present study suggest that digital screening can prevent maternal physical morbidity, contribute to psychosocial functioning, and enhance infant physical and cognitive health. (4) **Conclusions**: The research indicates that it is crucial to adopt and include a computerized screening practice to efficiently and immediately detect and clarify the signs of prenatal to neonatal depression. The introduction of digital screening has led to a decrease in scoring errors, an improvement in screening effectiveness, a decrease in administration times, the creation of clinical and patient reports, and the initiation of referrals for anxiety and depression therapy.

Keywords: screening; maternal mental health; digital training; diagnosis; perinatal depression; bibliometric analysis

Citation: Tzitiridou-Chatzopoulou, M.; Zournatzidou, G. Bibliometric Analysis on of the Impact of Screening to Minimize Maternal Mental Health on Neonatal Outcomes: A Systematic Review. *J. Clin. Med.* **2024**, *13*, 6013. https://doi.org/10.3390/jcm13196013

Academic Editors: Apostolos Mamopoulos and Ioannis Tsakiridis

Received: 20 August 2024
Revised: 1 October 2024
Accepted: 6 October 2024
Published: 9 October 2024

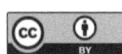

Copyright: © 2024 by the authors. Licensee MDPI, Basel, Switzerland. This article is an open access article distributed under the terms and conditions of the Creative Commons Attribution (CC BY) license (https:// creativecommons.org/licenses/by/ 4.0/).

1. Introduction

Perinatal depression, which is also referred to as perinatal depression, is a condition that affects approximately one in seven individuals during the perinatal period. Most of these patients, over 75%, do not receive any treatment for prenatal depression [1–3]. Perinatal depression may manifest during or prior to pregnancy and the postpartum period. Untreated perinatal depression is linked to an elevated risk of suicide and has adverse effects on the perinatal individual, the embryo (including premature birth and low birth weight), and the child (including poor attachment that can disrupt neurodevelopment). Additionally, it may have adverse effects on relationships with family members and social companions [4,5]. To diagnose perinatal depression, it is necessary to observe the presence of a minimum of five symptoms, including a despondent mood and a lack of interest or delight. These symptoms must be distinct from the individual's typical functioning and must endure for a minimum of two weeks [6]. Furthermore, clinicians should assess the frequency, severity, and duration of perinatal depression symptoms, as well as probe for suicidal ideation and prior suicide attempts; inquire about substance use, including alcohol and opioids; evaluate the impact of current medications that may contribute to, imitate, or exacerbate perinatal depression; and screen for indications of bipolar disorder [7,8]. Additionally, they should gather information about the individual's personal and family psychiatric histories; consider conducting tests for specific medical conditions, such as anemia and thyroid dysfunction; and inquire about substance use [9,10].

However, the absence of comprehensive data on the progression of symptoms associated with perinatal depression or any form of depression during pregnancy or the postpartum period has significantly restricted research on prenatal depression. Consequently, the development of new screening methods is essential and can contribute to the improvement and facilitation of therapies. Nevertheless, the digitalization of screening has occurred in recent years because of the integration of emergent technologies [11–14]. For instance, the quantity of and technological advancements in mobile phones have experienced unprecedented global surges. Mobile phones are significantly less likely to disrupt natural social behaviors than laboratory monitoring equipment because of their pervasive use, which renders them less noticeable [15,16]. Mobile phone applications are an effective aid in the continuous and frequent surveillance of mood states in women who are at a high risk of postpartum depression due to their broad appeal and immediate accessibility [17]. When patients are queried in a textual or in-app format, they are more likely to provide sensitive information in a comfortable environment, such as their own residence [18,19]. A study that was recently conducted examined the utilization of mobile applications to assess prenatal mental health [14].

Nevertheless, the global academic community is still in the process of identifying the field of digital screening and its significance in the prevention of perinatal depression symptoms. Consequently, the objective of the present study is to emphasize the transition from the conventional to the digital screening process and its impact on the enhancement of therapies that address perinatal depression symptoms. The research topic was addressed through the application of a bibliometric analysis using R Studio (4.4.0) and the bibliometric tools VOSviewer (1.6.20) and Biblioshiny (4.1). For this investigation, we obtained 197 documents from the Scopus and PubMed databases and employed Bibliometrix to analyze them. The results demonstrate a robust correlation between digital mental health and the screening of perinatal depression symptoms. Additionally, the findings underscore the significance of digital screening in the prevention of perinatal depression symptoms in refugee women, who are already at risk because of the circumstances and situations that force them to flee.

2. Perinatal Mental Health and Screening in the Digital Age

Perinatal mental health and psychosocial screening include gathering a number of responses from women related to queries about their present and past emotional and social well-being [20]. The objective is to ascertain the risk factors, symptoms, and indicators that are linked to the emergence of or advancement in a mental health disorder [9,10]. This may be accomplished as part of the standard prenatal and postoperative care that midwives, obstetricians, and other healthcare professionals provide. A critical component of perinatal mental health screening is the identification of women who are susceptible and may require additional support, as well as a comprehensive evaluation of their mental health. The failure to identify perinatal mental health problems during routine prenatal examinations is frequently the result of insufficient monitoring [21].

Screening may be performed using a structured questionnaire that offers predefined response options, or it can include a discussion with a healthcare practitioner in which open-ended questions are posed and answered. Screening is often performed using conventional techniques such as pen and paper, as well as contemporary digital technologies like the iCOPE digital prenatal mental health screening platform. Healthcare experts believe validated mental health and psychosocial screening devices to be credible. They provide a systematic method for addressing sensitive topics with mothers and improve the capacity to identify and provide timely treatment. The Australian clinical practice guidelines for mental healthcare during the perinatal period advocate for the use of many screening tools that have been designed and validated. These gadgets are often provided to women throughout pregnancy and after giving delivery. Their objective is to discern several facets of mental health and susceptibility to psychosocial challenges, including the likelihood of experiencing depression, anxiety, and other variables that provide protection [9,22].

According to national standards, it is advised that all women have regular screenings for depression and psychosocial risk factors at least two times during pregnancy and two times within the first year after giving birth. Within various prenatal and postnatal mental health settings, women may either neglect to receive regular tests or undergo screenings on many occasions. A range of approaches are used to provide healthcare during and after pregnancy, taking into account the woman's personal choices, medical needs, unique circumstances, and region of residency [2,23]. Local primary healthcare services, prenatal clinics, public hospitals, private hospitals, mother and child health services, and auxiliary home visits compose the settings. The way women are tested for perinatal mental health and psychosocial risk factors varies across various healthcare settings, regions, and states, despite the existence of national standards, in terms of approach, scheduling, and scope. Research suggests that certain demographics have historically been underrepresented in perinatal mental health screening. These women comprise First Nations women, women born outside of the country, solitary or separated women, private patients, and elderly mothers. These populations remain underrepresented, despite an increase in perinatal mental health screening over time.

Additionally, the utilization of screening technologies is contingent upon the precise metrics that are implemented. Most perinatal mental health screenings are conducted through clinical evaluations in clinics and home visits, or by evaluating validated measures using paper-based and pen-based assessments [24]. There are several structural obstacles that impede the screening process for prenatal mental health. These include insufficient resources, poor mental health education and training for midwives and obstetricians, time constraints, issues with patient-provider relations, and shortages of resources. However, introducing computerized mental health screening during pregnancy and after childbirth may successfully reduce errors in scoring, increase the number of referrals for treatment for mental health issues, and improve time management. The integration of digital health into global healthcare is becoming more prevalent. This integration facilitates the efficient transfer of health information between patients and healthcare professionals while also improving decision making via the use of integrated algorithms and local care pathways [25]. This systematic review provides a clear definition of digital screening as the use of dependable and precise screening instruments, such as mobile phones, tablets, laptops, or desktop computers, by women throughout pregnancy and the postpartum period via the usage of mobile applications or a web-based connection.

It is essential to acknowledge the challenges and limitations related to this issue before advancing, despite the significant benefits of digital screening in mitigating perinatal depression symptoms, which considerably affect neonatal health. The limits and problems include the lack of evidence-based standards, privacy issues, data governance challenges, and ethical dilemmas [26]. The sensitivity of health data is a major worry, since its digitization might lead to privacy issues. approval presents an extra ethical dilemma, since many users may not fully understand the conditions of the use agreement when they provide their approval. Moreover, there is a paucity of research about the effects of digital screening technologies on health outcomes, cost-effectiveness, and system efficiency. The effectiveness of telehealth platforms may also be affected by users' socioeconomic levels and incomes.

Mothers who move to low-income or rural areas may have difficulties in understanding and using digital health solutions due to their reduced health literacy [26–29].

At present, there are no exhaustive evaluations that investigate the utilization of digital screening for mental health during pregnancy and postpartum. Therefore, the objective of this study is to ascertain whether digital screenings for mental health during pregnancy and postpartum are more effective, acceptable, and feasible than conventional treatments. A reliable referral for further evaluation is provided by efficient screening, which identifies women who have a higher likelihood of concurrently having a mental health disorder or detects indicators of mental health conditions during pregnancy and postpartum. According to professional standards, anxiety and depression are the most prevalent mental health disorders during the perinatal period. This process typically entails the assessment of these criteria in real-world scenarios [5,30,31]. The following factors determine the level of feasibility: initiation of referrals for depression and anxiety treatments, production of personalized clinical and patient reports, utilization of accessible and user-friendly technology, improvement in screening capabilities, and minimization of scoring errors. Furthermore, the aim of this systematic review is to determine the factors that either facilitate or impede the implementation of digital screening for mental health during pregnancy and postpartum. Furthermore, it endeavors to provide recommendations for the most effective digital diagnostic methods for perinatal mental health [32].

3. Materials and Methods

The objective of this research was to identify areas of growth, deficiencies, and recurring themes by employing a bibliometric methodology to evaluate articles in a systematic manner. Bibliometric analysis can be employed to ascertain the status of research and to identify prominent academic journals, publishing houses, or authors in a specific field. By employing the bibliometric method to investigate digital screening toward the symptoms of perinatal depression, it is possible to enhance one's comprehension and acquire a comprehensive understanding of the academic subject. The inquiry evaluates aggregated literature data by employing the Scopus and PubMed, databases. In recent years, quantitative and bibliometric methodologies have become increasingly prevalent for the assessment of research output quality. An exhaustive examination is necessary to ascertain the efficacy, accuracy, and consistency of an assessment method.

The data for the present analysis were obtained from both Scopus and PubMed in June 2024. Furthermore, only articles published in English have been considered for the study of the specified document type. To provide more accurate bibliometric analysis findings, data from a whole year were assessed, resulting in the selection of publications published between 2011 and 2024. A prestigious bibliographic database, Scopus was established in 2004. Abstracts and citations from esteemed scientific journals compose the compilation. The database is composed of 36,377 titles that were acquired from 11,678 publishers. This investigation concentrates on the following four critical concepts: anguish, digital training, nurses, and postpartum depression. Also, the database of PubMed facilitated the exploration and recovery of biomedical and life sciences literature in order to enhance health outcomes on global and individual levels. The PubMed database has about 37 million citations and abstracts of the biological literature. Table 1 provides a comprehensive and detailed explanation of the keyword search procedure.

Table 1. Keyword search formula.

Step	Keyword Search
1	((("screening" AND "perinatal depression"))
2	((("screening" OR "digital screening") AND ("perinatal depression" OR "maternal perinatal depression"))
3	((("screening" OR "digital screening") AND ("perinatal depression" OR "maternal perinatal depression") AND ("maternal mental health"))
4	((("screening" OR "digital screening") AND ("perinatal depression" OR "maternal perinatal depression") AND ("maternal mental health" OR "maternal mental health disorders" OR "antenatal mental health"))
5	((("screening" OR "digital screening") AND ("perinatal depression" OR "maternal perinatal depression") AND ("maternal mental health" OR "maternal mental health disorders" OR "antenatal mental health") AND "neonates")
6	((("screening" OR "digital screening") AND ("perinatal depression" OR "maternal perinatal depression") AND ("maternal mental health" OR "maternal mental health disorders" OR "antenatal mental health") AND ("neonates" OR "infants"))
7	((("screening" OR "digital screening") AND ("perinatal depression" OR "maternal perinatal depression") AND ("maternal mental health" OR "maternal mental health disorders" OR "antenatal mental health" OR "anxiety") AND ("neonates" OR "infants"))
8	((("screening" OR "digital screening" OR "neonatal screening") AND ("perinatal depression" OR "maternal perinatal depression") AND ("maternal mental health" OR "maternal mental health disorders" OR "antenatal mental health" OR "anxiety") AND ("neonates" OR "infants"))
9	((("screening" OR "digital screening" OR "neonatal screening") AND ("perinatal depression" OR "maternal perinatal depression") AND ("maternal mental health" OR "maternal mental health disorders" OR "antenatal mental health" OR "anxiety" OR "psychological risk") AND ("neonates" OR "infants"))
10	((("screening" OR "digital screening" OR "neonatal screening") AND ("perinatal depression" OR "maternal perinatal depression") AND ("maternal mental health" OR "maternal mental health disorders" OR "antenatal mental health" OR "anxiety" OR "psychological risk") AND ("neonates" OR "infants")) AND (LIMIT-TO (DOCTYPE, "ar")) AND (LIMIT-TO (PUBSTAGE, "final") OR LIMIT-TO (PUBSTAGE, "aip")) AND (LIMIT-TO (SRCTYPE, "j"))

Furthermore, the PRISMA flow diagram visually illustrates the essential stages involved in choosing a dependable collection of publications for bibliometric analysis (Figure 1). The search query produced a grand total of 431 sources in the collection. Nevertheless, we limited the overall quantity of materials to 348 by only choosing periodicals. Following that, we carried out a comprehensive examination of a grand total of 223 papers, disregarding those that were too general or seemed unrelated to our current inquiry. The main objective of this inquiry is to highlight the significance of screening in reducing maternal and perinatal mental health symptoms, as well as the shift in screening methods to the digital age. Upon conducting a comprehensive analysis of the publications, we found that the title and keywords of numerous chosen sources did not explicitly mention the dimensions and qualities of the examined region. To exclude any extraneous references, we adjusted the search parameters to exclude articles that were not directly pertinent to the present study's inquiry. A total of 197 scholarly articles were chosen and included in the bibliometric study after using this screening process.

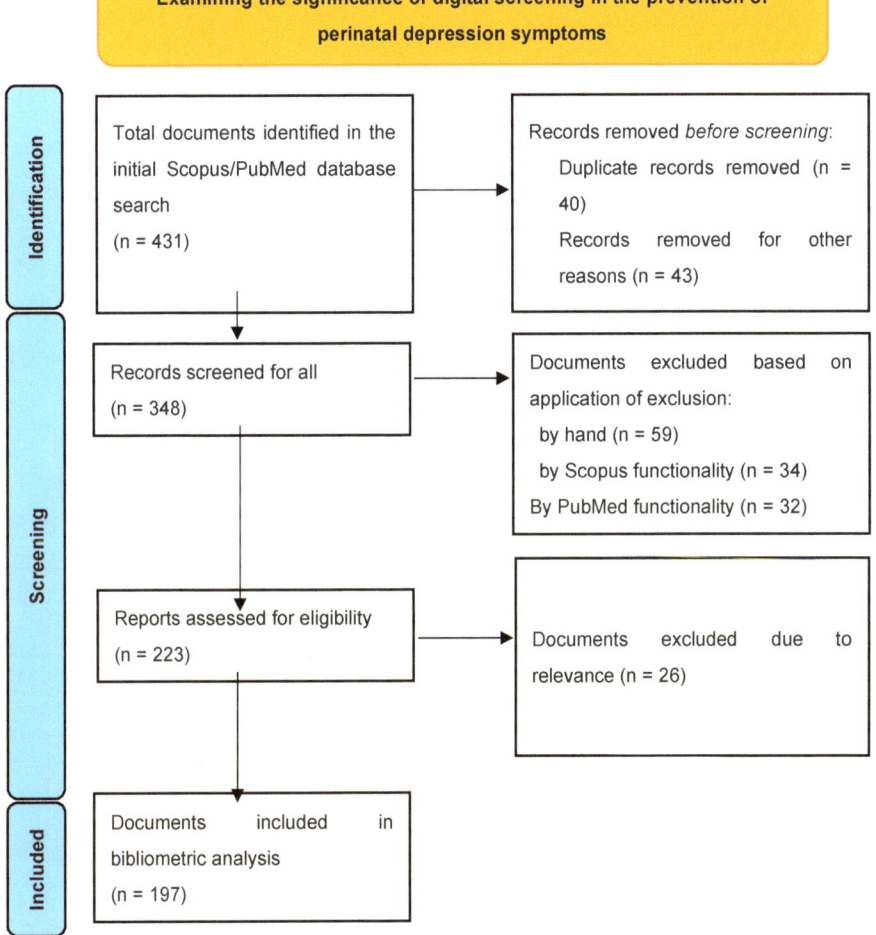

Figure 1. PRISMA flow diagram.

4. Results

4.1. Content Analysis

In recent years, the academic community has begun an investigation into the use of digital screening to prevent and mitigate the symptoms of maternal depression and its impact on the mental health of women and their infants. Figure 2 presents the scientific production in the field associated with the research topic spanning the years 2021 to 2024, as indicated by a query in the database of Scopus. The figure illustrates the exponential increase in the number of publications of this form of article over the past four years, culminating in a peak in the annual growth rate in 2022. The graph indicates a substantial increase in scientific production between 2021 and 2024, indicating an upward trend.

Table 2 and Figure 3 both display the sources (journals) that received the most research submissions on the study topic between 2019 and 2023. *Women and Birth* is the source with the greatest number of relevant publications (45 documents) on the subject of detecting and mitigating symptoms of perinatal depression. Furthermore, the *Archives of Women's Mental Health* ranked second among the sources for the greatest number of articles on the topic (34 documents). Additionally, the *Australian and New Zealand Journal of Psychiatry* is ranked third. This journal highlights the need of using digital screening to detect symptoms throughout the perinatal period, with a specific focus on refugee or migrant mothers.

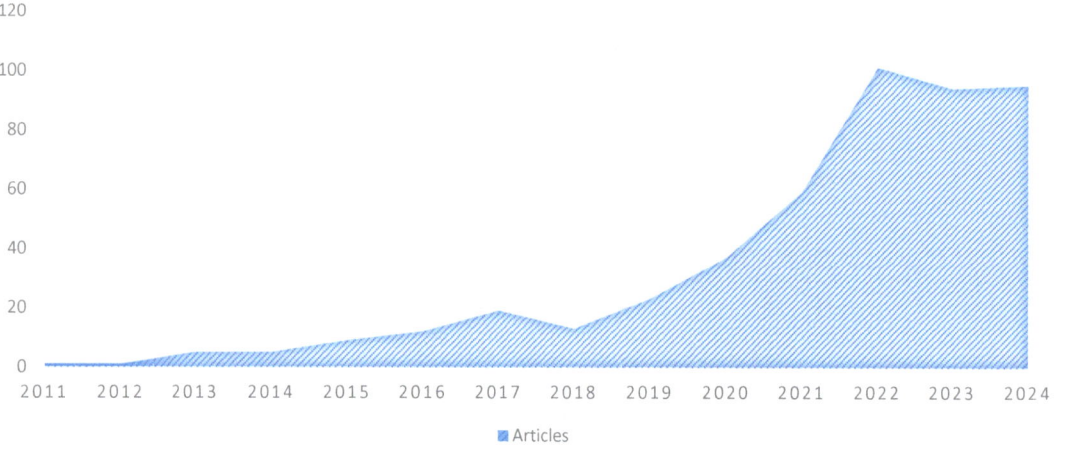

Figure 2. Annual production of scientific research in the field. Source: Scopus/Biblioshiny.

Table 2. Most relevant sources. Source: Scopus/PubMed/Biblioshiny.

Sources	Articles	Subject Area
Women and Birth	45	Maternity and Midwifery
Archives of Women's Mental Health	34	Obstetrics and Gynecology
Obstetrics & Gynecology	31	
Birth	24	Obstetrics and Gynecology
Bmc Pregnancy and Childbirth	19	Obstetrics and Gynecology
JAMA Pediatrics	17	
Health Expectations	10	Public Health, Environmental, and Occupational Health
Healthcare (Switzerland)	6	Health Policy
Journal of Midwifery & Women's Health	6	
Nursing for Women's Health	5	

Furthermore, Table 3 and Figure 4 provide a comprehensive analysis of the most significant articles on the subject, in addition to the bibliometric analysis. Research conducted by Willey et al. (2020), entitled "If you don't ask, you don't tell": Refugee women's attitudes on prenatal mental health screening", aims to assess the feasibility and acceptability of a digital perinatal mental health screening program for women with a refugee background. The research's findings highlighted the following three main topics: (i) women's encounters with perinatal mental health screenings while pregnant; (ii) obstacles to and facilitators for obtaining continuous mental healthcare; and (iii) enhancements to the implemented screening programs, such as the creation of audio versions, which women found to be more practical and agreeable. In addition, the second study, entitled "Implementing innovative evidence-based perinatal mental health screening for women of refugee background", agrees with the first paper. This is because the same authors who published the first study (Willey et al., 2019) authored this one as well, which may be seen as a preliminary version of the work entitled "If you don't ask, you don't tell: Refugee women's perspectives on perinatal mental health screening". A study entitled "Implementing innovative evidence-based perinatal mental health screening for women of refugee background" highlights the need of establishing national standards for regular screenings for depression and anxiety in all women throughout the perinatal period. The research contends that the effectiveness of regular pregnancy screenings is hindered by many obstacles at the service, community, and individual levels. Therefore, there is a pressing need to shift toward the utilization of digital screening methods [5,33].

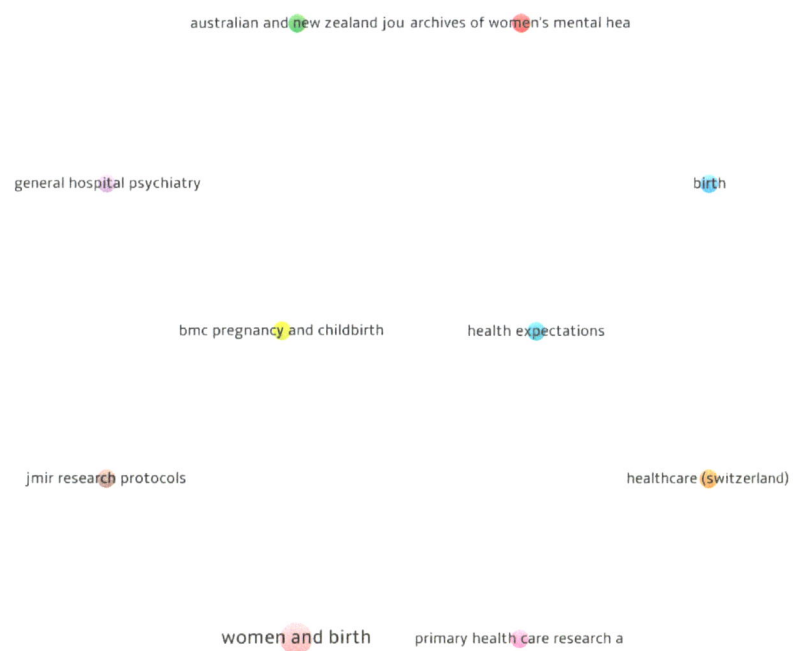

Figure 3. Most impactful sources in the field. Source: Scopus/VOSviewer.

Table 3. Most relevant documents in the field. Source: Scopus/Biblioshiny.

Paper	Total Citations	TC per Year
"If you don't ask . . . you don't tell": Refugee women's perspectives on perinatal mental health screening [33]	22	4.40
Implementing innovative evidence-based perinatal mental health screening for women of refugee background [5]	13	2.60
Perinatal mental health and psychosocial risk screening in a community maternal and child health setting: evaluation of a digital platform [23]	9	1.50
Introducing and integrating perinatal mental health screening: Development of an equity-informed evidence-based approach [9]	7	2.33
Improving Mental Health in Pregnancy for Refugee Women: Protocol for the Implementation and Evaluation of a Screening Program in Melbourne, Australia [34]	7	1.17
Validation of a Dari translation of the Edinburgh Postnatal Depression Scale among women of refugee background at a public antenatal clinic [35]	7	2.33
Digital screening for postnatal depression: mixed methods proof-of-concept study [14]	4	1.33
To screen or not to screen: Are we asking the right question? In response to considering de-implementation of universal perinatal depression screening [30]	1	0.50
Digital Training for Nurses and Midwives to Improve Treatment for Women with Postpartum Depression and Protect Neonates: A Dynamic Bibliometric Review Analysis [32]	0	0.00
Digital screening for mental health in pregnancy and postpartum: A systematic review [13]	0	0.00

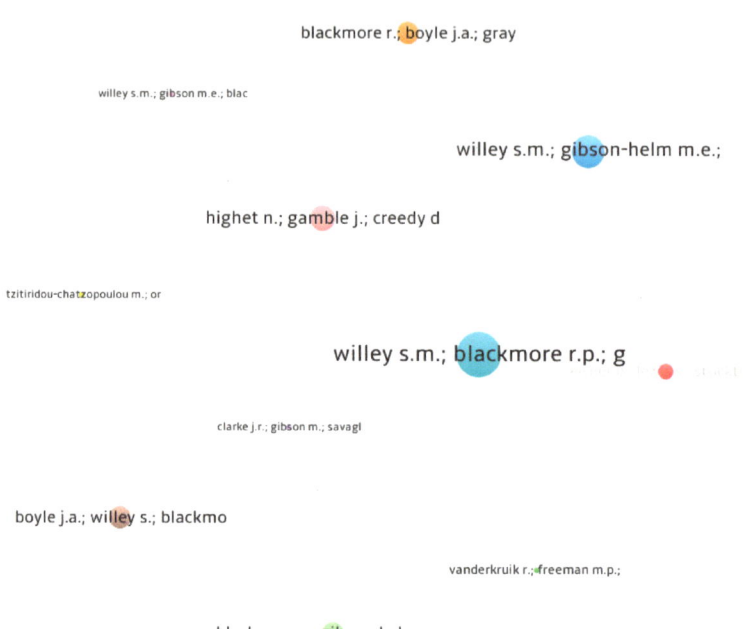

Figure 4. Most impactful documents in the field. Source: Scopus/VOSviewer.

Moreover, Figure 5 presents a map with the most impactful affiliations in the field. At the top of the list is the Department of Obstetrics & Gynecology at Monash University, which has an expertise on the screening technologies and outline the current evidence and best practice for managing the symptoms of perinatal depression. The Department of Obstetrics and Gynecology's clinical research endeavors are integrated within the Ritchie Centre, a renowned university research facility and a leading perinatal and women's health research cluster in Australia. The Ritchie Centre laboratories are located within Monash Health's Translational Research Facility and are primary research collaborators with Monash Children's Hospital and Monash Women's Services. The Ritchie Centre's objective is to promote the health of women and children by conducting innovative research that informs the development of more effective healthcare practices, such as digital screening.

4.2. Bibliometric Analysis

Figure 6 presents the three-field plot, or Sankey diagram, which visualizes multiple attributes at the same time. Based on the findings from the plots, perinatal mental health may be improved by the use of digital technologies to connect screening and therapy. An analysis of the English-language research found that, on average, a mere 22% of women who test positive for perinatal depression actually receive treatment, despite the importance of screening for this disease. The discrepancy between screening and treatment may be worsened by the need for an extra 4 million behavioral health practitioners, as stated in a 2020 workforce study by the Substance Abuse and Mental Health Services Administration (SAMHSA). Increasing the availability of treatment to a larger number of women is crucial, since the shortage of providers and limited access to care pose substantial challenges [7,8]. Therefore, innovation is necessary to overcome these constraints. When used correctly, mental health apps may provide evidence-based therapies to women who are waiting for a healthcare professional, enhance traditional care to reduce the need for visits, or even substitute traditional care with peer support or psychoeducation.

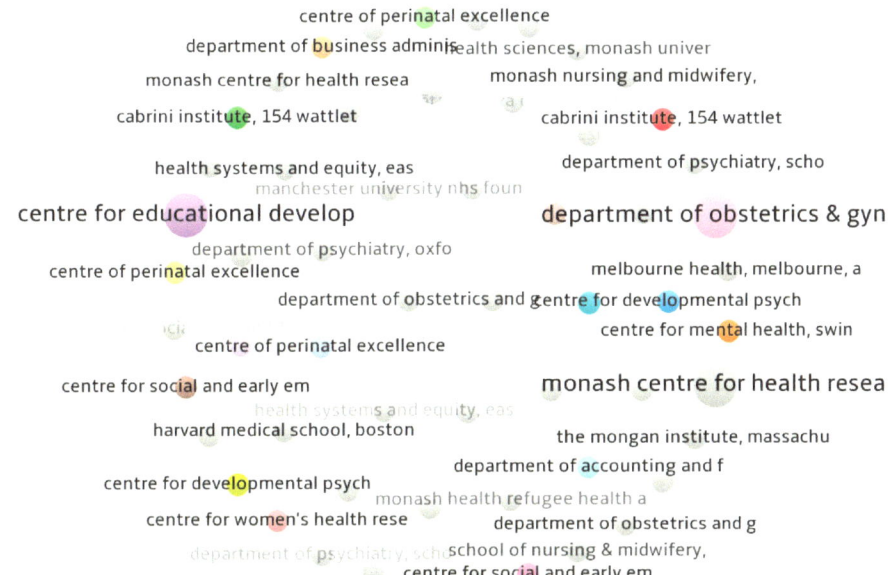

Figure 5. Most impactful affiliations in the field. Source: Scopus/VOSviewer.

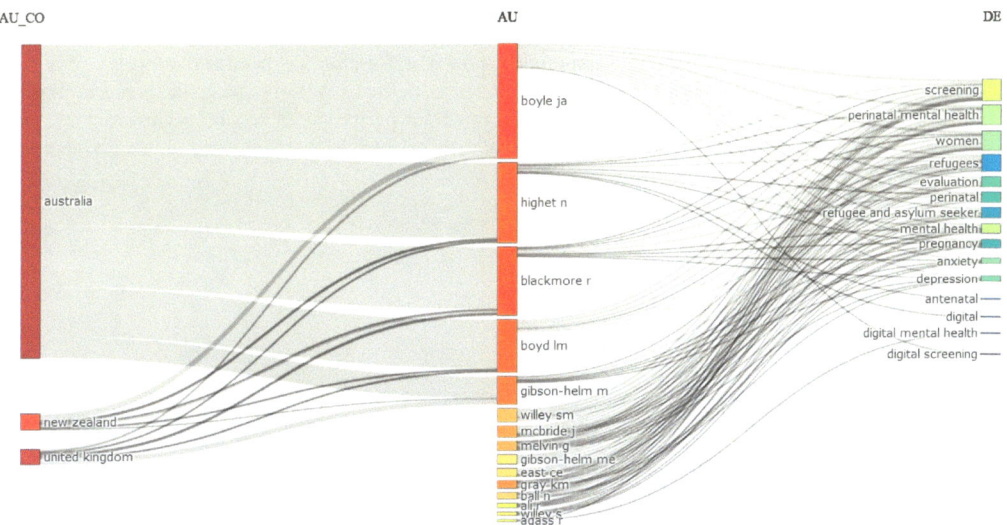

Figure 6. Three-field plot. Source: Scopus/PubMed/Biblioshiny.

Digital mental health solutions may also enhance accessibility for new moms. Amidst the pandemic, telemedicine has received favorable acknowledgment of its capacity to enhance accessibility for women in the postpartum period. These mothers may find that online medical treatment helps overcome challenges such as the need to arrange daycare or the hesitancy to bring young children to a medical facility. Considering that 85% of women own smartphones, the flexibility of apps to enhance care might make therapy more accessible compared to telemedicine alone. The ability to use an application at 4 AM while breastfeeding, instead of trying to rearrange a fragile sleep pattern to accommodate a doctor's visit, may be a boon for busy new parents [36]. Additionally, around 50%

of women have traumatic births [18], and the idea of revisiting a doctor's office where the trauma occurred might be stressful. Remote treatment might allow individuals to assimilate the event at their own pace, rather than experiencing emotional distress or avoiding critical medical attention. Furthermore, alternative methods that are currently being developed have the potential to empower postpartum women to take control of their mental well-being, which is an essential aspect of trauma-informed therapy [37,38].

An analysis of evidence-based therapies for postpartum mental health may demonstrate how several modalities can facilitate the establishment of a customized care system for new mothers and their teams, according to their specific needs and availability. By incorporating traditional appointments, like synchronous and asynchronous support interventions, it may be possible to create a personalized treatment plan for each new mother instead of expecting patients to follow a predetermined care model.

Furthermore, Figure 7 highlights the research trends in the domain from 2011 to 2024. The figure illustrates the present and future directions of digital screening, highlighting its significance in preventing and alleviating maternal depression symptoms and its effects on the mental health of mothers and their children via co-occurrence network mappings. The keywords suggest that the pandemic epidemic activated several elements that affected women's mental health. The myriad physical, emotional, and hormonal alterations linked to pregnancy and childbirth, alongside the forthcoming life transition and reconfiguration of the family unit, are significant factors contributing to the heightened vulnerability of women to depression and anxiety during and post-pregnancy. Nonetheless, the COVID-19 pandemic has had a significant influence. The quarantine, interruption of routine, and absence of social support have adversely affected new moms and their offspring. The confinement regulations significantly reduced the physical presence of the parental and social support network, which acts as a protective factor for mental health and, crucially, for suicide risk. The mental health of women, especially the most vulnerable, was significantly affected by the anxiety and worry stemming from the interplay of these causes and the widespread fear associated with the COVID-19 epidemic. Nevertheless, the data indicate that the screening approach for perinatal depression is clinically relevant, since any kind of sadness may profoundly affect a woman's interactions with her spouse and baby after delivery.

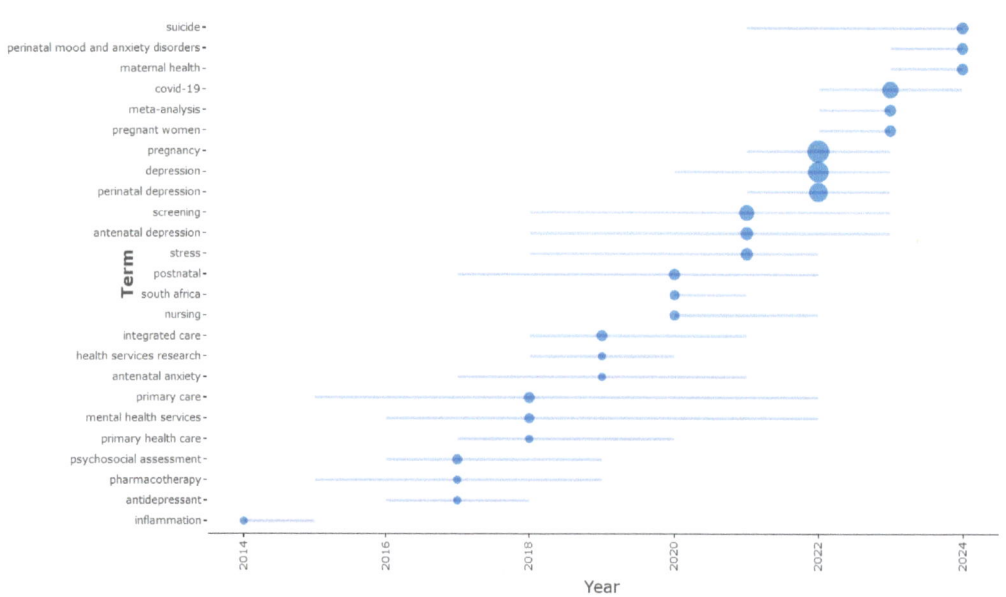

Figure 7. Research trends in the field. Source: Scopus/Biblioshiny.

4.3. Thematic Analysis

Furthermore, Figure 8 illustrates the research themes derived from the conceptual framework of the texts analyzed in the bibliometric study. The graph's clusters represent the primary disciplines of study, and each cluster's magnitude indicates the number of terms it encompasses. Each quadrant of the graph represents a distinctive concept. The image's upper-right quadrant prominently displays motor theme-related motifs, showcasing the high concentration and compactness levels. The upper-left quadrant of the thematic map illustrates the addressed niche subjects. The group stands out because of its high density and low centrality. Additionally, the thematic map highlights the development of concepts in the lower-left quadrant, characterized by their limited prominence and concentration, while also highlighting significant topics in the lower-right quadrant. Their dominance in this field underscores the importance of telehealth and telemedicine in alleviating tension for both parents and infants during perinatal disorders.

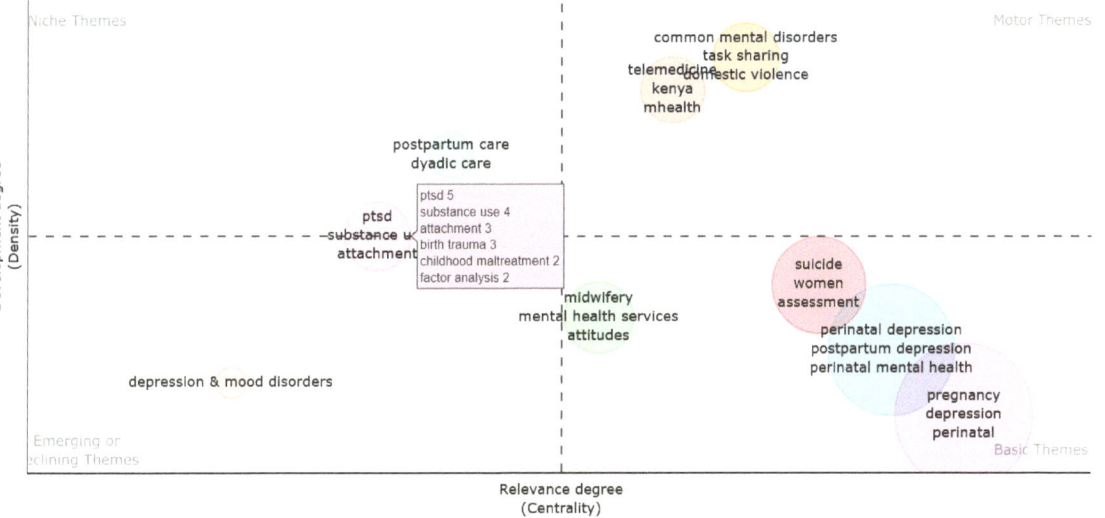

Figure 8. Thematic map. Source: Scopus/PubMed/Biblioshiny.

The study's thematic map reveals a significant association between the risk of post-traumatic stress disorder (PTSD), postpartum depression, and screening, all of which are distinct issues. Prenatal irritability significantly predicted heightened postpartum depressive symptoms, even when controlling for the following two robust predictors of postpartum depression: previous depression history and total trauma exposure. The research definitively indicates that a history of depression predicts postpartum depression; however, the relationship between trauma exposure and postpartum depressive symptoms is more intricate. The symptoms of PTSD, such as irritability, may function as critical indicators for assessment rather than only indicating the presence or absence of trauma. We should improve current screening methods for perinatal women by incorporating evaluations for both trauma and irritability to identify those at increased risk. We may modify depression screening instruments to include questions about irritability in addition to evaluating trauma history. A routine prenatal evaluation for trauma history and irritability may aid in identifying women at increased risk for postpartum depression before the likely onset of depressive symptoms.

The thematic mapping indicates that digital screening might be a very effective tool for aiding women in Africa in recognizing mental health issues associated with domestic abuse and pregnancy. During the perinatal period, symptoms of various mental illnesses, such as anxiety and depression, are notably widespread and associated with experiences of domestic abuse in Africa. Although research indicates that managing these symptoms throughout pregnancy improves health and economic outcomes for mothers and their children, pregnant women facing these challenges have limited access to regular screening and treatment. This is crucial for enhancing the welfare of perinatal moms and their children. The present theme analysis indicates that technology-based services are facilitating the alleviation of the mental health backlog for women suffering from pregnancy depression. Prior to the COVID-19 pandemic, pregnant women in need of mental health consultations were required to attend the hospital and arrange an appointment if necessary. Nonetheless, the revival of awareness has been necessitated by COVID-19. Although in-person consultations continue, the focus has shifted to enhancing access via digital screening techniques, since booking a virtual session has become quicker and more expedient than traditional methods.

Furthermore, Figure 9 illustrates that the VOSviewer application utilized a phrase co-occurrence analysis. Bibliometrix uses this form of analysis to highlight the importance of word co-occurrence clustering in digital screening, which helps to reduce symptoms of prenatal depression. In Figure 9, the font size and node area are determined by the weight value of the phrase. The frequency of the keyword's occurrence is directly proportional to the weight value. The relevant node and font size grow in direct proportion to the weight value. If there is a line connecting two nodes, it indicates that the two terms are often used. The level of co-occurrence between the two words is shown by the thickness of the connecting line. The thickness of the connecting line is directly correlated with the degree of co-occurrence, meaning that a thicker connecting line represents a higher frequency of co-occurrence between the two phrases. In Figure 9, the analysis reveals the presence of six separate groupings.

However, the cluster that has the highest number of items, shown in red, is associated with the subject of digital mental health [13]. This emphasizes the significance of using digital tools, such cellphones, for the screening process. Furthermore, the relationship between the previously indicated cluster and the yellow cluster, which represents prenatal mental health and screening, is of similar significance. Furthermore, the co-occurrence study serves as a reminder of the need for the use of digital screening to detect indications of prenatal depression in refugees and migrants. Migrant and refugee women have similar risk factors for mental health problems as the local population during the perinatal period, such as isolation, financial difficulties, and physical health concerns [39,40]. However, migrant and refugee women face a range of distinct and interconnected risk factors, including uncertain immigration status, limited social support, and gender-based violence. In addition, female refugees or migrants face significant barriers when trying to access prenatal mental healthcare. Barriers to accessing healthcare include the intricate nature of the healthcare system, the high costs of treatments, and the lack of culturally and linguistically appropriate services, especially for women on temporary visas who are not eligible for Medicare. Government policies and services have not been adequately designed to address the perinatal support requirements of migrant and refugee women, nor have they focused on their preferred support interventions. This is despite the evidence indicating that migrant and refugee women face higher rates of perinatal mental health issues. At the policy level, there is a tendency to treat migrant and refugee groups as a homogeneous group, disregarding the distinct needs of people and communities, as well as the impact of gender on mental well-being.

The obstacles that hinder migrant and refugee women from getting help include the financial burden of services and the lack of gender-specific, culturally acceptable, or suitable perinatal mental health treatments at the organizational and sector levels. Therefore, it is crucial to provide prenatal mental healthcare that is specifically tailored to the gender, cultural background, and fair treatment of migrant and refugee women [23]. In order to meet the needs of migrant and refugee women throughout the perinatal periods, it is crucial to perform a comprehensive analysis that takes into account many elements and is based on evidence. This analysis should include the intersecting factors that contribute to the mental health risks faced by these women. The findings from this analysis will inform the development of policy changes. Hence, it is crucial to examine the capacity of digital screening to mitigate prenatal depression symptoms in this specific cohort of women, considering the circumstances and the susceptibility of refugee women [41].

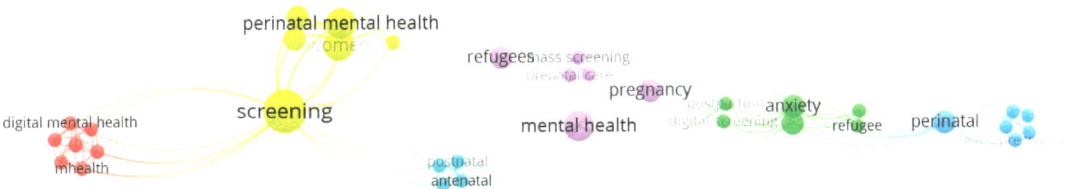

Figure 9. Keyword co-occurrence analysis. Source: Scopus/PubMed/VOSviewer.

5. Discussion

Symptoms of perinatal depression typically manifest within one to three weeks of the baby's birth. Nevertheless, they may commence at any point during the initial year following the birth of the child. The symptoms are more severe than the infant blues and may encompass a profound pessimism and a complete lack of interest in the neonate. The health and development of the infant may be impacted by postpartum depression. Although it is not a common consequence of delivery, postpartum depression is a frequent occurrence. This may be the result of a variety of factors. Hormone levels may undergo abrupt fluctuations after pregnancy. Sleep deprivation, stress resulting from new regimens, and other changes may also induce postpartum depression. The prompt identification and treatment of postpartum depression are made possible by a postpartum depression screening. Additionally, the prevention of chronic depression may be facilitated by the early commencement of therapy. Medicine and therapy may be effective treatments for most individuals. In severe cases, treatment may involve brain stimulation techniques, including electroconvulsive therapy (ECT), which is occasionally referred to as "shock therapy".

Nevertheless, the current research suggests that it is imperative to implement and integrate a computerized screening procedure to effectively and promptly identify and elucidate the symptoms of prenatal depression. The implementation of digital screening resulted in the reduction in scoring inaccuracies, an enhancement of screening efficiency, a reduction in the time required for administration, the generation of clinical and patient reports, and the commencement of referrals for anxiety and depression therapy. The selection of a user interface may influence the installation and adoption of digital screening. Nevertheless, these investigations were conducted on women who underwent screening at home at varying intervals, and it is uncertain whether these findings can be applied to clinical screening. The simplicity of instituting digital screening is facilitated by the information provided, capacity of the women to monitor their own actions and emotions, recommendation for social assistance, absence of scoring mistakes, and efficient self-completion. In general, women exhibited a high level of proficiency in the completion of digital screening, with minimal technical challenges. The screening was highly advantageous for them when it was conducted in their native language, as it was more efficient; they were able to comprehend the inquiries more readily, and they were more forthcoming with their responses. Digital screening has been demonstrated to effectively reduce humiliation, improve confidentiality, and promote equity among women and across various societies. Furthermore, women have demonstrated the ability to independently perform the operation in a sequestered clinic chamber by inputting their responses themselves using interactive voice response (IVR) technology.

The current research further demonstrates the need for digital screening in preventing prenatal depression symptoms in immigrant mothers [8,11,14,36]. Perinatal mental health concerns in migrant and refugee women are associated with social isolation, as well as a lack of adequate social support. Having a limited ability to speak English is a constant element that increases the likelihood of experiencing social isolation, especially for women who have moved as refugees or come from low-income and conflict-affected countries. The healthcare system may often be complex and difficult to navigate. Lack of culturally sensitive services and limited use of trained interpreters can create communication obstacles between healthcare providers and migrant and refugee women. These barriers can hinder the achievement of positive perinatal mental health outcomes and a safe pregnancy. Multiple studies have shown that the mental well-being of migrant and refugee women may be negatively impacted by health practitioners' insufficient understanding of cultural beliefs and practices related to pregnancy and the period after giving birth [6,42,43]. Migrant and refugee women may feel excluded from healthcare choices made by healthcare professionals throughout their prenatal period since culturally appropriate health services are not readily available [9,10]. As a result, migrant women may have a reduced inclination to use perinatal mental health services and seek help for their emotional difficulties throughout pregnancy and postpartum. Therefore, digital screening will positively affect refugee women.

During pregnancy and after giving birth, digital screening provides a new, feasible, well-received, and efficient method for screening women for mental health problems, such as anxiety and depression [44,45]. Both women and healthcare professionals have demonstrated the feasibility and positive reception of this approach in clinical treatment. Key factors contributing to the success of this initiative include the availability of technological aid and support to help women understand the purpose and advantages of screening. Additionally, it is crucial to provide education and training to HCPs on screening, digital technology, and risk management for women. Digital screening empowers women to actively participate in their mental healthcare, referral, and treatment by enabling them to independently monitor and control their behavior [8,36]. Ensuring the availability of appropriate organizational resources and staff is crucial for promoting widespread usage, fairness, and availability of mental health assistance for women globally throughout the prenatal and postpartum period.

Limitations

Certain limitations of the present study pertain to the use of bibliometric analysis. While bibliometric indicators may serve as a beneficial adjunct to the peer-review process, they are often misapplied and used without a comprehensive understanding of the underlying bibliometric research. Consequently, they are often used to assess metrics for which they were not designed or to draw comparisons that they are inherently incapable of facilitating.

6. Conclusions

The significance of digital screening in the prevention of prenatal depression symptoms is still being elucidated by the worldwide academic community. The objective of this inquiry is to highlight the importance of transitioning from conventional to digital screening processes and their impact on enhancing therapy for prenatal depression symptoms. The study topic was examined using bibliometric analysis with R Studio, together with the bibliometric applications VOSviewer and Biblioshiny. We used bibliometrix software to evaluate 197 papers acquired from the Scopus and PubMed databases for this study. The results demonstrate a significant association between the evaluation of prenatal depressive symptoms and digital mental health. Furthermore, the findings underscore the significance of digital screening in mitigating prenatal depression symptoms in refugee women, who are inherently vulnerable because of their precarious circumstances.

This research advocates for digital screening to mitigate prenatal depression among immigrant mothers. Social isolation and insufficient assistance are associated with prenatal mental health challenges in migrant and refugee women. Inadequate English proficiency increases the likelihood of social isolation, especially among women who are refugees or originate from low-income, conflict-affected nations. The healthcare system may be perplexing. In the absence of culturally relevant treatments and proficient interpreters, healthcare providers may have difficulties in communicating with migrant and refugee women. These impediments may hinder secure pregnancies and optimal perinatal health. Numerous studies have shown that health practitioners' insufficient understanding of cultural attitudes and practices around pregnancy and postpartum may adversely affect the mental health of migrant and refugee women. Migrant and refugee women may feel marginalized in prenatal healthcare choices because of the scarcity of culturally appropriate health treatments. Migrant women may exhibit reduced likelihoods of using perinatal mental health treatments for emotional support throughout pregnancy and the postpartum period. Consequently, digital screening will assist refugee women.

This bibliometric review has identified key screening tools and practices in order to help healthcare providers mitigate symptoms of perinatal depression, which can affect mothers' mental health and their neonates too, aid them in the implementation of digital screenings, and also provide recommendations for clinical practice. Future research and clinical practice should add to the literature by adapting current practices and implementing digital screenings for depression during pregnancy and postpartum in their specific healthcare settings worldwide, utilizing the theory-informed, best-practice recommendations presented in this systematic review, as well as various language translations and formats.

Author Contributions: Conceptualization, M.T.-C. and G.Z.; methodology, G.Z; software, M.T.-C. and G.Z; validation, M.T.-C. and G.Z; formal analysis, M.T.-C. and G.Z.; investigation, M.T.-C. and G.Z.; resources, G.Z.; data curation, M.T.-C. and G.Z.; writing—original draft preparation, M.T.-C. and G.Z.; writing—review and editing, M.T.-C. and G.Z.; visualization, M.T.-C. and G.Z.; supervision, M.T.-C. and G.Z.; project administration, G.Z. All authors have read and agreed to the published version of the manuscript.

Funding: This research received no external funding.

Institutional Review Board Statement: Not applicable. This study did not involve humans.

Informed Consent Statement: Not applicable. This study did not involve humans.

Data Availability Statement: Dataset available upon request from the authors.

Conflicts of Interest: The authors declare no conflicts of interest.

References

1. Castillo-Ruiz, A.; Mosley, M.; George, A.J.; Mussaji, L.F.; Fullerton, E.F.; Ruszkowski, E.M.; Jacobs, A.J.; Gewirtz, A.T.; Chassaing, B.; Forger, N.G. The microbiota influences cell death and microglial colonization in the perinatal mouse brain. *Brain Behav. Immun.* **2018**, *67*, 218–229. [CrossRef]
2. Thomas, E.B.K.; Miller, M.L.; Grekin, R.; O'Hara, M.W. Examining psychological inflexibility as a mediator of postpartum depressive symptoms: A longitudinal observational study of perinatal depression. *J. Context. Behav. Sci.* **2023**, *27*, 11–15. [CrossRef] [PubMed]
3. Lantigua-Martinez, M.; Trostle, M.E.; Torres, A.M.; Rajeev, P.; Dennis, A.; Silverstein, J.S.; Talib, M. Perinatal depression before and during the COVID-19 pandemic in New York City. *AJOG Glob. Rep.* **2023**, *3*, 100253. [CrossRef]
4. Kissler, K.; Thumm, E.B.; Smith, D.C.; Anderson, J.L.; Wood, R.E.; Johnson, R.; Roberts, M.; Carmitchel-Fifer, A.; Patterson, N.; Amura, C.R.; et al. Perinatal Telehealth: Meeting Patients where They Are. *J. Midwifery Women's Health* **2024**, *69*, 9–16. [CrossRef] [PubMed]
5. Willey, S.M.; Gibson-Helm, M.E.; Finch, T.L.; East, C.E.; Khan, N.N.; Boyd, L.M.; Boyle, J.A. Implementing innovative evidence-based perinatal mental health screening for women of refugee background. *Women Birth J. Aust. Coll. Midwives* **2020**, *33*, e245–e255. [CrossRef]
6. Hoffiz, Y.C.; Castillo-Ruiz, A.; Hall, M.A.L.; Hite, T.A.; Gray, J.M.; Cisternas, C.D.; Cortes, L.R.; Jacobs, A.J.; Forger, N.G. Birth elicits a conserved neuroendocrine response with implications for perinatal osmoregulation and neuronal cell death. *Sci. Rep.* **2021**, *11*, 2335. [CrossRef]
7. Gao, Y.; Bahl, M. Management of screening-detected lobular neoplasia in the era of digital breast tomosynthesis: A preliminary study. *Clin. Imaging* **2023**, *103*, 109979. [CrossRef]
8. Komanchuk, J.; Cameron, J.L.; Kurbatfinksi, S.; Duffett-Leger, L.; Letourneau, N. A realist review of digitally delivered child development assessment and screening tools: Psychometrics and considerations for future use. *Early Hum. Dev.* **2023**, *183*, 105818. [CrossRef]

9. Blackmore, R.; Boyle, J.A.; Gray, K.M.; Willey, S.; Highet, N.; Gibson-Helm, M. Introducing and integrating perinatal mental health screening: Development of an equity-informed evidence-based approach. *Health Expect. Int. J. Public Particip. Health Care Health Policy* **2022**, *25*, 2287–2298. [CrossRef]
10. Willey, S.M.; Gibson, M.E.; Blackmore, R.; Goonetilleke, L.; McBride, J.; Highet, N.; Ball, N.; Gray, K.M.; Melvin, G.; Boyd, L.M.; et al. Perinatal mental health screening for women of refugee background: Addressing a major gap in pregnancy care. *Birth* **2024**, *51*, 229–241. [CrossRef]
11. Linz, D.; Gawalko, M.; Betz, K.; Hendriks, J.M.; Lip, G.Y.H.; Vinter, N.; Guo, Y.; Johnsen, S. Atrial fibrillation: Epidemiology, screening and digital health. *Lancet Reg. Health-Eur.* **2024**, *37*, 100786. [CrossRef]
12. Odole, I.P.; Andersen, M.; Richman, I.B. Digital Interventions to Support Lung Cancer Screening: A Systematic Review. *Am. J. Prev. Med.* **2024**, *66*, 899–908. [CrossRef]
13. Clarke, J.R.; Gibson, M.; Savaglio, M.; Navani, R.; Mousa, M.; Boyle, J.A. Digital screening for mental health in pregnancy and postpartum: A systematic review. *Arch. Women's Ment. Health* **2024**, *27*, 489–526. [CrossRef]
14. Eisner, E.; Lewis, S.; Stockton-Powdrell, C.; Agass, R.; Whelan, P.; Tower, C. Digital screening for postnatal depression: Mixed methods proof-of-concept study. *BMC Pregnancy Childbirth* **2022**, *22*, 429. [CrossRef]
15. Shaffer, K.M.; Turner, K.L.; Siwik, C.; Gonzalez, B.D.; Upasani, R.; Glazer, J.V.; Ferguson, R.J.; Joshua, C.; Low, C.A. Digital health and telehealth in cancer care: A scoping review of reviews. *Lancet Digit. Health* **2023**, *5*, e316–e327. [CrossRef]
16. Tunis, R.; West, E.; Clifford, N.; Horner, S.; Radhakrishnan, K. Leveraging digital health technologies in heart failure self-care interventions to improve health equity. *Nurs. Outlook* **2024**, *72*, 102225. [CrossRef]
17. Tucker, L.; Villagomez, A.C.; Krishnamurti, T. Comprehensively addressing postpartum maternal health: A content and image review of commercially available mobile health apps. *BMC Pregnancy Childbirth* **2021**, *21*, 311. [CrossRef]
18. Tsai, Z.; Kiss, A.; Nadeem, S.; Sidhom, K.; Owais, S.; Faltyn, M.; Lieshout, R.J.V. Evaluating the effectiveness and quality of mobile applications for perinatal depression and anxiety: A systematic review and meta-analysis. *J. Affect. Disord.* **2022**, *296*, 443–453. [CrossRef]
19. Varma, D.S.; Mualem, M.; Goodin, A.; Gurka, K.K.; Wen, T.S.T.; Gurka, M.J.; Roussos-Ross, K. Acceptability of an mHealth App for Monitoring Perinatal and Postpartum Mental Health: Qualitative Study with Women and Providers. *JMIR Form. Res.* **2023**, *7*, e44500. [CrossRef] [PubMed]
20. Voit, F.A.C.; Kajantie, E.; Lemola, S.; Räikkönen, K.; Wolke, D.; Schnitzlein, D.D. Maternal mental health and adverse birth outcomes. *PLoS ONE* **2022**, *17*, e0272210. [CrossRef]
21. Chen, H.W.; Cheng, S.F.; Hsiung, Y.; Chuang, Y.H.; Liu, T.Y.; Kuo, C.L. Training perinatal nurses in palliative communication by using scenario-based simulation: A quasi-experimental study. *Nurse Educ. Pract.* **2024**, *75*, 103885. [CrossRef]
22. Green, S.M.; Donegan, E.; McCabe, R.E.; Streiner, D.L.; Furtado, M.; Noble, L.; Agako, A.; Frey, B.N. Cognitive Behavior Therapy for Women With Generalized Anxiety Disorder in the Perinatal Period: Impact on Problematic Behaviors. *Behav. Ther.* **2021**, *52*, 907–916. [CrossRef]
23. Highet, N.; Gamble, J.; Creedy, D. Perinatal mental health and psychosocial risk screening in a community maternal and child health setting: Evaluation of a digital platform. *Prim. Health Care Res. Dev.* **2019**, *20*, e58. [CrossRef]
24. Donegan, E.; Frey, B.N.; McCabe, R.E.; Streiner, D.L.; Green, S.M. Intolerance of Uncertainty and Perfectionistic Beliefs about Parenting as Cognitive Mechanisms of Symptom Change during Cognitive Behavior Therapy for Perinatal Anxiety. *Behav. Ther.* **2022**, *53*, 738–750. [CrossRef]
25. Leng, L.L.; Yin, X.C.; Chan, C.L.W.; Ng, S.M. Antenatal mobile-delivered mindfulness-based intervention to reduce perinatal depression risk and improve obstetric and neonatal outcomes: A randomized controlled trial. *J. Affect. Disord.* **2023**, *335*, 216–227. [CrossRef]
26. Koh, J.; Tng, G.Y.Q.; Hartanto, A. Potential and Pitfalls of Mobile Mental Health Apps in Traditional Treatment: An Umbrella Review. *J. Pers. Med.* **2022**, *12*, 1376. [CrossRef]
27. Al-Arkee, S.; Mason, J.; Lane, D.A.; Fabritz, L.; Chua, W.; Haque, M.S.; Jalal, Z. Mobile apps to improve medication adherence in cardiovascular disease: Systematic review and meta-analysis. *J. Med. Internet Res.* **2021**, *23*, e24190. [CrossRef]
28. Nicholas, J.; Fogarty, A.S.; Boydell, K.; Christensen, H. The reviews are in: A qualitative content analysis of consumer perspectives on apps for bipolar disorder. *J. Med. Internet Res.* **2017**, *19*, e105. [CrossRef]
29. Alqahtani, F.; Orji, R. Insights from user reviews to improve mental health apps. *Health Inform. J.* **2020**, *26*, 2042–2066. [CrossRef]
30. Vanderkruik, R.; Freeman, M.P.; Nonacs, R.; Jellinek, M.; Gaw, M.L.; Clifford, C.A.; Bartels, S.; Cohen, L.S. To screen or not to screen: Are we asking the right question? In response to considering de-implementation of universal perinatal depression screening. *Gen. Hosp. Psychiatry* **2023**, *83*, 81–85. [CrossRef]
31. Viveiros, C.J.; Darling, E.K. Perceptions of barriers to accessing perinatal mental health care in midwifery: A scoping review. *Midwifery* **2019**, *70*, 106–118. [CrossRef] [PubMed]
32. Tzitiridou-Chatzopoulou, M.; Orovou, E.; Zournatzidou, G. Digital Training for Nurses and Midwives to Improve Treatment for Women with Postpartum Depression and Protect Neonates: A Dynamic Bibliometric Review Analysis. *Healthcare* **2024**, *12*, 1015. [CrossRef] [PubMed]
33. Willey, S.M.; Blackmore, R.P.; Gibson-Helm, M.E.; Ali, R.; Boyd, L.M.; McBride, J.; Boyle, J.A. "If you don't ask … you don't tell": Refugee women's perspectives on perinatal mental health screening. *Women Birth* **2020**, *33*, e429–e437. [CrossRef] [PubMed]

34. Boyle, J.A.; Willey, S.; Blackmore, R.; East, C.; McBride, J.; Gray, K.; Melvin, G.; Fradkin, R.; Ball, N.; Highet, N.; et al. Improving Mental Health in Pregnancy for Refugee Women: Protocol for the Implementation and Evaluation of a Screening Program in Melbourne, Australia. *JMIR Res. Protoc.* **2019**, *8*, e13271. [CrossRef]
35. Blackmore, R.; Gibson-Helm, M.; Melvin, G.; Boyle, J.A.; Fazel, M.; Gray, K.M. Validation of a Dari translation of the Edinburgh Postnatal Depression Scale among women of refugee background at a public antenatal clinic. *Aust. N. Z. J. Psychiatry* **2021**, *56*, 525–534. [CrossRef]
36. Reading Turchioe, M.; Slotwiner, D. Screening for Atrial Fibrillation Using Digital Health: Moving from Promises to Reality. *JACC Adv.* **2023**, *2*, 100621. [CrossRef]
37. M.Ali, R.M.K.; Hogg, P. Eye radiation dose from breast cancer screening using full field digital mammography and digital breast tomosynthesis: A phantom study. *Radiography* **2024**, *30*, 141–144. [CrossRef]
38. Giorgi Rossi, P.; Mancuso, P.; Pattacini, P.; Campari, C.; Nitrosi, A.; Iotti, V.; Ponti, A.; Frigerio, A.; Correale, L.; Riggi, E.; et al. Comparing accuracy of tomosynthesis plus digital mammography or synthetic 2D mammography in breast cancer screening: Baseline results of the MAITA RCT consortium. *Eur. J. Cancer* **2024**, *199*, 113553. [CrossRef]
39. Javakhishvili, J.; Makhashvili, N.; Winkler, P.; Votruba, N.; van Voren, R. Providing immediate digital mental health interventions and psychotrauma support during political crises. *Lancet Psychiatry* **2023**, *10*, 727–732. [CrossRef]
40. Danese, A.; Martsenkovskyi, D.; Remberk, B.; Khalil, M.Y.; Diggins, E.; Keiller, E.; Masood, S.; Awah, I.; Barbui, C.; Beer, R.; et al. Scoping Review: Digital Mental Health Interventions for Children and Adolescents Affected by War. *J. Am. Acad. Child Adolesc. Psychiatry*, 2024; *In Press.* [CrossRef]
41. Grassi, M.; Defillo, A.; Daccò, S.; Caldirola, D.; Wolfy, Z.; Perna, G.; Young, T. A novel objective digital mental health platform based on machine learning for screening of current major depressive episode in sleep clinics. *Sleep Med.* **2024**, *115*, 403–404. [CrossRef]
42. Kumar, N.R.; Arias, M.P.; Leitner, K.; Wang, E.; Clement, E.G.; Hamm, R.F. Assessing the impact of telehealth implementation on postpartum outcomes for Black birthing people. *Am. J. Obstet. Gynecol. MFM* **2023**, *5*, 100831. [CrossRef]
43. Farias-Jofre, M.; Romero, R.; Galaz, J.; Xu, Y.; Miller, D.; Garcia-Flores, V.; Arenas-Hernandez, M.; Winters, A.D.; Berkowitz, B.A.; Podolsky, R.H.; et al. Blockade of IL-6R prevents preterm birth and adverse neonatal outcomes. *EBioMedicine* **2023**, *98*, 104865. [CrossRef] [PubMed]
44. Arias, M.P.; Wang, E.; Leitner, K.; Sannah, T.; Keegan, M.; Delferro, J.; Iluore, C.; Arimoro, F.; Streaty, T.; Hamm, R.F. The impact on postpartum care by telehealth: A retrospective cohort study. *Am. J. Obstet. Gynecol. MFM* **2022**, *4*, 100611. [CrossRef]
45. Hawkins, S.S. Telehealth in the Prenatal and Postpartum Periods. *JOGNN—J. Obstet. Gynecol. Neonatal Nurs.* **2023**, *52*, 264–275. [CrossRef]

Disclaimer/Publisher's Note: The statements, opinions and data contained in all publications are solely those of the individual author(s) and contributor(s) and not of MDPI and/or the editor(s). MDPI and/or the editor(s) disclaim responsibility for any injury to people or property resulting from any ideas, methods, instructions or products referred to in the content.

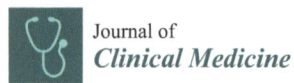 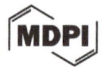

Systematic Review

Risk Factors of Velamentous Cord Insertion in Singleton Pregnancies—A Systematic Review and Meta-Analysis

Antonios Siargkas [1,*], Ioannis Tsakiridis [1], Athanasios Gatsis [1], Catalina De Paco Matallana [2,3], Maria Mar Gil [4,5,6], Petya Chaveeva [7,8] and Themistoklis Dagklis [1]

[1] Third Department of Obstetrics and Gynecology, School of Medicine, Faculty of Health Sciences, Aristotle University of Thessaloniki, Agiou Dimitriou, 54124 Thessaloniki, Greece; iotsakir@gmail.com (I.T.); athanasiosgatsis@gmail.com (A.G.); themistoklisdagklis@gmail.com (T.D.)

[2] Institute for Biomedical Research of Murcia, IMIB-Arrixaca, El Palmar, Faculty of Medicine, Universidad de Murcia, 30120 Murcia, Spain; katydepaco@gmail.com

[3] Maternal Fetal Medicine Unit, Department Obstetrics and Gynecology, Virgen de la Arrixaca, 30120 Murcia, Spain

[4] School of Medicine, Universidad Francisco de Vitoria, 28223 Madrid, Spain; mariadelmar.gil@ufv.es

[5] Department of Obstetrics and Gynecology, Hospital Universitario de Torrejón, 28850 Madrid, Spain

[6] Ultrasound and Fetal Medicine Unit, Obstetrics and Gynecology Department, Hospital Universitario La Paz, 28046 Madrid, Spain

[7] Department of Obstetrics and Gynecology, Faculty of Medicine, Medical University of Pleven, 5800 Pleven, Bulgaria; chaveevapetya@gmail.com

[8] Fetal Medicine Unit, Dr. Shterev Hospital, 1330 Sofia, Bulgaria

* Correspondence: antonis.siargkas@gmail.com; Tel.: +30-6940580900

Abstract: Objective: This meta-analysis aims to quantitatively summarize current data on various potential risk factors of velamentous cord insertion (VCI). A better understanding of these risk factors could enhance prenatal identification both in settings with routine screening and in those where universal screening for cord insertion anomalies is not yet recommended. **Methods:** A systematic search was conducted in MEDLINE, Cochrane Library, and Scopus from their inception until 7 February 2024. Eligible studies included observational studies of singleton pregnancies with VCI, identified either prenatally or postnatally, compared with pregnancies with central or eccentric cord insertion. Analyses were performed using DerSimonian and Laird random-effects models, with outcomes reported as risk ratios (RR) or mean differences with 95% confidence intervals (CI). **Results:** In total, 14 cohort and 4 case-control studies were included, reporting on 952,163 singleton pregnancies. Based on the cohort studies, the overall prevalence of VCI among singleton pregnancies was calculated to be 1.54%. The risk of VCI was significantly higher among pregnancies conceived using assisted reproductive technology (RR, 2.32; 95% CI: 1.77–3.05), nulliparous women (RR, 1.21; 95% CI: 1.15–1.28), women who smoked (RR, 1.14; 95% CI: 1.08–1.19), and pregnancies diagnosed with placenta previa (RR, 3.60; 95% CI: 3.04–4.28). **Conclusions:** This meta-analysis identified assisted reproductive technology, nulliparity, smoking, and placenta previa as significant risk factors of VCI among singleton pregnancies. These findings could inform screening policies in settings where universal screening for cord insertion is not routinely performed, suggesting a targeted approach for women with these specific risk factors.

Keywords: assisted reproductive technology; nulliparity; placenta previa; smoking; chronic hypertension; abnormal cord insertion

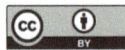

1. Introduction

In a velamentous cord insertion (VCI), the umbilical cord inserts into the fetal membranes (between the amnion and the chorion) away from the placental margin, and the vessels traverse between these membranes before reaching the placenta, as depicted in Figure 1 [1]. In cases of VCI, there may be an absence of the protective effect of Wharton's jelly, normally present around the vessels [2]. Placentas with non-central insertions may be less effective in supporting fetal growth despite their normal or even increased size. This decreased placental efficiency may be explained by a relative reduction in the chorionic vascular density of the placenta, as the cord is displaced from the center [3]. The reported occurrence of VCI among singleton pregnancies is 1.4%, and it was associated with several adverse perinatal outcomes including stillbirth, pre-eclampsia, placental abruption, small-for-gestational-age neonates, preterm delivery, emergency cesarean section (CS), reduced Apgar score and higher admission rate to the neonatal intensive care unit [4].

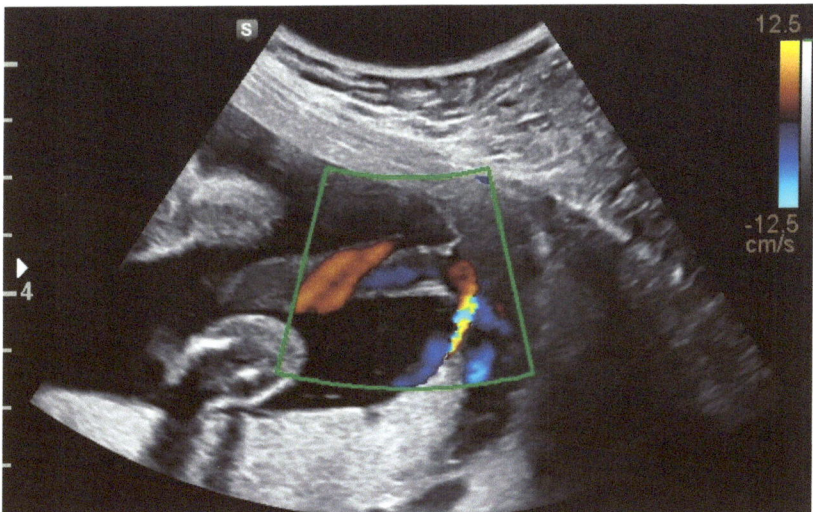

Figure 1. Ultrasound image depicting a velamentous cord insertion.

These findings, along with the feasibility of antenatal recognition of VCI, underscore the importance of a more systematic diagnostic approach; studies have shown that second-trimester sonographic identification of VCI is accurate, with an exceptionally high specificity of close to 100% but a lower sensitivity of about 70% [5]. Current recommendations vary regarding the need to identify a VCI antenatally. Thus, the American Institute of Ultrasound in Medicine recommends documenting abnormal cord insertions [6], whereas the International Society of Ultrasound in Obstetrics and Gynecology advises that an umbilical cord insertion assessment during mid-trimester scan is optional; however, an incidental finding of VCI should be documented [7].

A comprehensive understanding of risk factors for VCI may improve prenatal identification in settings with routine screening but also in settings where universal screening for cord insertion anomalies is not yet recommended and a targeted approach for women with specific risk factors should at least be considered. Published data have identified a variety of potential risk factors for VCI in singleton pregnancies, i.e., advanced maternal age, previous history of CS, Caucasian ethnicity, use of assisted reproductive technology (ART), smoking, placenta previa, nulliparity and chronic hypertension [8–10]. This meta-analysis aimed to conduct a rigorous evaluation and statistical analysis of the current evidence on possible risk factors for VCI.

2. Methods

This meta-analysis adhered to the Preferred Reporting Items for Systematic reviews and Meta-Analyses (PRISMA) [11] and Meta-analysis Of Observational Studies in Epidemiology (MOOSE) guidelines [12] and was registered with the International Prospective Register of Systematic Reviews (PROSPERO) with the protocol number: CRD42024512296.

Given its nature of synthesizing data from previously published literature, the study was exempt from the need for ethical approval and patient consent.

2.1. Search Strategy

The research question guiding this systematic search was, "Which population characteristics could serve as indicators of increased risk for VCI in singleton pregnancies". We crafted a search strategy employing keywords such as "umbilical cord insertion", "cord insertion", "insertion of the cord", "placental cord insertion", "velamentous", "abnormal" and "aberrant". The details of the search strategy can be found in the Supplementary Materials. We searched MEDLINE, Scopus and Cochrane databases from their inception until 7 February 2024. The identified records were managed using Rayyan (Rayyan Systems Inc., Cambridge, MA, USA), a web-based reference management tool. Further, we examined references from relevant articles and conducted manual searches online to identify additional studies. After removing duplicates, we screened titles and abstracts to exclude studies not pertinent to our question and then thoroughly reviewed the full texts of the remaining articles to determine their inclusion. This process was independently carried out by two reviewers (A.S. and A.G, both doctors) blind to each other's selections, with disagreements resolved through discussion or, if necessary, by a third reviewer (I.T., biostatistician).

2.2. Selection Criteria

Observational studies written in English, examining possible risk factors and population characteristics in singleton pregnancies identified with VCI either prenatally or following delivery, were considered eligible. The comparison group included pregnancies with central/eccentric cord insertion (CCI). In studies where the control groups included pregnancies with all types of non-velamentous umbilical cord insertions, adjustments were made, when possible, to ensure comparisons were exclusively with pregnancies having CCI. If such adjustments were not feasible, the studies were excluded. When the same database was utilized across two or more studies covering overlapping periods, we exclusively utilized data from the study encompassing the largest population. Raw data on perinatal outcomes were required. Abstracts and unpublished studies were not included.

2.3. Data Extraction

A standardized data collection template was prepared ahead of the study selection. This template captured study characteristics such as author, publication year, journal, study location, methodology, criteria for inclusion and exclusion, timing and definition of VCI diagnosis, study demographics and investigated risk factors. A second part of the template was dedicated to collecting data on predetermined outcomes, including raw data and, where available, adjusted odds ratios or adjusted risk ratios. Our protocol specified that outcomes reported in at least three studies would be considered for analysis, even if not initially outlined. We reached out to authors for missing data or clarifications and selected the most comprehensive report for studies with multiple publications on the same cohort.

2.4. Outcomes of Interest

Outcomes of interest included every risk factor reported by three or more studies, including ART, maternal age, prior CS, smoking, placenta previa, nulliparity, chronic hypertension and any other possible risk factor with adequate data as stipulated by our protocol.

2.5. Quality and Bias Assessment

The quality of the included studies was independently assessed by two researchers (A.S. and A.G) using the Newcastle–Ottawa scale [13], which evaluates the selection of the study groups, comparability of the groups, and ascertainment of the outcome/risk factor, employing a star system that assigns up to 9 points for high quality. Additionally, the Quality In Prognosis Studies (QUIPS) tool [14] was used to evaluate the risk of bias across six domains: study participation, attrition, prognostic factor measurement, outcome measurement, study confounding and statistical analysis/reporting, with studies rated on a three-point scale (low, moderate, high). Discrepancies in the assessment of quality or bias were reviewed and resolved by a third reviewer (I.T.).

2.6. Statistical Analysis

In our primary analysis, the cumulative raw data were analyzed to calculate the various risk factors' effect on the VCI prevalence. This data synthesis involved computing effect sizes and their 95% confidence intervals (CI) via Review Manager software, version 5.4.1. We determined risk ratios (RR) for binary outcomes using the Mantel–Haenszel technique and mean differences (MD) for continuous variables through the inverse variance method. Due to the significant variability in observational studies, we followed the Cochrane Handbook's recommendation to employ the DerSimonian and Laird random-effects model as the default analytical method. To evaluate the heterogeneity of the included studies, we utilized two approaches. The I^2 statistic was employed to quantify the proportion of the total variance in the observed effect sizes that was due to differences between studies rather than chance. I^2 values of up to 40% might be unimportant, 30–60% moderate, 50–90% substantial and 75–100% considerable [15]. Additionally, we applied the Cochran Q test to examine the homogeneity of the effect sizes across studies, with a *p*-value threshold of 0.10 for statistical significance. In R version 2.15.1 (R Foundation for Statistical Computing, Vienna, Austria) [16], the package meta [17] was employed to generate the funnel plot and the package dmetar [18] to perform the Egger's test. These methods were used to assess publication bias only for the outcome with the higher number of published studies.

2.7. Sensitivity Analysis

As per our established methodology, we carried out a sensitivity analysis that only included cases identified prenatally. This was based upon the premise that our end goal is a better and more focused prenatal diagnosis of VCI. Furthermore, we conducted another sensitivity review that considered only those studies deemed as having a low or moderate risk of bias, as per the QUIPS tool criteria. The objective here was to filter the data less likely to be affected by bias and verify if these refined results would align with our initial findings. Notably, a sensitivity analysis was only deemed feasible if data from three or more studies were available for evaluation.

3. Results

Initially, 1559 records were identified from the Medline, Scopus, and Cochrane databases, while other methods like Web search and citation searching contributed nine additional records. After removing 69 duplicates, we screened 1490 records and excluded 1311 for various reasons. Upon assessing for eligibility, we evaluated 175 full texts, and 18 studies met the eligibility criteria for the review. The other search methods resulted in nine relevant reports, none of which was eligible (Figure 2). The two reviewers achieved an excellent coefficient of agreement on article selection (Cohen's kappa, 0.932), resulting in the retention of 14 cohort [8–10,19–29] and 4 case-control studies [30–33] for the final analysis. The characteristics of the included studies are presented in Table 1.

Table 1. Characteristics of the included studies.

First Author, Year	Country	Study Period	Study Type	Inclusion Criteria	Exclusion Criteria	Cord Insertion Site Diagnosis	Risk Factors
Aragie et al., 2022 [28]	Ethiopia	2021	retrospective cohort	singleton pregnancies	marginal cord insertion, placenta specimens without intact umbilical cord, placenta with externally identifiable pathology, and bifurcated umbilical cord before its insertion	postnatally (inspection of cord insertion during the delivery)	chronic hypertension
Curtin et al., 2019 [30]	USA	2002–2015	retrospective case-control	singleton pregnancies	multiple pregnancies	postnatally (identification of cord insertion through pathology reports)	ART, maternal age, nulliparity, smoking, hypertension
Ebbing et al., 2013 [8]	Norway	1999–2009	retrospective cohort	singleton pregnancies delivered at 16–45 wk	multiple pregnancies	postnatally (form completed by the attending midwife or physician shortly after delivery)	smoking, pre-existing diabetes, placenta previa, chronic hypertension
Ebbing et al., 2015 [19]	Norway	1999–2011	retrospective cohort	singleton pregnancies delivered at 16–45 wk	multiple pregnancies	postnatally (inspection of cord insertion during the delivery)	prior CS
Ebbing et al., 2016 [20]	Norway	1999–2013	retrospective cohort	singleton pregnancies delivered at 16–45 wk	multiple pregnancies	postnatally (inspection of cord insertion during the delivery)	ART, nulliparity
Fukuda et al., 2023 [29]	Japan	2020–2022	retrospective cohort	singleton pregnancies	Intrauterine fetal death, multiple pregnancies, unknown method of conception, multiple-lobed and/or accessory placentas, undelivered placentas due to adhesion, and incomplete entry	postnatally (inspection of cord insertion during the delivery)	ART
Gavriil et al., 1993 [33]	Belgium		retrospective case-control	ART and intrauterine embryo transfer pregnancies	includes twin pregnancies but reports separate raw data for singleton pregnancies	postnatally through pathologic examination	ART

Table 1. Cont.

First Author, Year	Country	Study Period	Study Type	Inclusion Criteria	Exclusion Criteria	Cord Insertion Site Diagnosis	Risk Factors
Hasegawa et al., 2006 [22]	Japan	2002–2004	retrospective cohort	singleton pregnancies	women who first visited the hospital after 20 weeks of gestation	postnatally (inspection of cord insertion during the delivery)	maternal age
Hasegawa et al., 2009 [21]	Japan	2005–2006	retrospective cohort	singleton pregnancies delivered at 22–41 wk	multiple pregnancies	postnatally (inspection of cord insertion during the delivery)	maternal age
Heinonen et al., 1996 [23]	Finland	1989–1993	retrospective cohort	singletons pregnancies delivered after 24 wk	multiple pregnancies and pregnancies with fetal chromosomal abnormalities or structural malformations	postnatally (inspection of cord insertion during the delivery)	prior CS, smoking, unmarried, placenta previa
Jauniaux et al., 1990 [32]	Belgium	1985–1988	retrospective case-control	singleton pregnancies conceived and delivered at term in ART clinic	multiple pregnancies and pregnancies with early vanishing twin phenomenon	postnatal macroscopic examination	ART
Larcher et al., 2023 [27]	Italy	2019–2021	prospective cohort	singleton pregnancies	prior CS-unmatched pregnancies and delivery at gestation age <32 weeks	prenatally (transvaginal/transabdominal) US examination at 11–14, 19–22 and 32–35 weeks	ART
O'Quinn et al., 2020 [25]	Canada	2012–2015	retrospective cohort	singleton pregnancies with completed anatomic survey, delivered >24^{+6} wk,	multiple pregnancies, placenta previa, vasa previa, no documented cord insertion type, or fetal anomalies	prenatally (at the 18–21-week anatomy ultrasound scan)	ART, maternal age, nulliparity, smoking, pre-existing diabetes, chronic hypertension
Raisanen et al., 2012 [24]	Finland	2000–2011	retrospective population-based registerstudy	singleton pregnancies, live-born and stillborn infants delivered afterthe 22 wk or weighing 500 g or more	multiple pregnancies	postnatally (inspection of cord insertion during the delivery)	ART, prior CS, pre-existing diabetes, smoking, placenta previa, nulliparity

Table 1. *Cont.*

First Author, Year	Country	Study Period	Study Type	Inclusion Criteria	Exclusion Criteria	Cord Insertion Site Diagnosis	Risk Factors
Sinkin et al., 2017 [31]	USA	2005–2015	retrospective case-control	singleton pregnancies and at least one ultrasound examination by the maternal-fetal medicine service	fetal anomalies, gestational age at delivery <23 weeks, and vasa previa.	postnatally (according to placenta pathology records)	maternal age, maternal BMI, prior CS, nulliparity, chronic hypertension
Tsakiridis et al., 2021 [9]	Greece	2016–2020	retrospective cohort	singleton pregnancies with a second trimester anomaly scan at 20^{+0}–23^{+6} wk	fetal abnormalities, vasa previa, and single umbilical artery	prenatally (anomaly scan at 20^{+0}–23^{+6} wk)	ART, maternal age, nulliparity, smoking
Visentin et al., 2021 [10]	Italy	2016–2017	retrospective cohort	singleton pregnancies delivered >24 wk	multiple pregnancies, miscarriages and voluntary abortions.	postnatally (according to placenta pathology records)	ART, maternal age, nulliparity, placenta previa
Yang et al., 2020 [26]	China	2004–2014	retrospective cohort	singleton pregnancies	multiple pregnancies	prenatally (color Doppler ultrasonography)	ART, maternal age, nulliparity, smoking, prior CS, placenta previa

Abbreviations: ART, assisted reproductive technology; CS, cesarean section; wk, gestational week.

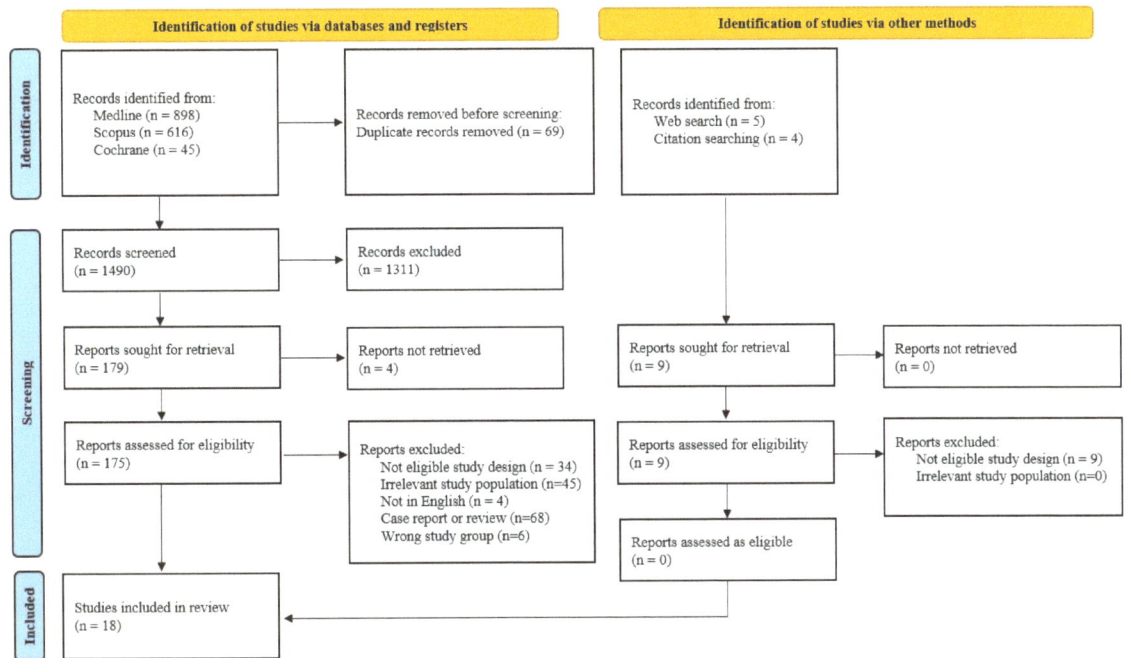

Figure 2. Study selection flow diagram.

3.1. Quality and Risk of Bias Assessment of the Studies

The quality of the studies assessed using the Newcastle–Ottawa Scale varied, with six achieving the top score of nine stars [8,9,19,20,24,26], indicating excellent methodology. Five studies earned eight stars [23,25,27,29,32] and five received seven stars [10,21,22,28,33], reflecting solid research approaches, while two studies scored six stars [30,31], suggesting some methodological concerns. The commonest weakness of the studies was the comparability category. No other significant deficits were noted (Table 2). A risk of bias visualization according to QUIPS was constructed for each study next to every forest plot. The QUIPS tool's domains were each assigned a corresponding letter, ranging from A for study participation, B for study attrition, C for the measurement of prognostic factors, D for outcome measurement, E for study confound, and F for statistical analysis and reporting. This systematic approach facilitated a comprehensive evaluation of each study's methodological quality and potential biases.

Table 2. Quality assessment of the included studies according to the Newcastle.

First Author, Year	Study Type	S1	S2	S3	S4	C	O1	O2	O3	Total
Aragie et al., 2022 [28]	retrospective cohort	b *	a *	b *	a *	-	b *	a *	a *	7
Curtin et al., 2019 [30]	retrospective case-control	b	a *	a *	a *	-	a *	a *	a *	6
Ebbing et al., 2013 [8]	retrospective cohort	a *	a *	a *	a *	a *, b *	b *	a *	a *	9
Ebbing et al., 2015 [19]	retrospective cohort	a *	a *	a *	a *	a *, b *	b *	a *	a *	9
Ebbing et al., 2016 [20]	retrospective cohort	a *	a *	a *	a *	a *, b *	b *	a *	a *	9
Fukuda et al., 2023 [29]	retrospective cohort	b *	a *	a *	a *	a *	b *	a *	a *	8

Table 2. *Cont.*

First Author, Year	Study Type	S1	S2	S3	S4	C	O1	O2	O3	Total
Gavriil et al., 1993 [33]	retrospective case control	a *	b	a *	a *	a *	b *	a *	a *	7
Hasegawa et al., 2006 [22]	retrospective cohort	b *	a *	a *	a *	-	b *	a *	a *	7
Hasegawa et al., 2009 [21]	retrospective cohort	b *	a *	a *	a *	-	b *	a *	a *	7
Heinonen et al., 1996 [23]	retrospective cohort	b *	a *	a *	a *	a *	b *	a *	a *	8
Jauniaux et al., 1990 [32]	retrospective case control	b *	a *	a *	a *	a *	a *	a *	a *	8
Larcher et al., 2023 [27]	prospective cohort	b *	a *	a *	a *	a *	b *	a *	a *	8
O'Quinn et al., 2020 [25]	retrospective cohort	a *	a *	a *	a *	b *	b *	a *	a *	8
Raisanen et al., 2012 [24]	retrospective cohort	b *	a *	a *	a *	a *, b *	b *	a *	a *	9
Sinkin et al., 2017 [31]	retrospective case-control	b	a *	a *	a *	-	a *	a *	a *	6
Tsakiridis et al., 2021 [9]	retrospective cohort	b *	a *	a *	a *	a *, b *	b *	a *	a *	9
Visentin et al., 2021 [10]	retrospective cohort	c	a *	a *	a *	a *	b *	a *	a *	7
Yang et al., 2020 [26]	retrospective cohort	a *	a *	a *	a *	a *, b *	b *	a *	a *	9

Abbreviations: a, first answer according to NOS; b, second answer according to NOS; c, third answer according to NOS; S, selection; C, comparability; O, outcome; *, attribution of a star according to NOS.

3.2. Raw Data Analysis

We included 14 relevant cohort studies and, based on their data (951,343 singleton pregnancies), the prevalence of VCI was calculated to be 1.54% (95% CI 1.52% to 1.57%).

3.3. Risk Factors' Analyses

In a composite analysis of eight cohort [9,10,20,24–27,29] and three case-control [30,32,33] studies, 692 cases of VCI were reported among the ART group, accounting for approximately 3.48% of the pregnancies, while the control group had 13,800 VCI cases, representing approximately 1.52% of the pregnancies. The occurrence of VCI in pregnancies with ART was significantly higher than those in the control group, with an RR of 2.32 (95% CI 1.77 to 3.05). Substantial heterogeneity was observed across the studies ($p = 0.007$; $I^2 = 59\%$) (Figure 3).

In a composite analysis of six cohort [9,10,21,22,25,26] and two case-control [30,31] studies, the mean maternal age was assessed. The mean difference in maternal age between the VCI and CCI groups was +0.40 (95% CI −0.09 to 0.90)—not significantly different. There was low-to-moderate heterogeneity observed across the studies ($p = 0.18$; $I^2 = 31\%$) (Figure 4).

In a composite analysis of six cohort [9,10,20,24–26] and two case-control [30,31] studies, 6682 cases of VCI were reported among the pregnancies of nulliparous women, accounting for approximately 1.73% of the pregnancies, while the control group had 7818 cases, representing approximately 1.44% of the pregnancies. The occurrence of VCI among nulliparous women was significantly higher compared to those in the multiparous group, with an RR of 1.21 (95% CI 1.15 to 1.28). There was low heterogeneity observed across the studies ($p = 0.39$; $I^2 = 6\%$) (Figure 5).

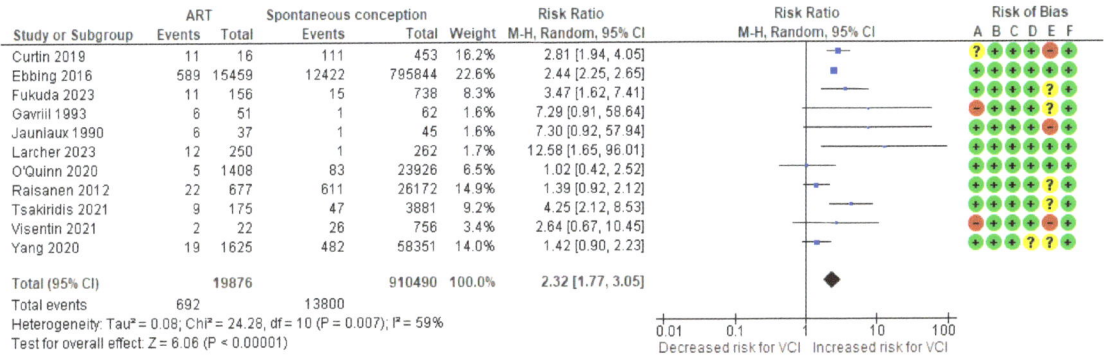

Figure 3. Forest plot demonstrating the risk for VCI in singleton pregnancies relative to the use of ART. Abbreviations: ART, assisted reproductive technology; CI, confidence interval; M–H, Mantel–Haenszel method; VCI, velamentous cord insertion.

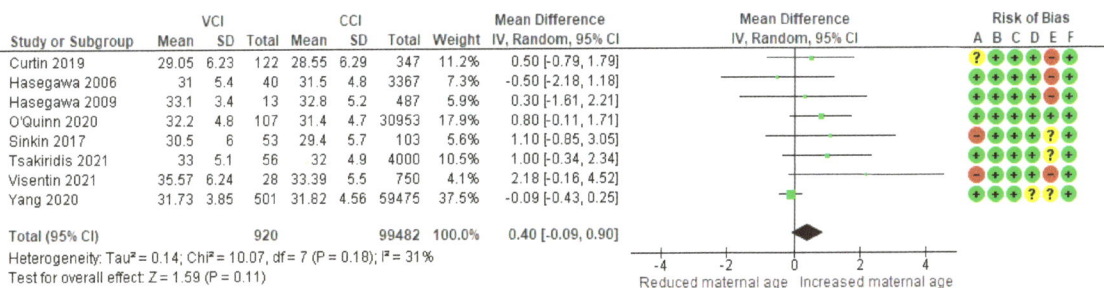

Figure 4. Forest plot demonstrating the risk for VCI in singleton pregnancies relative to mean maternal age. Abbreviations: CCI, central/eccentric cord insertion; CI, confidence interval; IV, weighted mean difference; SD, standard deviation; VCI, velamentous cord insertion.

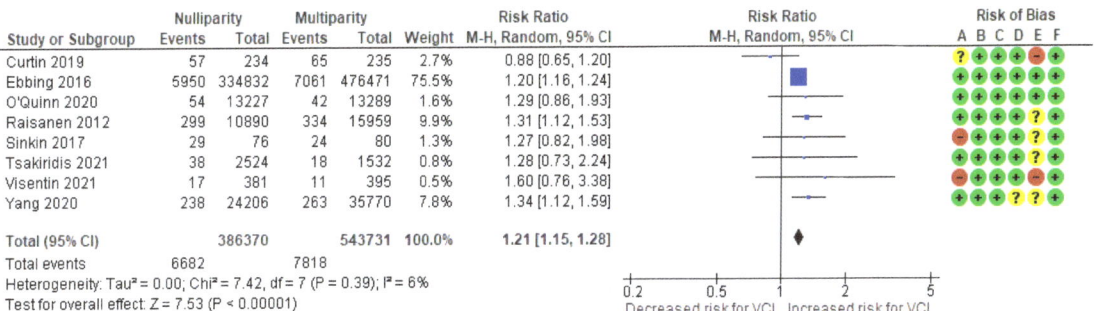

Figure 5. Forest plot demonstrating the risk for VCI in singleton pregnancies relative to parity. Abbreviations: CI, confidence interval; M–H, Mantel–Haenszel method; VCI, velamentous cord insertion.

In a composite analysis of six cohort [8,9,23–26] and one case-control [30] study, 1941 cases of VCI were reported among the group of smokers, accounting for approximately 1.87% of the pregnancies, while the control group had 7878 cases, representing approximately 1.57% of the pregnancies. The occurrence of VCI among women who smoked was significantly different from those in the non-smoking group, with an RR of 1.14 (95% CI 1.08 to 1.19). No heterogeneity was observed across the studies ($p = 0.50$; $I^2 = 0\%$) (Figure 6).

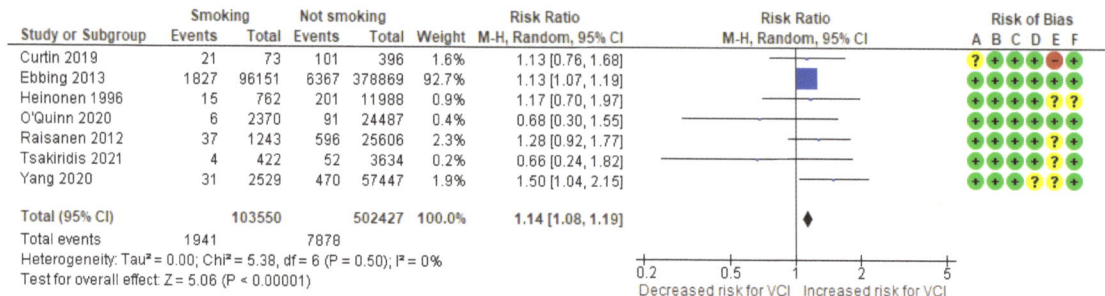

Figure 6. Forest plot demonstrating the risk for VCI in singleton pregnancies relative to smoking. Abbreviations: CI, confidence interval; M−H, Mantel−Haenszel method; VCI, velamentous cord insertion.

In a composite analysis of four cohort [19,23,24,26] and one case-control study [31], 2635 cases with VCI were reported among the group with prior CS, accounting for approximately 2.39% of the pregnancies, while the control group had 10,175 cases, representing approximately 1.51% of the pregnancies. The occurrence of VCI in pregnancies with prior CS was not significantly different from those in the control group, with an RR of 0.92 (95% CI 0.58 to 1.47). There was considerable heterogeneity observed across the studies ($p < 0.001$; $I^2 = 92\%$) (Figure 7).

In a composite analysis of five cohort studies [8,10,23,24,26], 125 cases of VCI were reported among the pregnancies complicated by placenta previa, accounting for approximately 5.59% of the pregnancies, while the control group had 10,753 cases of VCI, representing approximately 1.60% of the pregnancies. The occurrence of VCI in pregnancies with placenta previa was significantly different from those in the control group, with an RR of 3.60 (95% CI 3.04 to 4.28). No heterogeneity was observed across the studies ($p = 0.54$; $I^2 = 0\%$) (Figure 8).

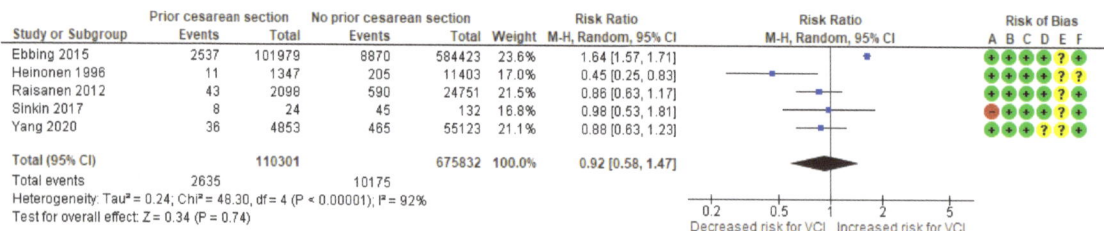

Figure 7. Forest plot demonstrating the risk for VCI in singleton pregnancies relative to having a prior cesarean section. Abbreviations: CI, confidence interval; M−H, Mantel−Haenszel method; VCI, velamentous cord insertion.

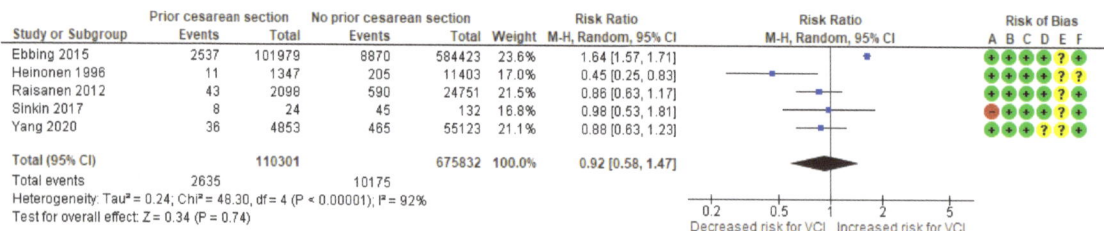

Figure 8. Forest plot of risk for VCI in singleton pregnancies relative to placenta previa. Abbreviations: CI, confidence interval; M−H, Mantel−Haenszel method; VCI, velamentous cord insertion.

In a composite analysis of three cohort [8,25,28] and one case-control study [31], 78 cases of VCI were reported among the women diagnosed with chronic hypertension, accounting for approximately 2.23% of the pregnancies, while the control group had 9594 cases, representing approximately 1.59% of the pregnancies. The occurrence of VCI in pregnancies with chronic hypertension was not significantly different from those in the control group, with an RR of 1.488 (95% CI 0.998 to 2.219). There was low heterogeneity observed across the studies ($p = 0.29$; $I^2 = 20\%$) (Figure 9).

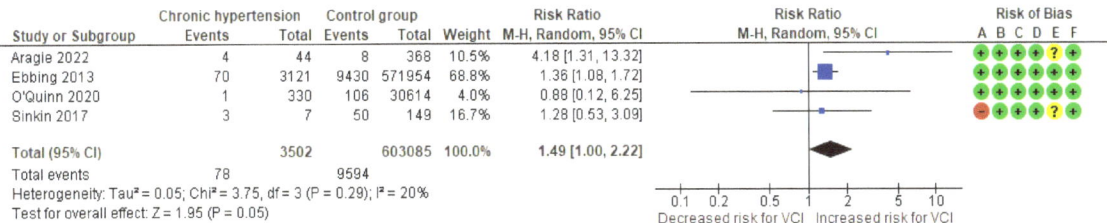

Figure 9. Forest plot demonstrating the risk for VCI in singleton pregnancies relative to chronic hypertension. Abbreviations: CI, confidence interval; M−H, Mante−Haenszel method; VCI, velamentous cord insertion.

In a composite analysis of three cohort studies [8,24,25], 91 cases of VCI were reported among pregnancies with pre-existing diabetes mellitus, accounting for approximately 2.03% of the pregnancies, while the control group had 10,137 cases, representing approximately 1.61% of the pregnancies. The occurrence of VCI in pregnancies of women with a diagnosis of diabetes was not significantly different from those in the control group, with an RR of 1.23 (95% CI 0.84 to 1.79). There was low heterogeneity observed across the studies ($p = 0.31$; $I^2 = 14\%$) (Figure 10).

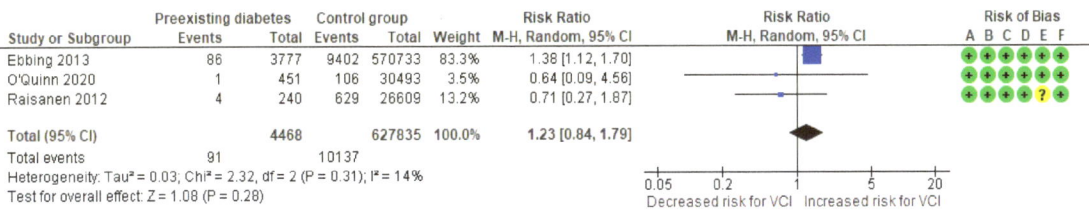

Figure 10. Forest plot demonstrating the risk for VCI in singleton pregnancies relative to pre-existing diabetes. Abbreviations: CI, confidence interval; M−H, Mante−Haenszel method; VCI, velamentous cord insertion.

The cumulative results of our primary analysis are compiled and displayed in Table 3.

Table 3. Results of the meta-analysis regarding risk factors of velamentous cord insertion in singleton pregnancies.

Risk Factor	Number of Studies	VCI Cases/Total Cases (Exposed to Risk Factor)	VCI Cases/Total Cases (Not Exposed to Risk Factor)	RR	95% CI	I^2; p-Value
Assisted reproductive technology	11	692/19,876 (3.48%)	13,800/910,490 (1.52%)	2.32	1.77–3.05	59%; 0.007
Maternal age	8	920 (VCI cases)	99,482 (CCI cases)	0.40 (MD)	−0.09 to 0.90	31%; 0.18

Table 3. Cont.

Risk Factor	Number of Studies	VCI Cases/Total Cases (Exposed to Risk Factor)	VCI Cases/Total Cases (Not Exposed to Risk Factor)	RR	95% CI	I^2; p-Value
Nulliparity	8	6682/386,370 (1.73%)	7818/543,731 (1.44%)	1.21	1.15–1.28	6%; 0.39
Smoking	7	1941/103,550 (1.87%)	7878/502,427 (1.57%)	1.14	1.08–1.19	0%; 0.50
Prior cesarean section	5	2635/110,301 (2.39%)	10,175/675,832 (1.51%)	0.92	0.58–1.47	92%; <0.001
Placenta previa	5	125/2234 (5.59%)	10,753/672,194 (1.60%)	3.60	3.04–4.28	0%; 0.54
Chronic hypertension	4	78/3502 (2.23%)	9594/603,085 (1.59%)	1.488	0.998–2.219	20%; 0.29
Pre-existing diabetes	3	91/4468 (2.03%)	10,137/627,835 (1.61%)	1.23	0.84–1.79	14%; 0.31

Abbreviations: CI, confidence interval; I^2 (Heterogeneity in meta-analysis); MD, mean difference; p-value, Cochran Q test's p-value; RR, relative risk; VCI, velamentous cord insertion.

3.4. Sensitivity Analyses Regarding Prenatal Diagnosis and Risk of Bias

Limiting our analysis to studies that provided data on prenatal diagnosis of umbilical cord insertion, we examined 18 studies, with 4 involving prenatal identification of VCI, and we could sufficiently assess three risk factors: ART, mean maternal age and nulliparity. The updated findings were consistent with the main results (Table 4 and Supplementary Figures S1–S3).

Subsequently, the studies identified as a high risk of bias were removed. Within the scope of ten analyses, seven were affected by the presence of high-risk bias studies. Following their exclusion, six out of seven analyses maintained comparable results to the initial findings. The updated findings were consistent with the main results (Table 4 and Supplementary Figures S4–S10).

Table 4. Confidence intervals from all the analyses performed.

Risk Factor	Overall Analysis		Prenatally Diagnosed		RoB Sensitivity Analysis	
	RR	95% CI	RR	95% CI	RR	95% CI
Assisted reproductive technology	2.32	1.77–3.05	3.18	1.10–9.21	2.14	1.49–3.08
Maternal age	0.40	−0.09 to 0.90	0.40	−0.35 to 1.15	0.40	−0.35 to 1.15
Nulliparity	1.21	1.15–1.28	1.33	1.14–1.55	1.21	1.17–1.25
Smoking	1.14	1.08–1.19			1.15	1.05–1.26
Prior cesarean section	0.92	0.58–1.47			0.91	0.53–1.55
Placenta previa	3.60	3.04–4.28			3.56	2.94–4.30
Chronic hypertension	1.488	0.998–2.219			1.73	0.81–3.70

Abbreviations: CI, confidence interval; RR, relative risk; RoB, risk of bias.

3.5. Publication Bias

The risk factor with the most included studies was ART, which was tested for publication bias. Neither the funnel plot nor the Egger's test demonstrated any indication of publication bias (Figure 11).

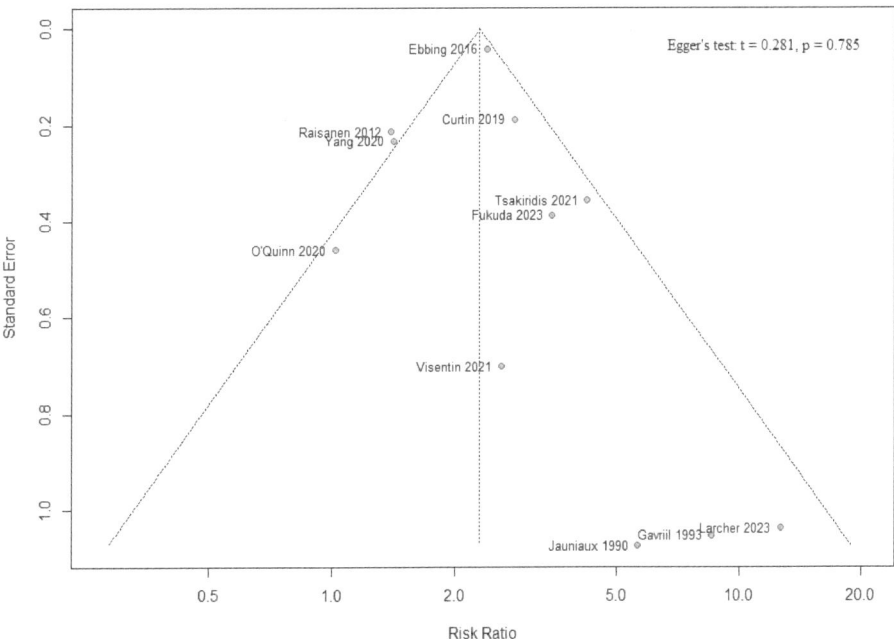

Figure 11. Funnel plot and Egger's test regarding our most investigated outcome—assisted reproductive technology.

4. Discussion

4.1. Principal Findings

Our analysis found that first, the reported prevalence of VCI in singleton pregnancies is 1.54%, and second, the factors associated with an increased risk of VCI include ART, nulliparity, smoking and placenta previa.

4.2. Interpretation of the Findings

The largest investigated population was in the ART-VCI analysis, which incorporated 11 studies. The analysis demonstrated that ART is associated with a two-fold higher risk for VCI among singleton pregnancies and this association persisted in cases prenatally diagnosed with VCI and after excluding studies at high risk of bias. Our findings are consistent with those of a recent meta-analysis, which reported an OR of 2.14; however, this study included twin gestations in the analysis and the control group was broadly defined [34]. Our results support earlier epidemiological findings that pregnancies conceived via ART are associated with a higher incidence of umbilico-placental abnormalities [35–37]. The mechanism that ART could disrupt placentation has not been established; nevertheless, interventions such as controlled ovarian hyperstimulation, intrauterine insemination, gamete or embryo freezing, in-vitro fertilization, embryo culture, cell biopsy and blastocyst or embryo transfer may exercise oxidative, thermal, and mechanical stresses, and changes in DNA methylation that could alter the natural biological processes of reproduction [38,39]. Finally, related surgical procedures, such as septum excision, myomectomy, and other surgical treatments of uterine anomalies, may also contribute to the elevated risk of VCI, underscoring the need for further investigation in this area.

The analysis of maternal age in relation to the risk of VCI encompassed eight studies and revealed no significant increase in risk; only one study that categorized maternal age found that women aged over 35 years exhibited a higher risk of developing VCI (RR, 1.61) [23]. Moreover, two additional studies that were excluded from our meta-analysis due to the inclusion of cases with marginal cord insertion in the control group similarly identified maternal age above 35 years as a risk factor for VCI [40,41]. These findings suggest that the relationship between maternal age and VCI may be more nuanced, with significant risks manifesting particularly after the age of 35. This association could be partially attributed to the increased utilization of ART among this age group.

Nulliparity was identified as a significant risk factor for VCI, even when focusing on prenatally diagnosed pregnancies and studies with low risk of bias. While most small studies did not report a statistically significant association between nulliparity and VCI [9,10,25,30,31], the three larger studies [20,24,26], which made up over 90% of the pooled data, showed a strong association. No relevant studies explaining the pathophysiological cause were found, but we hypothesize that the lack of physiological adaptations that occur in the uterus and placenta during subsequent pregnancies may be a plausible explanation.

Regarding smoking, although most individual studies did not establish a significant relationship with VCI, the aggregated analysis indicated a 14% increased risk of VCI among smokers. Maternal smoking has been documented to adversely impact both the local immune response and microcirculation within decidual tissues [42]. It is conceivable that these alterations in the decidual environment during the implantation and the embryogenesis phase may play a role in the formation of VCI. A study of 83,708 women utilizing multiple regression models observed that exposure to fine particulate matter was positively associated with VCI and described two possible mechanisms: ischemia of the endometrium and intrauterine inflammation [43].

Prior CS was not associated with VCI in our meta-analysis. It seems that contrary to the low placental implantation, which is strongly associated with prior CS, abnormal cord insertion is not associated with them. However, placenta previa was identified as a significant risk factor for VCI, increasing its incidence fourfold [44].

Finally, no association was detected with chronic hypertension or pre-existing diabetes and VCI. However, it is noteworthy that chronic hypertension had a high RR of 1.49, indicating a potential 50% increase in the risk of VCI. The marginal lack of statistical significance is likely due to the sample size and the use of random effect models. Therefore, additional data are required to make a definitive conclusion about this matter.

4.3. Clinical and Research Implications

Currently, there is no consensus on the usefulness of universal screening for cord insertion anomalies. Therefore, our findings on the risk factors for VCI may inform the development of a more targeted screening approach for women exhibiting these risk factors. Given that isolated VCI is a primary risk factor for various adverse perinatal outcomes, including stillbirth [4], while also being the main risk factor for vasa previa [45]—a condition associated with significant perinatal mortality if prenatally undiagnosed [46] but preventable if diagnosed [47]—the importance of identifying VCI cannot be overstated [1,48]. Furthermore, recent studies have linked VCI with a twofold increased risk of cerebral palsy, suggesting that early detection of VCI could be crucial in identifying fetuses at a higher risk for this condition [49].

4.4. Strengths and Limitations

Our study's main strength lies in its comprehensive design, which allowed us to include numerous studies and explore a wide array of possible risk factors. We maintained strict selection criteria, which led to more reliable estimates of effects and potentially reduced variability among the included studies. Our focus was to provide additional information on the prenatal diagnosis of VCI. To this end, our sensitivity analysis specifically targeting pregnancies with prenatal diagnosis of VCI may enhance the broader applicability of our findings.

The primary limitation of our meta-analysis stems from the nature of the included studies, all of which were observational, including case-control designs. Additionally, most of these studies focused primarily on the perinatal outcomes of VCI rather than investigating risk factors, making them susceptible to selection and recall biases. Furthermore, we were unable to examine the association between prenatally diagnosed VCI and all its risk factors, as not every study provided the necessary data. A further limitation is that in the studies with prenatally diagnosed cases, there was no systematic postnatal confirmation. Finally, none of the studies reported adjusted effect measures, preventing us from accounting for significant confounding variables.

5. Conclusions

This meta-analysis identified ART, nulliparity, smoking and placenta previa as significant risk factors for VCI. These findings may assist the screening policy in settings where cord insertion is not universally offered. Additionally, this may enhance the antenatal detection of vasa previa, a condition that poses significant risks to pregnancies, as VCI is the primary risk factor for its development. Furthermore, the findings may also induce further high-quality research that addresses potential confounding variables to substantiate these associations. The exploration into the pathophysiological mechanisms underlying these relationships is imperative to enhance our understanding and further guide obstetric policies.

Supplementary Materials: The following supporting information can be downloaded at: https://www.mdpi.com/article/10.3390/jcm13185551/s1, Figure S1: Forest plot demonstrating the risk for prenatally diagnosed VCI in singleton pregnancies relative to the use of ART; Figure S2: Forest plot demonstrating the risk for prenatally diagnosed VCI in singleton pregnancies relative to mean maternal age; Figure S3: Forest plot demonstrating the risk for prenatally diagnosed VCI in singleton pregnancies relative to parity; Figure S4: Risk of bias sensitivity analysis regarding ART—VCI association in singleton pregnancies; Figure S5: Risk of bias sensitivity analysis regarding mean maternal age—VCI association in singleton pregnancies; Figure S6: Risk of bias sensitivity analysis regarding nulliparity—VCI association in singleton pregnancies; Figure S7: Risk of bias sensitivity analysis regarding smoking—VCI association in singleton pregnancies; Figure S8: Risk of bias sensitivity analysis regarding prior cesarean section—VCI association in singleton pregnancies; Figure S9: Risk of bias sensitivity analysis regarding placenta previa—VCI association in singleton pregnancies; Figure S10: Risk of bias sensitivity analysis regarding chronic hypertension—VCI association in singleton pregnancies.

Author Contributions: Conceptualization, I.T. and T.D.; methodology, A.S., I.T. and M.M.G.; data collection, A.S., A.G. and I.T.; software, A.S.; meta-analysis, A.S. and A.G.; writing—original draft preparation, A.S. and I.T.; writing—review and editing, C.D.P.M., M.M.G., P.C. and T.D.; supervision, T.D. All authors have read and agreed to the published version of the manuscript.

Funding: This research received no external funding.

Institutional Review Board Statement: Given its nature of synthesizing data from previously published literature, the study was exempt from the need for ethical approval and patient consent.

Informed Consent Statement: Given its nature of synthesizing data from previously published literature, the study was exempt from the need for ethical approval and patient consent.

Data Availability Statement: Not applicable.

Conflicts of Interest: The authors declare no conflict of interest.

Abbreviations

ART	assisted reproductive technology
CCI	central/eccentric cord insertion
CI	confidence interval
CS	cesarean section
MD	mean difference
QUIPS	Quality In Prognosis Studies
RR	risk ratio
VCI	velamentous cord insertion

References

1. Jauniaux, E.; Ebbing, C.; Oyelese, Y.; Maymon, R.; Prefumo, F.; Bhide, A. European association of perinatal medicine (EAPM) position statement: Screening, diagnosis and management of congenital anomalies of the umbilical cord. *Eur. J. Obstet. Gynecol. Reprod. Biol.* **2024**, *298*, 61–65. [CrossRef] [PubMed]
2. Sherer, D.M.; Al-Haddad, S.; Cheng, R.; Dalloul, M. Current Perspectives of Prenatal Sonography of Umbilical Cord Morphology. *Int. J. Women's Health* **2021**, *13*, 939–971. [CrossRef] [PubMed]
3. Yampolsky, M.; Salafia, C.M.; Shlakhter, O.; Haas, D.; Eucker, B.; Thorp, J. Centrality of the umbilical cord insertion in a human placenta influences the placental efficiency. *Placenta* **2009**, *30*, 1058–1064. [CrossRef] [PubMed]
4. Siargkas, A.; Tsakiridis, I.; Pachi, C.; Mamopoulos, A.; Athanasiadis, A.; Dagklis, T. Impact of velamentous cord insertion on perinatal outcomes: A systematic review and meta-analysis. *Am. J. Obstet. Gynecol. MFM* **2023**, *5*, 100812. [CrossRef] [PubMed]
5. Buchanan-Hughes, A.; Bobrowska, A.; Visintin, C.; Attilakos, G.; Marshall, J. Velamentous cord insertion: Results from a rapid review of incidence, risk factors, adverse outcomes and screening. *Syst. Rev.* **2020**, *9*, 147. [CrossRef]
6. American Institute of Ultrasound in Medicine. AIUM Practice Guideline for the Performance of Obstetric Ultrasound Examinations. *J. Ultrasound Med.* **2013**, *32*, 1083–1101. [CrossRef]
7. Coutinho, C.M.; Sotiriadis, A.; Odibo, A.; Khalil, A.; D'Antonio, F.; Feltovich, H.; Salomon, L.J.; Sheehan, P.; Napolitano, R.; Berghella, V.; et al. ISUOG Practice Guidelines: Role of ultrasound in the prediction of spontaneous preterm birth. *Ultrasound Obstet. Gynecol. Off. J. Int. Soc. Ultrasound Obstet. Gynecol.* **2022**, *60*, 435–456. [CrossRef]
8. Ebbing, C.; Kiserud, T.; Johnsen, S.L.; Albrechtsen, S.; Rasmussen, S. Prevalence, risk factors and outcomes of velamentous and marginal cord insertions: A population-based study of 634,741 pregnancies. *PLoS ONE* **2013**, *8*, e70380. [CrossRef]
9. Tsakiridis, I.; Dagklis, T.; Athanasiadis, A.; Dinas, K.; Sotiriadis, A. Impact of Marginal and Velamentous Cord Insertion on Uterine Artery Doppler Indices, Fetal Growth, and Preeclampsia. *J. Ultrasound Med. Off. J. Am. Inst. Ultrasound Med.* **2022**, *41*, 2011–2018. [CrossRef]
10. Visintin, S.; Londero, A.P.; Santoro, L.; Pizzi, S.; Andolfatto, M.; Venturini, M.; Saraggi, D.; Coati, I.; Sacchi, D.; Rugge, M.; et al. Abnormal umbilical cord insertions in singleton deliveries: Placental histology and neonatal outcomes. *J. Clin. Pathol.* **2022**, *75*, 751–758. [CrossRef]
11. Page, M.J.; Moher, D.; Bossuyt, P.M.; Boutron, I.; Hoffmann, T.C.; Mulrow, C.D.; Shamseer, L.; Tetzlaff, J.M.; Akl, E.A.; Brennan, S.E.; et al. PRISMA 2020 explanation and elaboration: Updated guidance and exemplars for reporting systematic reviews. *BMJ (Clin. Res. Ed.)* **2021**, *372*, n160. [CrossRef] [PubMed]
12. Stroup, D.F.; Berlin, J.A.; Morton, S.C.; Olkin, I.; Williamson, G.D.; Rennie, D.; Moher, D.; Becker, B.J.; Sipe, T.A.; Thacker, S.B. Meta-analysis of observational studies in epidemiology: A proposal for reporting. Meta-analysis Of Observational Studies in Epidemiology (MOOSE) group. *JAMA* **2000**, *283*, 2008–2012. [CrossRef] [PubMed]
13. Wells, G.; Shea, B.; O'Connell, D.; Peterson, J.; Welch, V.; Losos, M.; Tugwell, P. The Newcastle–Ottawa Scale (NOS) for Assessing the Quality of Non-Randomized Studies in Meta-Analysis. 2000.
14. Hayden, J.A.; van der Windt, D.A.; Cartwright, J.L.; Côté, P.; Bombardier, C. Assessing bias in studies of prognostic factors. *Ann. Intern. Med.* **2013**, *158*, 280–286. [CrossRef] [PubMed]
15. Higgins, J.; Thomas, J.; Chandler, J.; Cumpston, M.; Li, T.; Page, M.; Welch, V. (Eds.) *Cochrane Handbook for Systematic Reviews of Interventions Version 6.4*; Cochrane: Chichester, UK, 2023.
16. R Core Team. *R: A Language and Environment for Statistical Computing*; R Foundation for Statistical Computing: Vienna, Austria, 2013; ISBN 3-900051-07-0. Available online: http://www.R-project.org/ (accessed on 28 May 2024).
17. Balduzzi, S.; Rücker, G.; Schwarzer, G. How to perform a meta-analysis with R: A practical tutorial. *Evid. -Based Ment. Health* **2019**, *22*, 153–160. [CrossRef]
18. Harrer, M.; Cuijpers, P.; Furukawa, T.; Ebert, D.D. dmetar: Companion R Package for the Guide 'Doing Meta-Analysis in R'. R Package Version 0.0.9000. 2019. Available online: http://dmetar.protectlab.org/ (accessed on 28 May 2024).
19. Ebbing, C.; Kiserud, T.; Johnsen, S.L.; Albrechtsen, S.; Rasmussen, S. Third stage of labor risks in velamentous and marginal cord insertion: A population-based study. *Acta Obstet. Et Gynecol. Scand.* **2015**, *94*, 878–883. [CrossRef]
20. Ebbing, C.; Johnsen, S.L.; Albrechtsen, S.; Sunde, I.D.; Vekseth, C.; Rasmussen, S. Velamentous or marginal cord insertion and the risk of spontaneous preterm birth, prelabor rupture of the membranes, and anomalous cord length, a population-based study. *Acta Obstet. Et Gynecol. Scand.* **2017**, *96*, 78–85. [CrossRef]
21. Hasegawa, J.; Matsuoka, R.; Ichizuka, K.; Kotani, M.; Nakamura, M.; Mikoshiba, T.; Sekizawa, A.; Okai, T. Atypical variable deceleration in the first stage of labor is a characteristic fetal heart-rate pattern for velamentous cord insertion and hypercoiled cord. *J. Obstet. Gynaecol. Res.* **2009**, *35*, 35–39. [CrossRef]
22. Hasegawa, J.; Matsuoka, R.; Ichizuka, K.; Sekizawa, A.; Farina, A.; Okai, T. Velamentous cord insertion into the lower third of the uterus is associated with intrapartum fetal heart rate abnormalities. *Ultrasound Obstet. Gynecol. Off. J. Int. Soc. Ultrasound Obstet. Gynecol.* **2006**, *27*, 425–429. [CrossRef]
23. Heinonen, S.; Ryynänen, M.; Kirkinen, P.; Saarikoski, S. Perinatal diagnostic evaluation of velamentous umbilical cord insertion: Clinical, Doppler, and ultrasonic findings. *Obstet. Gynecol.* **1996**, *87*, 112–117. [CrossRef]
24. Räisänen, S.; Georgiadis, L.; Harju, M.; Keski-Nisula, L.; Heinonen, S. Risk factors and adverse pregnancy outcomes among births affected by velamentous umbilical cord insertion: A retrospective population-based register study. *Eur. J. Obstet. Gynecol. Reprod. Biol.* **2012**, *165*, 231–234. [CrossRef]

25. O'Quinn, C.; Cooper, S.; Tang, S.; Wood, S. Antenatal Diagnosis of Marginal and Velamentous Placental Cord Insertion and Pregnancy Outcomes. *Obs. Gynecol* **2020**, *135*, 953–959. [CrossRef] [PubMed]
26. Yang, M.; Zheng, Y.; Li, M.; Li, W.; Li, X.; Zhang, X.; Wang, R.; Zhang, J.; Zhou, F.; Yang, Q.; et al. Clinical features of velamentous umbilical cord insertion and vasa previa: A retrospective analysis based on 501 cases. *Medicine* **2020**, *99*, e23166. [CrossRef] [PubMed]
27. Larcher, L.; Jauniaux, E.; Lenzi, J.; Ragnedda, R.; Morano, D.; Valeriani, M.; Michelli, G.; Farina, A.; Contro, E. Ultrasound diagnosis of placental and umbilical cord anomalies in singleton pregnancies resulting from in-vitro fertilization. *Placenta* **2023**, *131*, 58–64. [CrossRef] [PubMed]
28. Aragie, H.; Kibret, A.A.; Teshager, N.W.; Adugna, D.G. Velamentous cord insertion at the University of Gondar Comprehensive Specialized Hospital, Northwest Ethiopia. *Clin. Epidemiol. Glob. Health* **2022**, *18*, 101180. [CrossRef]
29. Fukuda, E.; Hamuro, A.; Kitada, K.; Kurihara, Y.; Tahara, M.; Misugi, T.; Nakano, A.; Tamaue, M.; Shinomiya, S.; Yoshida, H.; et al. The Impact of Assisted Reproductive Technology on Umbilical Cord Insertion: Increased Risk of Velamentous Cord Insertion in Singleton Pregnancies Conceived through ICSI. *Medicina* **2023**, *59*, 1715. [CrossRef]
30. Curtin, W.M.; Hill, J.M.; Millington, K.A.; Hamidi, O.P.; Rasiah, S.S.; Ural, S.H. Accuracy of fetal anatomy survey in the diagnosis of velamentous cord insertion: A case-control study. *Int. J. Women's Health* **2019**, *11*, 169–176. [CrossRef]
31. Sinkin, J.A.; Craig, W.Y.; Jones, M.; Pinette, M.G.; Wax, J.R. Perinatal Outcomes Associated With Isolated Velamentous Cord Insertion in Singleton and Twin Pregnancies. *J. Ultrasound Med.* **2018**, *37*, 471–478. [CrossRef]
32. Jauniaux, E.; Englert, Y.; Vanesse, M.; Hiden, M.; Wilkin, P. Pathologic features of placentas from singleton pregnancies obtained by in vitro fertilization and embryo transfer. *Obstet. Gynecol.* **1990**, *76*, 61–64.
33. Gavriil, P.; Jauniaux, E.; Leroy, F. Pathologic examination of placentas from singleton and twin pregnancies obtained after in vitro fertilization and embryo transfer. *Pediatr. Pathol.* **1993**, *13*, 453–462. [CrossRef]
34. Matsuzaki, S.; Ueda, Y.; Matsuzaki, S.; Nagase, Y.; Kakuda, M.; Lee, M.; Maeda, M.; Kurahashi, H.; Hayashida, H.; Hisa, T.; et al. Assisted Reproductive Technique and Abnormal Cord Insertion: A Systematic Review and Meta-Analysis. *Biomedicines* **2022**, *10*, 1722. [CrossRef]
35. Yanaihara, A.; Hatakeyama, S.; Ohgi, S.; Motomura, K.; Taniguchi, R.; Hirano, A.; Takenaka, S.; Yanaihara, T. Difference in the size of the placenta and umbilical cord between women with natural pregnancy and those with IVF pregnancy. *J. Assist. Reprod. Genet.* **2018**, *35*, 431–434. [CrossRef] [PubMed]
36. Ruiter, L.; Kok, N.; Limpens, J.; Derks, J.B.; de Graaf, I.M.; Mol, B.W.; Pajkrt, E. Systematic review of accuracy of ultrasound in the diagnosis of vasa previa. *Ultrasound Obstet. Gynecol. Off. J. Int. Soc. Ultrasound Obstet. Gynecol.* **2015**, *45*, 516–522. [CrossRef] [PubMed]
37. Nagata, C.; Konishi, K.; Wada, K.; Tamura, T.; Goto, Y.; Koda, S.; Mizuta, F.; Iwasa, S. Maternal Acrylamide Intake during Pregnancy and Sex Hormone Levels in Maternal and Umbilical Cord Blood and Birth Size of Offspring. *Nutr. Cancer* **2019**, *71*, 77–82. [CrossRef] [PubMed]
38. Vrooman, L.A.; Xin, F.; Bartolomei, M.S. Morphologic and molecular changes in the placenta: What we can learn from environmental exposures. *Fertil. Steril.* **2016**, *106*, 930–940. [CrossRef] [PubMed]
39. Furuya, S.; Kubonoya, K.; Yamaguchi, T. Incidence and risk factors for velamentous umbilical cord insertion in singleton pregnancies after assisted reproductive technology. *J. Obstet. Gynaecol. Res.* **2021**, *47*, 1772–1779. [CrossRef] [PubMed]
40. Esakoff, T.F.; Cheng, Y.W.; Snowden, J.M.; Tran, S.H.; Shaffer, B.L.; Caughey, A.B. Velamentous cord insertion: Is it associated with adverse perinatal outcomes? *J. Matern. Fetal Neonatal Med. Off. J. Eur. Assoc. Perinat. Med. Fed. Asia Ocean. Perinat. Soc. Int. Soc. Perinat. Obs.* **2015**, *28*, 409–412. [CrossRef]
41. Eddleman, K.A.; Lockwood, C.J.; Berkowitz, G.S.; Lapinski, R.H.; Berkowitz, R.L. Clinical significance and sonographic diagnosis of velamentous umbilical cord insertion. *Am. J. Perinatol.* **1992**, *9*, 123–126. [CrossRef]
42. Prins, J.R.; Hylkema, M.N.; Erwich, J.J.; Huitema, S.; Dekkema, G.J.; Dijkstra, F.E.; Faas, M.M.; Melgert, B.N. Smoking during pregnancy influences the maternal immune response in mice and humans. *Am. J. Obstet. Gynecol.* **2012**, *207*, 76.e1–76.e14. [CrossRef]
43. Michikawa, T.; Morokuma, S.; Takeda, Y.; Yamazaki, S.; Nakahara, K.; Takami, A.; Yoshino, A.; Sugata, S.; Saito, S.; Hoshi, J.; et al. Maternal exposure to fine particulate matter over the first trimester and umbilical cord insertion abnormalities. *Int. J. Epidemiol.* **2022**, *51*, 191–201. [CrossRef]
44. Santana, E.F.M.; Castello, R.G.; Rizzo, G.; Grisolia, G.; Araujo Júnior, E.; Werner, H.; Lituania, M.; Tonni, G. Placental and Umbilical Cord Anomalies Diagnosed by Two- and Three-Dimensional Ultrasound. *Diagnostics* **2022**, *12*, 2810. [CrossRef]
45. Gross, A.; Markota Ajd, B.; Specht, C.; Scheier, M. Systematic screening for vasa previa at the 20-week anomaly scan. *Acta Obstet. Et Gynecol. Scand.* **2021**, *100*, 1694–1699. [CrossRef] [PubMed]
46. Zhang, W.; Geris, S.; Al-Emara, N.; Ramadan, G.; Sotiriadis, A.; Akolekar, R. Perinatal outcome of pregnancies with prenatal diagnosis of vasa previa: Systematic review and meta-analysis. *Ultrasound Obstet. Gynecol. Off. J. Int. Soc. Ultrasound Obstet. Gynecol.* **2021**, *57*, 710–719. [CrossRef] [PubMed]
47. Conyers, S.; Oyelese, Y.; Javinani, A.; Jamali, M.; Zargarzadeh, N.; Akolekar, R.; Hasegawa, J.; Melcer, Y.; Maymon, R.; Bronsteen, R.; et al. Incidence and causes of perinatal death in prenatally diagnosed vasa previa: A systematic review and meta-analysis. *Am. J. Obstet. Gynecol.* **2024**, *230*, 58–65. [CrossRef] [PubMed]

48. Oyelese, Y.; Javinani, A.; Gudanowski, B.; Krispin, E.; Rebarber, A.; Akolekar, R.; Catanzarite, V.; D'Souza, R.; Bronsteen, R.; Odibo, A.; et al. Vasa previa in singleton pregnancies: Diagnosis and clinical management based on an international expert consensus. *Am. J. Obstet. Gynecol.* **2024**, *in press*. [CrossRef]
49. Ebbing, C.; Rasmussen, S.; Kessler, J.; Moster, D. Association of placental and umbilical cord characteristics with cerebral palsy: National cohort study. *Ultrasound Obstet. Gynecol. Off. J. Int. Soc. Ultrasound Obstet. Gynecol.* **2023**, *61*, 224–230. [CrossRef]

Disclaimer/Publisher's Note: The statements, opinions and data contained in all publications are solely those of the individual author(s) and contributor(s) and not of MDPI and/or the editor(s). MDPI and/or the editor(s) disclaim responsibility for any injury to people or property resulting from any ideas, methods, instructions or products referred to in the content.

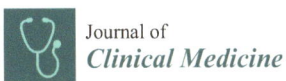

Article

Association between Subclinical Hypothyroidism and Adverse Pregnancy Outcomes in Assisted Reproduction Technology Singleton Pregnancies: A Retrospective Study

Yuichiro Narita, Hiroyuki Tsuda *, Eri Tsugeno, Yumi Nakamura, Miho Suzuki, Yumiko Ito, Atsuko Tezuka and Tomoko Ando

Department of Obstetrics and Gynecology, Japanese Red Cross Aichi Medical Center Nagoya Daiichi Hospital, Nagoya 453-8511, Japan; yuichiro0202@gmail.com (Y.N.); eri.uchiyama.56@gmail.com (E.T.); yuim0201@gmail.com (Y.N.); miho418miho@gmail.com (M.S.); yum.ito.jrc@gmail.com (Y.I.); a_atsuko_sadaka@yahoo.co.jp (A.T.); ando-tm@nagoya-1st.jrc.or.jp (T.A.)
* Correspondence: hirotty7099@yahoo.co.jp; Tel.: +81-52-481-5111

Abstract: Background/Objectives: Women with subclinical hypothyroidism (SCH) were reported to be at an increased perinatal risk. We aimed to investigate the relationship between SCH and perinatal outcomes in singleton pregnancies resulting from assisted reproduction technology (ART). **Methods**: We retrospectively examined the perinatal outcomes of ART singleton pregnancies in women who underwent thyroid function screening before conception and delivered at our hospital from January 2020 to July 2023. We defined SCH as thyroid-stimulating hormone (TSH) levels > 2.5 mU/L and normal free T_4 levels. The patients were categorized into three groups: normal thyroid function (group A), SCH without levothyroxine therapy (group B), and SCH with levothyroxine therapy (group C). The risks of preterm birth, preeclampsia, fetal growth restriction, manual placental removal, and blood loss at delivery were compared among the three groups. **Results**: Out of the 650 ART singleton deliveries, 581 were assigned to group A, 34 to group B, and 35 to group C. The preterm birth rate at <34 weeks was significantly higher in group B and significantly lower in group C than in group A. The rate of preterm delivery at <34 weeks increased in correlation with TSH levels. Levothyroxine therapy was the significant preventive factor for preterm birth at <34 weeks. **Conclusions**: The preterm birth rate before 34 weeks was significantly higher in the SCH group. Levothyroxine therapy is a significant protective factor against preterm birth before 34 weeks. Universal screening for thyroid function and appropriate hormone therapy in pregnant women may help reduce perinatal risks, including preterm birth.

Keywords: ART; preterm birth; subclinical hypothyroidism; thyroid stimulating hormone; levothyroxine therapy

Citation: Narita, Y.; Tsuda, H.; Tsugeno, E.; Nakamura, Y.; Suzuki, M.; Ito, Y.; Tezuka, A.; Ando, T. Association between Subclinical Hypothyroidism and Adverse Pregnancy Outcomes in Assisted Reproduction Technology Singleton Pregnancies: A Retrospective Study. *J. Clin. Med.* **2024**, *13*, 5137. https://doi.org/10.3390/jcm13175137

Academic Editors: Ioannis Tsakiridis and Apostolos Mamopoulos

Received: 26 July 2024
Revised: 22 August 2024
Accepted: 27 August 2024
Published: 29 August 2024

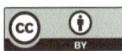

Copyright: © 2024 by the authors. Licensee MDPI, Basel, Switzerland. This article is an open access article distributed under the terms and conditions of the Creative Commons Attribution (CC BY) license (https:// creativecommons.org/licenses/by/ 4.0/).

1. Introduction

Thyroid function studies using the Japanese adult general health examination system documented thyroid dysfunction in approximately 10% of cases, with subclinical hypothyroidism (SCH) accounting for half of the cases [1]. This finding suggests that many pregnant women may have undiagnosed SCH. SCH is defined as normal free T_4 levels and elevated serum thyroid-stimulating hormone (TSH) levels. It is observed in 2.0–2.5% of screened pregnant women, according to reports from iodine-sufficient areas of the United States [2,3].

Some [4–7], but not all [8,9], studies have demonstrated that women with SCH have a higher perinatal risk of severe preeclampsia, preterm delivery, placental abruption, neonatal respiratory distress syndrome, and/or pregnancy loss than do euthyroid women. One meta-analysis from 19 cohort studies reported an odds ratio (OR) of 1.29 (95% confidence interval [CI], 1.01–1.64) for preterm birth [10], and another meta-analysis reported an OR of 1.53 (95% CI, 1.09–2.15) for preeclampsia [6]. Interestingly, preterm delivery rates increase with TSH levels as follows: 5.4% of pregnancies with TSH levels between 4 and 6 mU/L, 7.8% between 6 and 10 mU/L, and 11.4% with >10 mU/L [11]. Furthermore, limited data suggest that perinatal outcomes are worse in women undergoing in vitro fertilization (IVF) if their preconception TSH levels are >2.5 mU/L. In one study of pregnancies after IVF, 150 deliveries with a preconception TSH level < 2.5 mU/L resulted in higher gestational age and birth weight than 45 deliveries with a TSH level > 2.5 mU/L [12].

Because overt or SCH is thought to be associated with pregnancy complications and thyroid testing is common and easy to perform, attention has been focused on the utility of screening for thyroid dysfunction in all pregnant women. To our knowledge, no high-quality studies have used a universal screening for thyroid function in pregnant women. The advantages and disadvantages of screening thyroid function in all pregnant women in early pregnancy remain inconclusive. This is because there are insufficient data to show not only the effects of thyroid disease on pregnancy but also the benefits of hormone therapy [13,14]. In Japan, universal screening for thyroid dysfunction in asymptomatic pregnant women is rare; however, universal screening for thyroid dysfunction is common in women initiating fertility treatment. This study aimed to examine the association between the presence of SCH and perinatal outcomes in assisted reproduction technology (ART) pregnancies using preconception thyroid function screening and the effects of thyroid hormone replacement (levothyroxine sodium hydrate) during pregnancy.

2. Materials and Methods

2.1. Participants

In this retrospective cohort study, we analyzed the perinatal outcomes of pregnancies delivered at the Japanese Red Cross Nagoya Daiichi Hospital, Nagoya, Japan, between January 2020 and July 2023. This study included ART singleton pregnancies in which thyroid function screening was performed before conception (n = 687). Among them, we excluded 22 cases of overt thyroid disease (n = 22) and 15 cases of placenta previa (n = 15) (Figure 1).

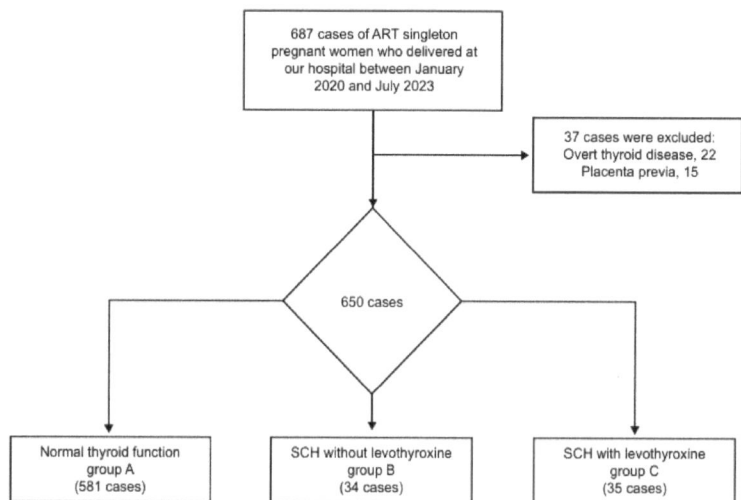

Figure 1. Study flowchart of patient enrollment.

This study was approved by the Ethics Committee of our hospital (approval number: 2023-070).

2.2. Data Collection and Definition

In this study, we defined SCH as preconception TSH levels > 2.5 mU/L and normal free T_4 levels. Patients with preconception TSH levels < 2.5 mU/L were assigned to group A (normal group). Patients with SCH were categorized into two groups: women who took levothyroxine sodium hydrate before and throughout pregnancy (group C) and those who did not (group B). In group C, after diagnosing SCH, patients were treated by an endocrinologist with levothyroxine sodium hydrate (approximately 0.5 μg/kg/day) and followed up regularly (every 2–4 weeks) for TSH and free T4 levels. Doses were increased (12–25 μg/day) until the TSH level fell below 2.5 mU/L. Once the target level was achieved, the maintenance dose was continued until the end of pregnancy (TSH and free T4 levels were monitored every 4–6 weeks). Moreover, all patients in group C had normalized TSH levels at the time of pregnancy. The following maternal and perinatal data were obtained from medical records: age, parity, body mass index before pregnancy, history of abortion, history of previous cesarean deliveries, gestational weeks at delivery, preterm birth (at <37 weeks, <34 weeks, <32 weeks, and <28 weeks), preeclampsia, fetal growth restriction (FGR), blood loss at delivery, transfusion, manual placental removal, and the value of TSH before pregnancy. We also obtained the birth weight of the newborns. Preeclampsia was defined as the appearance of gestational hypertension, proteinuria, and/or signs of end-organ impairment during pregnancy [15]. FGR was defined as neonatal body weight at birth <−1.5 than the standard deviation for gestational age in Japan [16].

2.3. Statistical Analyses

All statistical analyses were performed using EZR (v. 1.37, Saitama, Japan). The Shapiro–Wilk test was used to analyze the normality of the data. Continuous variables among the three groups were compared using the Kruskal–Wallis test. The Mann–Whitney U test was used for nonparametric comparisons during the post hoc analysis. Nominal data were analyzed using Fisher's exact test. In multivariate analysis, maternal age, body mass index, parity, preeclampsia, FGR, history of abortion, levothyroxine therapy, and TSH levels were selected as variables associated with preterm birth. $p < 0.05$ was considered statistically significant.

3. Results

Among the 650 ART singleton deliveries in this study, 581 were assigned to group A, 34 to group B, and 35 to group C (Figure 1). The three groups did not significantly differ in terms of age, body mass index, history of previous cesarean deliveries, blood loss at delivery, manual placental removal, transfusion, preeclampsia, FGR, history of abortion, and neonatal body weight (Table 1).

Expectedly, the TSH levels were significantly lower in group A than in groups B and C ($p < 0.001$). After the initiation of levothyroxine therapy in group C, the TSH levels were 1.11 (±0.60) mU/L. The rate of preterm birth at <34 weeks was significantly higher in group B (14.7%) and significantly lower in group C (0%) than in group A ($p = 0.046$). Group C had no cases of preterm delivery under 34 weeks. The preterm birth rate at <37 weeks was lower in group C (5.7%) than in groups A and B; however, the difference was not significant ($p = 0.059$) (Table 1).

When 69 patients diagnosed with SCH (groups B and C) were examined for the rate of preterm delivery at <34 weeks per TSH level, the rates were 1/30 (3.3%) at TSH levels of 2.5–3 mU/L, 2/22 (9.1%) at 3–4 mU/L, and 2/17 (11.8%) at >4 mU/L. The rate of preterm delivery at <34 weeks increased according to the TSH levels, but the difference was not statistically significant.

Table 1. Maternal characteristics and perinatal outcomes of this study.

	Group A (n = 581)	Group B (n = 34)	Group C (n = 35)	p-Value
Maternal age (years) *	36.5 (±4.3)	36.6 (±4.7)	36.5 (±3.8)	0.988
Pre-pregnant BMI (kg/m^2) *	21.5 (±3.4)	22.0 (±2.6)	21.8 (±2.8)	0.634
History of abortion	218/581 (37.5%)	11/34 (32.4%)	8/35 (22.9%)	0.194
Preterm birth at <37 weeks	106/581 (18.2%)	9/34 (26.5%)	2/35 (5.7%)	0.059
Preterm birth at <34 weeks	36/581 (6.2%)	5/34 (14.7%)	0/35 (0%)	0.046
Preterm birth at <32 weeks	32/581 (5.5%)	1/34 (2.9%)	0/35 (0%)	0.411
Preterm birth at <28 weeks	16/581 (2.8%)	0/34 (0%)	0/35 (0%)	1
Preeclampsia	56/581 (9.6%)	3/34 (8.8%)	4/35 (11.4%)	0.945
Fetal growth restriction	23/581 (4.0%)	1/34 (2.9%)	0/35 (0%)	0.768
Cesarean delivery	272/581 (46.8%)	15/34 (44.1%)	19/34 (54.3%)	0.641
Blood loss at delivery (mL) *	812 (±676)	970 (±716)	788 (±406)	0.393
Manual placental removal	53/581 (9.1%)	3/34 (8.8%)	5/35 (14.3%)	0.591
Transfusion	33/581 (5.7%)	1/34 (2.9%)	0/35 (0%)	0.374
Neonatal birth weight (g) *	2901 (±1339)	2819 (±640)	3064 (±475)	0.705
TSH value (mU/L) *	1.36 (±0.57)	4.02 (±2.47)	3.55 (±1.07)	<0.001

BMI, body mass index; TSH, thyroid-stimulating hormone. * Median (range).

The results of multivariate analysis of the risk of preterm birth at <37 weeks are shown in Table 2.

Table 2. Multivariate logistic regression analysis for preterm birth at <37 weeks.

	Adjusted OR	95% CI	p-Value
Maternal age	1.00	0.956–1.05	0.880
Pre-pregnant BMI	1.00	0.939–1.07	0.991
Nulliparous	0.95	0.602–1.50	0.822
History of abortion	0.97	0.621–1.52	0.899
Preeclampsia	4.98	2.81–8.81	<0.001
Fetal growth restriction	3.31	1.31–8.34	0.011
Levothyroxine therapy	1.36	0.378–1.36	0.230
TSH value	1.05	0.485–2.29	0.895

BMI, body mass index; TSH, thyroid-stimulating hormone; OR, odds ratio; CI, confidence interval.

When performing the multivariate analysis, we included maternal age, body mass index, parity, preeclampsia, FGR, history of abortion, levothyroxine therapy, and TSH levels as variables to calculate the OR. Preeclampsia (OR = 4.98) and FGR (OR = 3.31) were significant risk factors for preterm birth at <37 weeks; however, levothyroxine therapy and TSH levels did not affect the risk of preterm birth at <37 weeks.

The results of the multivariate analysis of the risk of preterm birth at <34 weeks are shown in Table 3.

Table 3. Multivariate logistic regression analysis for preterm birth at <34 weeks.

	Adjusted OR	95% CI	p-Value
Maternal age	1.00	0.926–1.07	0.915
Pre-pregnant BMI	1.03	0.942–1.13	0.506
Nulliparous	1.20	0.567–2.53	0.638
History of abortion	1.20	0.606–2.40	0.595
Preeclampsia	3.65	1.65–8.09	0.001
Fetal growth restriction	2.92	0.877–9.74	0.081
Levothyroxine therapy	0.117	0.015–0.948	0.044
TSH value	2.18	0.750–6.36	0.152

BMI, body mass index; TSH, thyroid-stimulating hormone; OR, odds ratio; CI, confidence interval.

In the multivariate analysis, we included maternal age, body mass index, parity, preeclampsia, FGR, history of abortion, levothyroxine therapy, and TSH level as variables to calculate the OR. The significant risk factor for preterm birth at <34 weeks was preeclampsia (OR = 3.65; 95% CI, 1.65–8.09), and the significant preventive factor was levothyroxine therapy (OR = 0.117; 95% CI, 0.015–0.948).

Of the 69 patients with TSH levels > 2.5 mU/L in this study, thyroid peroxidase (TPO) antibodies were measured in 44 patients (63.8%). TPO antibodies were positive in 4 out of 19 patients (21.1%) in group B and 6 out of 25 patients (24%) in group C, with no significant difference between the two groups ($p = 0.817$).

The results of multivariate analysis assessing the impact of TSH on perinatal outcomes are shown in Table S1. TSH levels were not identified as an independent risk factor for various perinatal complications, including preterm birth, preeclampsia, FGR, cesarean delivery, and the need for transfusion.

4. Discussion

We investigated the effects of SCH and its preconception treatment on the perinatal outcomes of ART singleton pregnancies, all of which were screened for thyroid function prior to conception. The preterm birth rate at <34 weeks was significantly higher in patients with SCH; however, it was significantly lower in patients with SCH treated with levothyroxine therapy before pregnancy. The rate of preterm delivery at <34 weeks increased according to TSH levels. The multivariate analysis revealed that levothyroxine therapy was a significant protective factor against preterm birth at <34 weeks.

Women with SCH have a higher risk of preeclampsia and preterm delivery than euthyroid women [5,6,10]. However, in the present study, we found that the rate of preterm birth at <34 weeks was significantly higher in patients with SCH and was not significantly different for preterm birth (<37, <32, and <28 weeks) and preeclampsia. The results may be because our study was limited to cases of singleton ART pregnancies. In general, women undergoing infertility treatment appear to have a small but statistically significant increase in risk for preterm birth, low birth weight, and severe maternal morbidity (such as preeclampsia, antepartum hemorrhage, need for transfusion, thrombotic embolism, and disseminated intravascular coagulation) [17–19]. Therefore, the background factors of ART pregnancy may have influenced these results. Limited data also suggest that in women undergoing IVF, cases with preconception TSH levels > 2.5 mU/L may result in a lower gestational age at delivery and a lower birth weight [12]. However, other pregnancy outcomes, such as the rate of preterm birth, the rate of FGR, preeclampsia, blood loss during delivery, and the need for transfusion, may not have been examined. To our knowledge, there are no other studies on the association between SCH and adverse outcomes in ART pregnancies, and we believe that the present study provides new insights. In addition, the rate of preterm delivery at <34 weeks increased according to the TSH level but was not significant in the present study. The results are significantly interesting, but the limited number of cases did not allow for significant differences. Previous studies have reported that TSH levels correlate with preterm birth rates [11], but there are no high-quality data stratified by cutoff of the TSH level, presence of antithyroid antibodies, or treatment for SCH. Thus, future studies are required.

Screening for hypothyroidism in asymptomatic pregnant women during early pregnancy remains controversial. In prospective trials, even with universal screening for thyroid function, there was no improvement in pregnancy outcomes compared with a targeted or no screening group [20]. In a randomized trial, >4500 women in their first trimester of pregnancy participated. They were randomly assigned to either a universal screening group or a case-finding group [21]. Overall, the total number of adverse outcomes was similar between the case-finding and universal screening groups. However, secondary analysis revealed that low-risk women diagnosed with SCH and treated with thyroid hormone therapy in the universal screening group had 57% fewer adverse outcomes (preterm birth, preeclampsia, gestational diabetes, and miscarriage) than low-risk women diagnosed with

SCH but not treated in the case-finding group [21]. In addition, it has been suggested that universal screening may show higher cost-effectiveness [22,23]. As mentioned above, universal screening of thyroid function in pregnant women has its advantages and disadvantages, but the results of our study suggest that, although limited to ART pregnancies, preconception screening and treatment for SCH may contribute to improved perinatal outcomes. In the future, universal screening for thyroid function and proper hormone therapy in pregnant women may contribute to reducing perinatal risks, including preterm birth.

There are no established criteria for the indications for SCH treatment in pregnant women. In a multicenter trial, 677 pregnant women with SCH (median TSH, 4.4 mU/L; free T4, normal) were randomized to levothyroxine therapy or placebo group [24]. Levothyroxine treatment had no significant effect on maternal or fetal outcomes, such as preterm delivery, preeclampsia, gestational hypertension, and miscarriage, and there was no interaction effect with TPO antibody positivity. In a meta-analysis of nine randomized controlled trials and 13 cohort studies, there was no benefit of SCH treatment on pregnancy outcomes [9]. However, evaluation of antithyroid antibodies is also important in women diagnosed with SCH [4]. In a systematic review by the American Thyroid Association (ATA) regarding pregnancy-specific complications, although there is clearly a higher risk in TPO-positive women with TSH > 2.5 mU/L, the risk was not constant in TPO-negative women, even at significantly higher TSH levels (>5–10 mU/L) [25]. In a trial of 131 TPO antibody-positive women diagnosed with SCH, levothyroxine replacement significantly reduced the rate of preterm delivery, especially in women with TSH $\geq$ 4 mU/L [26]. At present, it is uncertain whether thyroid hormone replacement therapy reduces perinatal risk in women with SCH. A recent meta-analysis suggested that high levels of TPO antibodies, even in euthyroid pregnant women, could adversely influence pregnancy outcomes after ART [27]. In contrast, no significant differences were observed in pregnancy outcomes following fresh or frozen embryo transfer in euthyroid patients with TPO and/or antithyroglobulin antibodies [28]. Therefore, the perinatal risk of antithyroid antibodies alone in euthyroid patients remains inconclusive. In the present study, we demonstrated that levothyroxine therapy could reduce the risk of preterm birth at <34 weeks among SCH patients with TSH $\geq$ 2.5 mU/L. However, complete data on anti-TPO antibodies were not available; therefore, further studies are required in the future.

Furthermore, in the present study, the diagnostic criterion for SCH was defined as TSH level > 2.5 mU/L for the following reasons. First, the study included ART pregnancies. Pregnancy outcomes for women undergoing IVF may be worse among those with preconception TSH levels > 2.5 mU/L [12]. Second, the treatment goal for SCH should be to achieve a TSH level of $\leq$2.5 mU/L. Finally, according to the ATA guidelines, levothyroxine therapy should be considered for TPO antibody-positive women with TSH levels > 2.5 mU/L. Moreover, we decided to use the cutoff of 2.5 mU/L because complete data on TPO antibodies were not available. Therefore, the interpretation of our findings is that levothyroxine therapy with TSH levels > 2.5 mU/L, regardless of the presence of autoantibodies, can reduce the risk of preterm birth at <34 weeks.

This study included cases of ART singleton pregnancies in which thyroid function screening was performed before fertility treatment. The SCH rate was higher in the infertile women than in the control women (healthy women with confirmed fertility) (13.9% vs. 3.9%) [29]. A recent study demonstrated that pregnant women with singleton ART with a history of abortion or spontaneous abortion were more likely to have thyroid-related diseases [30]. In Japan, universal screening of thyroid function is commonly performed before fertility treatment. In addition, all patients in group C were already receiving appropriate levothyroxine therapy by an endocrinologist at the time of conception and were appropriately managed for SCH throughout their pregnancy. The strength of this study is that the patients' backgrounds were well-established. Second, because it is a single-center study, there is consistency in pregnancy management and treatment policies, and a certain quality of care is maintained. Our institution follows the Guidelines for Obstetrical Practice in Japan and provides standardized care. The limitations of this study include the following: inclusion of only singleton data from ART pregnancies; the absence of data on placental abruption, neonatal respiratory distress syndrome, and/or pregnancy loss among adverse pregnancy outcomes; the absence of data on the prognosis of the child, such as respiratory disorders and cognitive function; and the absence of data on anti-TPO antibodies. Another limitation is that the criteria for levothyroxine therapy (groups B and C) in patients with SCH are unknown. Finally, the number of cases examined in this study was limited, especially in the SCH groups (34 and 35 cases in groups B and C, respectively); therefore, it is possible that statistical differences could not be detected. This study has the following inherent limitations: limitations inherent to the study design, the potential for selection bias, and the inability to generalize the findings to different populations. Therefore, large-scale studies are required in the future.

In conclusion, the rate of preterm birth at <34 weeks is significantly higher in patients with SCH; however, it is significantly lower in patients with SCH treated with levothyroxine therapy before and during pregnancy. Moreover, levothyroxine therapy is a significant protective factor against preterm birth at <34 weeks. These data provide valuable information for future clinical practice. Universal screening of thyroid function and proper hormone therapy in all pregnant women may reduce perinatal risks, including preterm birth. Further large-scale studies are warranted to estimate the perinatal risk of SCH, including data on antithyroid antibodies and the effects of levothyroxine therapy on perinatal risk, and to set cutoff values for appropriate therapeutic interventions.

Supplementary Materials: The following supporting information can be downloaded at: https://www.mdpi.com/article/10.3390/jcm13175137/s1, Table S1: Multivariate logistic regression analysis assessing the impact of TSH on perinatal outcomes.

Author Contributions: All authors contributed to the conception and design of this study. Material preparation, data collection, and analysis, Y.N. (Yuichiro Narita), E.T., Y.N. (Yumi Nakamura), M.S., Y.I., A.T., and T.A.; writing of the first draft of the manuscript, H.T.; and all authors commented on the previous versions of the manuscript. All authors have read and agreed to the published version of the manuscript.

Funding: This research was funded by the Japanese Red Cross, Aichi Medical Center, Nagoya Daiichi Hospital (Research Grant NFRCH 24-0008). The funding body had no role in the study design, data collection, analysis, interpretation, or the writing of the manuscript.

Institutional Review Board Statement: This study was conducted in accordance with the principles outlined in the 1964 Declaration of Helsinki. This study was approved by the Ethics Committee of the Japanese Red Cross Aichi Medical Center Nagoya Daiichi Hospital, Nagoya, Japan (approval number: 2023-070 date of approval: 2 June 2023). Data were compiled and analyzed so that personal information could not be identified.

Informed Consent Statement: Patient informed consent was waived as this study used anonymous clinical data.

Data Availability Statement: The data in the manuscript will not be deposited. However, upon request, we will submit data (deidentified participant data) that support the findings of this study.

Acknowledgments: We thank Atsushi Kubo for collecting data from the medical records.

Conflicts of Interest: The authors declare no conflicts of interest. The authors alone are responsible for the content and writing of this manuscript.

References

1. Kasagi, K.; Takahashi, N.; Inoue, G.; Honda, T.; Kawachi, Y.; Izumi, Y. Thyroid function in Japanese adults as assessed by a general health checkup system in relation with thyroid-related antibodies and other clinical parameters. *Thyroid* **2009**, *19*, 937–944. [CrossRef]
2. Allan, W.C.; Haddow, J.E.; Palomaki, G.E.; Williams, J.R.; Mitchell, M.L.; Hermos, R.J.; Faix, J.D.; Klein, R.Z. Maternal thyroid deficiency and pregnancy complications: Implications for population screening. *J. Med. Screen.* **2000**, *7*, 127–130. [CrossRef] [PubMed]

3. Klein, R.Z.; Haddow, J.E.; Faix, J.D.; Brown, R.S.; Hermos, R.J.; Pulkkinen, A.; Mitchell, M.L. Prevalence of thyroid deficiency in pregnant women. *Clin. Endocrinol.* **1991**, *35*, 41–46. [CrossRef]
4. Liu, H.; Shan, Z.; Li, C.; Mao, J.; Xie, X.; Wang, W.; Fan, C.; Wang, H.; Zhang, H.; Han, C.; et al. Maternal subclinical hypothyroidism, thyroid autoimmunity, and the risk of miscarriage: A prospective cohort study. *Thyroid* **2014**, *24*, 1642–1649. [CrossRef] [PubMed]
5. Lee, S.Y.; Cabral, H.J.; Aschengrau, A.; Pearce, E.N. Associations between maternal thyroid function in pregnancy and obstetric and perinatal outcomes. *J. Clin. Endocrinol. Metab.* **2020**, *105*, e2015–e2023. [CrossRef]
6. Toloza, F.J.K.; Derakhshan, A.; Männistö, T.; Bliddal, S.; Popova, P.V.; Carty, D.M.; Chen, L.; Taylor, P.; Mosso, L.; Oken, E.; et al. Association between maternal thyroid function and risk of gestational hypertension and pre-eclampsia: A systematic review and individual-participant data meta-analysis. *Lancet Diabetes Endocrinol.* **2022**, *10*, 243–252. [CrossRef] [PubMed]
7. Breathnach, F.M.; Donnelly, J.; Cooley, S.M.; Geary, M.; Malone, F.D. Subclinical hypothyroidism as a risk factor for placental abruption: Evidence from a low-risk primigravid population. *Aust. N. Z. J. Obstet. Gynaecol.* **2013**, *53*, 553–560. [CrossRef]
8. Cleary-Goldman, J.; Malone, F.D.; Lambert-Messerlian, G.; Sullivan, L.; Canick, J.; Porter, T.F.; Luthy, D.; Gross, S.; Bianchi, D.W.; D'Alton, M.E. Maternal thyroid hypofunction and pregnancy outcome. *Obstet. Gynecol.* **2008**, *112*, 85–92. [CrossRef]
9. Jiao, X.F.; Zhang, M.; Chen, J.; Wei, Q.; Zeng, L.; Liu, D.; Zhang, C.; Li, H.; Zou, K.; Zhang, L.; et al. The impact of levothyroxine therapy on the pregnancy, neonatal and childhood outcomes of subclinical hypothyroidism during pregnancy: An updated systematic review, meta-analysis and trial sequential analysis. *Front. Endocrinol.* **2022**, *13*, 964084. [CrossRef] [PubMed]
10. Consortium on Thyroid and Pregnancy—Study Group on Preterm Birth—Study Group on Preterm Birth; Korevaar, T.I.M.; Derakhshan, A.; Taylor, P.N.; Meima, M.; Chen, L.; Bliddal, S.; Carty, D.M.; Meems, M.; Vaidya, B.; et al. Association of thyroid function test abnormalities and thyroid autoimmunity with preterm birth: A systematic review and meta-analysis. *JAMA* **2019**, *322*, 632–641. [CrossRef] [PubMed]
11. Knøsgaard, L.; Andersen, S.; Hansen, A.B.; Vestergaard, P.; Andersen, S.L. Maternal hypothyroidism and adverse outcomes of pregnancy. *Clin. Endocrinol.* **2023**, *98*, 719–729. [CrossRef]
12. Baker, V.L.; Rone, H.M.; Pasta, D.J.; Nelson, H.P.; Gvakharia, M.; Adamson, G.D. Correlation of thyroid stimulating hormone (TSH) level with pregnancy outcome in women undergoing in vitro fertilization. *Am. J. Obstet. Gynecol.* **2006**, *194*, 1668–1674, discussion 1674. [CrossRef] [PubMed]
13. Blatt, A.J.; Nakamoto, J.M.; Kaufman, H.W. National status of testing for hypothyroidism during pregnancy and postpartum. *J. Clin. Endocrinol. Metab.* **2012**, *97*, 777–784. [CrossRef]
14. Vaidya, B.; Hubalewska-Dydejczyk, A.; Laurberg, P.; Negro, R.; Vermiglio, F.; Poppe, K. Treatment and screening of hypothyroidism in pregnancy: Results of a European survey. *Eur. J. Endocrinol.* **2012**, *166*, 49–54. [CrossRef]
15. Watanabe, K.; Matsubara, K.; Nakamoto, O.; Ushijima, J.; Ohkuchi, A.; Koide, K.; Makino, S.; Mimura, K.; Morikawa, M.; Naruse, K.; et al. Outline of the new definition and classification of "hypertensive disorders of pregnancy (HDP)"; a revised JSSHP statement of 2005. *Hypertens. Res. Pregnancy* **2018**, *6*, 33–37. [CrossRef]
16. Yoshida, S.; Unno, N.; Kagawa, H.; Shinozuka, N.; Kozuma, S.; Taketani, Y. Prenatal detection of a high-risk group for intrauterine growth restriction based on sonographic fetal biometry. *Int. J. Gynaecol. Obstet.* **2000**, *68*, 225–232. [CrossRef]
17. Jaques, A.M.; Amor, D.J.; Baker, H.W.G.; Healy, D.L.; Ukoumunne, O.C.; Breheny, S.; Garrett, C.; Halliday, J.L. Adverse obstetric and perinatal outcomes in subfertile women conceiving without assisted reproductive technologies. *Fertil. Steril.* **2010**, *94*, 2674–2679. [CrossRef] [PubMed]
18. Declercq, E.; Luke, B.; Belanoff, C.; Cabral, H.; Diop, H.; Gopal, D.; Hoang, L.; Kotelchuck, M.; Stern, J.E.; Hornstein, M.D. Perinatal outcomes associated with assisted reproductive technology: The Massachusetts Outcomes Study of Assisted Reproductive Technologies (MOSART). *Fertil. Steril.* **2015**, *103*, 888–895. [CrossRef]
19. Murugappan, G.; Li, S.; Lathi, R.B.; Baker, V.L.; Luke, B.; Eisenberg, M.L. Increased risk of severe maternal morbidity among infertile women: Analysis of US claims data. *Am. J. Obstet. Gynecol.* **2020**, *223*, 404.e1–404.e20. [CrossRef]
20. Lazarus, J.H.; Bestwick, J.P.; Channon, S.; Paradice, R.; Maina, A.; Rees, R.; Chiusano, E.; John, R.; Guaraldo, V.; George, L.M.; et al. Antenatal thyroid screening and childhood cognitive function. *N. Engl. J. Med.* **2012**, *366*, 493–501. [CrossRef]
21. Negro, R.; Schwartz, A.; Gismondi, R.; Tinelli, A.; Mangieri, T.; Stagnaro-Green, A. Universal screening versus case finding for detection and treatment of thyroid hormonal dysfunction during pregnancy. *J. Clin. Endocrinol. Metab.* **2010**, *95*, 1699–1707. [CrossRef] [PubMed]
22. Thung, S.F.; Funai, E.F.; Grobman, W.A. The cost-effectiveness of universal screening in pregnancy for subclinical hypothyroidism. *Am. J. Obstet. Gynecol.* **2009**, *200*, 267.e1–267.e7. [CrossRef] [PubMed]
23. Dosiou, C.; Barnes, J.; Schwartz, A.; Negro, R.; Crapo, L.; Stagnaro-Green, A. Cost-effectiveness of universal and risk-based screening for autoimmune thyroid disease in pregnant women. *J. Clin. Endocrinol. Metab.* **2012**, *97*, 1536–1546. [CrossRef] [PubMed]
24. Casey, B.M.; Thom, E.A.; Peaceman, A.M.; Varner, M.W.; Sorokin, Y.; Hirtz, D.G.; Reddy, U.M.; Wapner, R.J.; Thorp, J.M., Jr.; Saade, G.; et al. Treatment of subclinical hypothyroidism or hypothyroxinemia in pregnancy. *N. Engl. J. Med.* **2017**, *376*, 815–825. [CrossRef]
25. Alexander, E.K.; Pearce, E.N.; Brent, G.A.; Brown, R.S.; Chen, H.; Dosiou, C.; Grobman, W.A.; Laurberg, P.; Lazarus, J.H.; Mandel, S.J.; et al. 2017 Guidelines of the American Thyroid Association for the diagnosis and management of thyroid disease during pregnancy and the postpartum. *Thyroid* **2017**, *27*, 315–389. [CrossRef] [PubMed]

26. Nazarpour, S.; Ramezani Tehrani, F.; Simbar, M.; Tohidi, M.; Alavi Majd, H.; Azizi, F. Effects of levothyroxine treatment on pregnancy outcomes in pregnant women with autoimmune thyroid disease. *Eur. J. Endocrinol.* **2017**, *176*, 253–265. [CrossRef]
27. Zhang, S.; Yang, M.; Li, T.; Yang, M.; Wang, W.; Chen, Y.; Ding, Y.; Liu, J.; Xu, X.; Zhang, J.; et al. High level of thyroid peroxidase antibodies as a detrimental risk of pregnancy outcomes in euthyroid women undergoing ART: A meta-analysis. *Mol. Reprod. Dev.* **2023**, *90*, 218–226. [CrossRef]
28. Yang, X.; Qiu, S.; Jiang, W.; Huang, Z.; Shi, H.; Du, S.; Sun, Y.; Zheng, B. Impact of thyroid autoimmunity on pregnancy outcomes in euthyroid women following fresh/frozen–thawed embryo transfer. *Clin. Endocrinol.* **2023**, *99*, 113–121. [CrossRef] [PubMed]
29. Abalovich, M.; Mitelberg, L.; Allami, C.; Gutierrez, S.; Alcaraz, G.; Otero, P.; Levalle, O. Subclinical hypothyroidism and thyroid autoimmunity in women with infertility. *Gynecol. Endocrinol.* **2007**, *23*, 279–283. [CrossRef]
30. Sun, H.; Su, X.; Liu, Y.; Li, G.; Liu, X.; Du, Q. Association between abortion history and perinatal and neonatal outcomes of singleton pregnancies after assisted reproductive technology. *J. Clin. Med.* **2022**, *12*, 1. [CrossRef]

Disclaimer/Publisher's Note: The statements, opinions and data contained in all publications are solely those of the individual author(s) and contributor(s) and not of MDPI and/or the editor(s). MDPI and/or the editor(s) disclaim responsibility for any injury to people or property resulting from any ideas, methods, instructions or products referred to in the content.

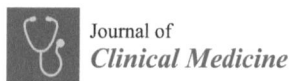

Article

Association between Flexibility, Measured with the Back-Scratch Test, and the Odds of Oxytocin Administration during Labour and Caesarean Section

Virginia A. Aparicio [1,2,3], Nuria Marín-Jiménez [2,4,5,*], Jose Castro-Piñero [4,5], Marta Flor-Alemany [6,*], Irene Coll-Risco [2] and Laura Baena-García [2,7,8]

1. Department of Physiology, Institute of Nutrition and Food Technology, University of Granada, 18003 Granada, Spain; virginiaaparicio@ugr.es
2. Sport and Health University Research Institute (iMUDSmuds), University of Granada, 18007 Granada, Spain; irecollrisco@gmail.com (I.C.-R.); lbaenagarcia@ugr.es (L.B.-G.)
3. Glzartea, Kirola eta Arikera Fisikoa Ikerkuntza Taldea (GIKAFIT), Society Sports and Exercise Research Group, Department of Physical Education and Sport, Faculty of Education and Sport, Physical Activity and Sport Sciences Section, University of the Basque Country (UPV/EHU), 01006 Vitoria-Gasteiz, Spain
4. GALENO Research Group, Department of Physical Education, Faculty of Education Sciences, University of Cadiz, 11519 Puerto Real, Spain; jose.castro@uca.es
5. Instituto de Investigación e Innovación Biomédica de Cádiz (INiBICA), 11009 Cadiz, Spain
6. Department of Health and Biomedical Sciences, Faculty of Health Sciences, University of Loyola Andalucia, Campus Sevilla, Avda. de las Universidades S/N, 41704 Dos Hermanas, Spain
7. Department of Nursing, Faculty of Health Sciences, University of Granada, 18071 Granada, Spain
8. Biosanitary Research Institute, IBS, University of Granada, 18012 Granada, Spain
* Correspondence: nmjimenez@ual.es (N.M.-J.); mdelaflor@uloyola.es (M.F.-A.)

Abstract: Objective: This study explored whether assessing flexibility levels in clinical settings might predict the odds of oxytocin administration and caesarean section to stimulate labour. **Methods:** Pregnant women from the GESTAFIT Project (n = 157), participated in this longitudinal study. Maternal upper-body flexibility was assessed at 16 gestational weeks (g.w.) through the Back-scratch test. Clinical data, including oxytocin administration and type of birth, were registered from obstetric medical records. **Results:** Pregnant women who required oxytocin administration or had caesarean sections showed lower flexibility scores ($p < 0.05$ and $p < 0.01$, respectively). The receiver operating characteristic curve analysis showed that the Back-scratch test was able to detect the need for oxytocin administration ((area under the curve [AUC] = 0.672 (95% confidence interval [CI]: 0.682 (95% CI: 0.59–0.78, $p = 0.001$)). The AUC to establish the ability of flexibility to discriminate between vaginal and caesarean section births was 0.672 (95% CI: 0.60–0.77, $p = 0.002$). A Back-scratch test worse than 4 centimetres was associated with a ~5 times greater increased odds ratio of requiring exogenous oxytocin administration (95% CI: 2.0–11.6, $p = 0.001$) and a ~4 times greater increased odds ratio of having a caesarean section (95% CI: 1.7–10.2, $p = 0.002$). **Conclusions:** These findings suggest that lower flexibility levels at the 16th g.w. discriminates between pregnant women who will require oxytocin and those who will not, and those with a greater risk of a caesarean section than those with a vaginal birth. Pregnant women below the proposed Back-scratch test cut-offs at 16th g.w. might specifically benefit from physical therapies that include flexibility training.

Keywords: pregnant woman; physical fitness; flexibility; oxytocin; labour; obstetric risk

Citation: Aparicio, V.A.; Marín-Jiménez, N.; Castro-Piñero, J.; Flor-Alemany, M.; Coll-Risco, I.; Baena-García, L. Association between Flexibility, Measured with the Back-Scratch Test, and the Odds of Oxytocin Administration during Labour and Caesarean Section. *J. Clin. Med.* **2024**, *13*, 5245. https://doi.org/10.3390/jcm13175245

Academic Editors: Ioannis Tsakiridis and Apostolos Mamopoulos

Received: 17 July 2024
Revised: 28 August 2024
Accepted: 29 August 2024
Published: 4 September 2024

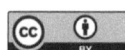

Copyright: © 2024 by the authors. Licensee MDPI, Basel, Switzerland. This article is an open access article distributed under the terms and conditions of the Creative Commons Attribution (CC BY) license (https://creativecommons.org/licenses/by/4.0/).

1. Introduction

Events related to the labour process have important implications for both the mother and the new-born [1–4]. Therefore, it is clinically relevant to explore and identify factors that might be associated with a lower risk of common interventions that should be avoided during labour [2,5], such as the exogenous administration of oxytocin [2,4–6] and caesarean sections [7].

In this context, we previously observed that greater physical fitness was associated with better labour-related outcomes, such as less need for oxytocin administration to induce or stimulate labour [8] and lower caesarean incidence [9]. Previous studies have shown that muscle stretching exercises during pregnancy are associated with better maternal and neonatal birth outcomes (such as less pelvic pain, greater mobility, better maternal mental state, and lower rate of obstetric complications) [10,11]. In this regard, a randomised clinical trial showed that women who undertook a yoga programme during pregnancy had lower rates of labour induction and caesarean sections [12]. The dimension of physical fitness that tends to increase with this type of intervention is flexibility. However, the role of this variable in relation to induction and/or stimulation of labour and type of birth has not been explored so far. Notwithstanding, most of the tests employed for measuring physical fitness require large spaces, special equipment such as a treadmill, or excessive time for assessment in clinical settings. Consequently, the election of time-efficient measuring tools adapted to health professionals, who usually have less than five minutes of consultation time [13], is mandatory. In this sense, the Back-scratch test, a quick and easy tool for measuring the range of motion that only requires a standard ruler, could be an excellent option. Furthermore, this tool has demonstrated a powerful capacity to predict key health outcomes such as cardiometabolic risk in several populations [14,15], an association with better mental health in healthy women and women with fibromyalgia, and even a role in predicting the risk of fibromyalgia and its severity [16]. Furthermore, within the GESTAtion and FITness (GESTAFIT) project, we have observed that this test is associated with improved maternal and neonatal birth-related outcomes [9].

Consequently, the aims of the present study were (i) to identify whether flexibility levels during the early second trimester of pregnancy may predict the need for oxytocin administration to induce or stimulate labour and the type of birth (i.e., vaginal or caesarean section) and (ii) to establish Back-scratch test cut-off points able to improve the accuracy of the need for oxytocin administration and the prognosis of caesarean section as a clinician tool for identifying pregnant women who could benefit from physical therapy programs that include flexibility training.

2. Materials and Methods

2.1. Study Sample and Design

The detailed procedures and inclusion and exclusion criteria (see Supplementary Table S1) of the GESTAFIT project were previously published [17]. Briefly, pregnant women between 18 and 45 years old with a normal pregnancy course who were able to walk without assistance, write and read properly, and signed an informed consent were eligible for selection. In addition, twin pregnancies, women with acute or terminal illnesses and gestations with foetal pathologies were excluded. This study is a secondary analysis that is part of a larger project in which a concurrent physical exercise program (aerobic plus strength training) was carried out in the intervention group from the 17th gestational week (g.w.) until birth. A total of 384 pregnant women were informed about this study during their 12th g.w. visits to the gynaecologist at the University Hospital. A final number of 159 women were interested in participating and signed an informed consent. Finally, 137 women had complete and valid data in relation to the specific aims of this study. The GESTAFIT project was approved by the Ethics Committee on Clinical Research (CEIC) of Granada, Regional Government of Andalusia, Spain (code: GESFIT-0448-N-15).

2.2. Procedures

The first evaluation of this study was carried out during the 16th g.w. The research team was present at all times to provide any explanations or instructions as needed. The pregnant women completed a self-reported questionnaire, anthropometric assessment, and the Back-scratch test. Height and weight were also assessed. Obstetric and gynaecological histories and birth outcomes were collected through the Pregnancy Health Document and digital medical records.

2.3. Maternal Sociodemographic and Clinical Data

Sociodemographic (age, number of children and marital, educational, and working status), reproductive history, and clinical (suffering or having suffered specific diseases and drug consumption) data were assessed with a self-reported questionnaire.

2.4. Anthropometric Assessment

Height and weight were measured using a stadiometer (Seca 22, Hamburg, Germany) and a scale (InBody R20; Biospace, Seoul, Republic of Korea), respectively. The body mass index was calculated as weight (kg)/height (m^2).

2.5. Pregnancy Health Document: Obstetric during Pregnancy and Pregnancy History

The "Pregnancy Health Document" is given to all pregnant women by the Andalusian regional government, and it contains obstetric and medical data recorded during the whole pregnancy. In this way, information about previous pregnancies and births and gynaecological antecedents were obtained. Gestational age was calculated by the date of last menstruation corrected for cycles of 28 days.

2.6. Labour Outcomes

All data related to the type of birth (vaginal or caesarean), gestational week at birth, use of epidural analgesia, offspring sex, neonatal weight, and the Apgar test were obtained from perinatal obstetric records (partogram) from the hospital after birth.

Oxytocin Administration before or during Labour

Information about the use of oxytocin was collected from the partogram. In this document, midwives usually record whether oxytocin is administered or not, but the dose and administration time are not frequently collected, so these data were not assessed in the present study. Moreover, we considered that oxytocin was administered both by induction of labour and uterine stimulation, but we did not consider the administration of this drug during placenta birth.

2.7. The Back-Scratch Test

The Back-scratch test [18] was used to assess upper-body flexibility (Figure 1). The test consists of measuring the overall shoulder range of motion by measuring the distance between (or overlap of) the middle fingers as they come together behind the back. This test was performed twice with both hands, alternatively; the final score in centimetres (cm) was calculated as the mean value of the best attempts for both arms.

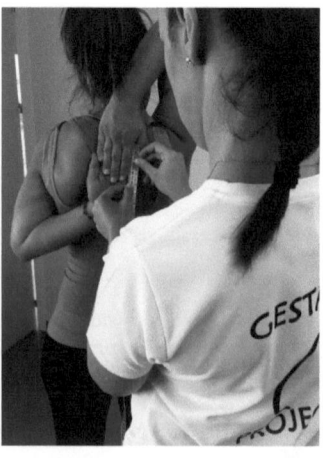

Figure 1. "Back-scratch" test assessment.

2.8. Statistical Analyses

Descriptive statistics were summarized as mean (standard deviation) for quantitative variables and frequency (%) for categorical variables.

The comparisons of the Back-scratch test between pregnant women with and without oxytocin administration and with and without caesarean section were performed by the T-student test and one-way analysis of covariance (ANCOVA) after adjustment for maternal age and weight, parity, the exercise intervention, epidural analgesia, and birth place. Planned caesarean sections were excluded from the analyses (n = 5, Figure 2). Furthermore, standardized effect size statistics were estimated for these comparisons through Cohen's *d* and its exact confidence interval (CI). The effect size was interpreted as small (~0.2), medium (~0.5) or large (~0.8 or greater).

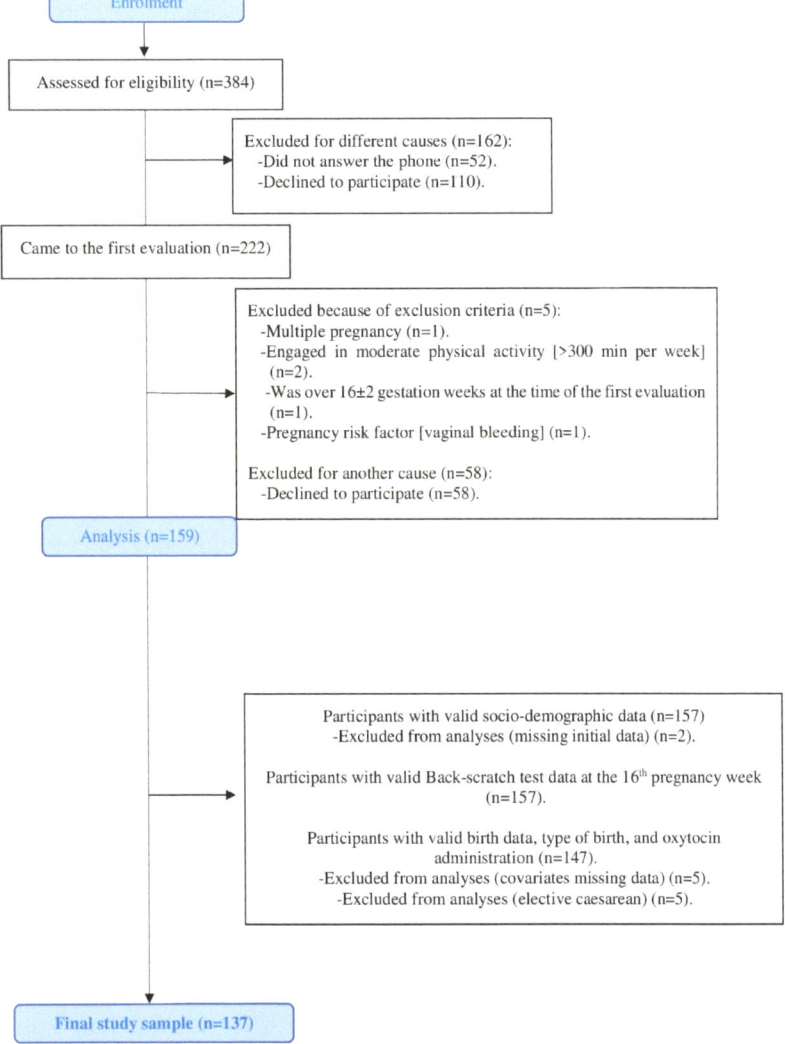

Figure 2. Flow diagram of the study participants.

The Back-scratch test thresholds that best prognosticated the subjects as having vs. not having oxytocin administration and as having vs. not having a caesarean section were determined by using receiver operating characteristic (ROC) curve analysis [19].

The ROC curve is a plot of all the sensitivity/specificity pairs resulting from varying the decision threshold [19]. To identify the best threshold, the distance between the perfect test and each sensitivity and 1-specificity pair was calculated, and then, the pair closest to 1 was chosen. We also calculated the area under the curve (AUC) and the 95% CI. The AUC represents the ability of the Back-scratch test to correctly classify subjects as having vs. not having oxytocin administration and having vs. not having a caesarean section as having vs. not having oxytocin administration. The values of AUC range between 1 (perfect test) and 0.5 (worthless test).

Binary logistic regression was used to further study the relationship among the Back-scratch test-derived cut-offs, oxytocin administration, and the presence/absence of caesarean section. Maternal age and weight, parity, maternal, exercise intervention, epidural analgesia, and birth place were also additionally included as covariates to test their potential confounder effects on upper-body flexibility and the risk of oxytocin administration and caesarean section.

All the analyses were performed using the Statistical Package for Social Sciences (IBM SPSS Statistics for Windows, version 26.0; Armonk, NY, USA), and the level of significance was set at $p < 0.05$.

3. Results

Of the 159 women who met the eligibility criteria and completed the first assessment, 157 women had complete and valid sociodemographic data. However, data on birth type and oxytocin administration were missing for 15 participants, and five pregnant women were excluded from the analyses because they had elective caesarean sections (see Figure 2).

The sociodemographic and clinical characteristics of the study participants are shown in Table 1. The final sample size was composed of 137 Caucasian pregnant women (aged 32.9 ± 4.6 years old, 66.7 ± 11.9 kg of mean weight at the 16th g.w.). Most of the participants lived with their partners (97%), had University degrees (57%), and worked full time. Approximately 61% of the sample were nulliparous, and 23% had a caesarean section. More than half of the caesarean sections (55%) were due to failure of labour progression (prolonged labour). Births took place around 39.6 ± 1.3 g.w., with a mean neonate body weight of 3.3 ± 0.5 kg. The mean value of the Back-scratch test was 4.1 ± 6 cm.

Table 1. Sociodemographic and clinical characteristics of the study participants (n = 137).

Maternal Outcome	Mean (SD)
Age, years	32.9 (4.6)
Body mass index at 16th gestational week, kg/m^2	24.9 (4.1)
Weight at 16th gestational week, kg	66.7 (11.9)
	n (%)
Living with a partner, yes	133 (97.1)
Educational status	
Primary or highschool	33 (24.1)
Specialized training	26 (18.9)
University degree	78 (56.9)
Working status	
Homework/unemployed	41 (29.9)
Partial-time employed/student	37 (27)
Full-time employed	59 (43.1)

Table 1. *Cont.*

Maternal Outcome	Mean (SD)
Oxytocin administration to induce or stimulate labour	44 (32.1)
Epidural analgesia, yes	94 (72.9)
Type of birth	
Vaginal	106 (77.4)
Non-planned caesarean section	31 (22.6)
Reason of caesarean section	n (%)
Risk of loss of foetal well-being	9 (29)
Failed induction	2 (6.5)
Failure to progress	17 (54.8)
Suspected Cephalopelvic Disproportion	3 (9.7)
Birth place	
Public hospital	131 (95.6)
Private hospital	5 (3.6)
Home	1 (0.7)
Parity	
Nulliparous	84 (61.3)
Multiparous	53 (38.7)
Back-scratch test	Mean (SD)
	4.1 (6.2)
16th gestational week	Median
	4.7
Neonatal outcome	
Sex (female, n (%))	68 (50.7)
Gestational age at birth, weeks	39.6 (1.3)
Birth weight, grams	3314 (482.8)
Apgar Test 1 min	8.6 (1.0)
Apgar Test 5 min	9.6 (0.7)

Differences in the Back-scratch test of the pregnant women at the 16th g.w. by oxytocin administration and type of birth are shown in Table 2. The mean scores in the Back-scratch test were +1.8 cm in women who needed oxytocin administration compared with +5.4 cm in women who did not require its administration ($p = 0.001$ for the unadjusted model and $p = 0.004$ for the adjusted model, Cohen's $d = 0.59$, 95% CI: 0.2–0.95). The mean cm values in the Back-scratch test were +1.6 cm in women who had caesarean sections compared with +5.0 cm in women who had vaginal births ($p = 0.004$ for the unadjusted model and $p = 0.017$ for the adjusted model, Cohen's $d = 0.55$, 95% CI: 0.2–0.9).

Table 2. Differences in the Back-scratch test of the pregnant women at the 16th gestational week by oxytocin administration and type of birth.

Oxytocin Was Not Administered (n = 93)	Oxytocin Was Administered (n = 44)	p	p *	Effect Size *d*-Cohen (95% CI)
5.40 (0.68)	1.76 (0.89)	0.001	0.004	0.59 (0.23, 0.95)
Vaginal Birth (n = 106)	Caesarean Section (n = 31)	p	p *	Effect Size *d*-Cohen (95% CI)
5.04 (0.63)	1.61 (0.89)	0.004	0.017	0.55 (0.21, 0.89)

Values are shown as mean (standard error of the mean). CI, confidence interval. * Model adjusted for maternal age, parity, maternal weight, exercise intervention, epidural analgesia, and birth place.

Figure 3 shows the capacity of the Back-scratch test to discriminate between the need for oxytocin administration before or during labour (Figure 3A) and presence/absence of caesarean section (Figure 3B). The AUC to establish the ability of the Back-scratch test to detect the need for oxytocin administration was 0.682 (95% CI: 0.59, 0.78, $p = 0.001$). The AUC to establish the ability of the Back-scratch test to detect the odds of caesarean section was 0.672 (95% CI: 0.60, 0.77, $p = 0.002$).

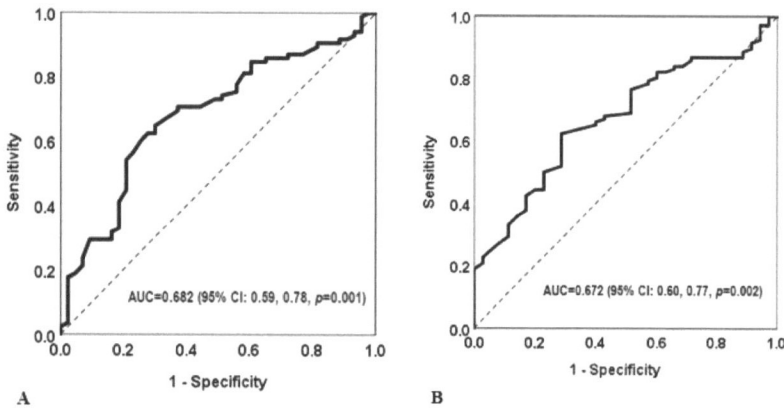

Figure 3. (**A**) Capacity of the Back-scratch test to discriminate the need (or not) for oxytocin administration before or during labour. (**B**) Capacity of the Back-scratch test to discriminate between vaginal birth and caesarean section.

The thresholds derived from the ROC analysis for the need for oxytocin administration and the presence/absence of caesarean section are shown in Table 3. The optimal cut-off to discriminate the need for oxytocin administration was +3.6 cm (OR = 4.2; 95% CI: 1.9–9.3 for the unadjusted model, and OR: 4.8; 95% CI: 2.0–11.6.7 for the adjusted model). The cut-off points, ORs, and 95% CIs of the Back-scratch test to identify caesarean presence were tested in an unadjusted model after adjusting for maternal age and weight, parity, exercise intervention, epidural analgesia, and birth place. The optimal cut-off point to discriminate between the presence and absence of a caesarean section was +4.1 cm (OR: 4.1; 95% CI: 1.8–9.5 for the unadjusted model, and OR: 4.2; 95% CI: 1.7–10.2 for the model adjusted for the abovementioned potential confounders).

Table 3. Binary logistic regression statistics testing the predictive capacity of the Back-scratch test thresholds derived from the receiver operating characteristics curve analysis for the need for oxytocin administration before or during labour and the presence/absence of caesarean section.

	Low Back-Scratch Test (Based on the Cut-Off)						
	Cut-Off Point (cm)	Unadjusted Model			Adjusted Model *		
		OR	95% CI	p	OR	95% CI	p
Oxytocin administration	<3.6	4.23	1.92–9.31	<0.001	4.79	1.97–11.6	0.001
Caesarean section	<4.1	4.13	1.80–9.50	0.001	4.15	1.70–10.2	0.002

High Back-scratch test was used as reference; OR, odds ratio; CI, confidence interval; * Model adjusted for maternal age, parity, maternal weight, exercise intervention, epidural analgesia, and birth place.

4. Discussion

The main findings of the present study indicate that lower flexibility levels during the early second trimester of pregnancy may be indicators of the need for oxytocin administration before or during labour and caesarean section.

At the 16th g.w., a Back-scratch test score < 3.6 cm was associated with a ~5 times greater increased odds ratio for requiring exogenous oxytocin administration to induce or stimulate labour. A Back-scratch test score < 4.1 cm was associated with a ~4 times greater increased odds ratio for having a caesarean section. The proposed cut-offs provide useful information for clinical settings that can be used to recommend a potential tailored prescription of flexibility training programs during pregnancy.

Within the GESTAFIT project, our group previously showed that maternal physical fitness is a key factor related to maternofoetal health and birth outcomes [8,9]. The present results support our previous findings and highlight the importance of implementing physical fitness testing as a complementary tool for the screening of healthy pregnancies. Therefore, considering that the Back-scratch test is efficient in terms of time and equipment, we propose its use as a powerful test to be implemented in routine clinical practice.

Since women who required oxytocin administration showed lower flexibility during the early second trimester of pregnancy, this physical fitness component might be key in preventing the need for this intervention. According to the Spanish Ministry of Health, Social Services, and Equality, the prevalence of the use of exogenous oxytocin during spontaneous labour in Spanish public hospitals is 53%, which is much higher than the recommended standards of 5–10% [20]. In the present study, 34% of women were provided with this hormone during labour, which represents almost four times the recommendations. Synthetic oxytocin is extensively employed as a method to induce labour [21,22] and a treatment for dystocia of uterine dynamics [22]. However, its use has been related to increased risk of uterine hyperactivity, alterations in the foetal heart rate, and postpartum haemorrhage [7]. In addition, other studies have associated the use of oxytocin with sucking problems and early cessation of breastfeeding [4], among other neonatal complications [6].

It was previously shown that maternal flexibility was associated with a lower incidence of caesarean sections [8], and modalities of exercise widely recommended during pregnancy that prioritize flexibility training, such as yoga, have been related to higher rates of vaginal births [12]. To note, caesarean sections are clearly associated with greater postpartum complications for the mother and new-born [1–3]. In our study sample, 25% of the births were caesarean sections, a much higher rate than the one recommended by the World Health Organization, which establishes that rates above 15% do not reduce maternal and neonatal morbidity and mortality [23]. It should also be taken into account that in Spanish private hospitals, the caesarean ratio is higher than in public hospitals, which we considered by including the place of birth as a potential confounder.

Several mechanisms might partially explain the role of flexibility in the type of delivery and the need for oxytocin administration. First, overall bodily flexibility levels may be related to the status of the connective tissue (i.e., ligaments) during pregnancy, which may present greater ligament laxity, which is necessary for the correct maintenance of pregnancy and labour progression. Second, pregnant women with greater flexibility might also present greater serum relaxin concentrations [23], which are also naturally increased during pregnancy [24]. Relaxin is a key hormone during pregnancy that also powerfully increases ligament laxity [25] and, consequently, body flexibility. Third, relaxin also provides vasodilator effects [26], which promote enhanced blood flow to the foetus and reduce potential alterations in foetal well-being. Moreover, since relaxin has endothelium-dependent vasodilation effects in the uterine artery [26], it seems feasible that the uteroplacental flow was more efficient during labour in women with greater relaxin concentrations—and probably also higher body flexibility. In this line, in a previous study [9], we found that greater maternal flexibility at the 16th gestational week was associated with a more alkaline pH, higher PO_2, higher arterial oxygen saturation, and lower PCO_2 in the arterial umbilical cord blood. Fourth, it seems that high levels of relaxin might also have a determinant role in the appearance of uterine contractions [27,28]. Finally, although more studies are needed to confirm this hypothesis, it is possible that women with better cardiometabolic status—which has been highly associated with the Back-scratch test scores in several populations [14,15]—showed greater cardiorespiratory fitness [29] and, therefore, experienced less fatigue during labour. Less fatigue promotes better uterine dynamic [30], and fatigue is also one of the main clinical reasons for providing this hormone during labour [23].

This study has several clinical implications to highlight. The high capacity of the Back-scratch test to establish the odds of the need for oxytocin administration and caesarean section, and the fact that it is a very accessible tool, reinforces that it should be included as a new complementary pregnancy screening tool. Particularly, the Back-scratch test has great potential in a clinical setting for the following reasons: (i) a measuring tape or a ruler is all the equipment needed to perform this test, so it is extremely cheap; (ii) the procedures for this test are simple and do not require any particular training; (iii) typically, physical fitness tests require larger spaces, while the Back-scratch test can be performed in any room without any special requirement; and (iv) this test is time-efficient, requiring just one minute, which is a fundamental issue for clinicians who are usually under time constraints.

As our intention is the prompt detection of these common obstetric risks, we encourage clinicians to assess this test around the 16th g.w. in order to initiate prevention strategies focused on flexibility early. From the GESTAFIT project team, we highly recommend those preventive interventions focused on physical exercise [8,9,31], as it exerts strong positive effects on birth-related outcomes such as the prevalence of caesarean sections, gestational age, length of labour stages, birth weight, Apgar test scores, and umbilical cord blood gases, among others [8,9,31]. We also recommend incorporating flexibility training in pregnant women below the cut-offs. Future studies are warranted to check the influence of specific flexibility programs (e.g., yoga, stretching) on women below the proposed cut-offs in order to explore their potential positive influences on birth outcomes through flexibility gains.

Some limitations must be highlighted. The study sample was relatively small, and we have missing data for different reasons, so studies with larger sample sizes are needed to establish more robust cut-off points. Moreover, because of the relatively small sample size, we could not further establish age-specific cut-off points (e.g., for women aged more or less than 30 years old).

This study also has several strengths to note. As far as we know, this is the first study establishing simple physical flexibility test cut-off points for the monitoring of pregnancies in clinical settings. Further, this test might also provide a powerful preventive tool for clinicians. Moreover, we confirmed the potential of the Back-scratch test after the adjustment for relevant potential confounders that could affect flexibility or the risk of caesarean section and complicated births, such as maternal age and weight, parity, birth place or the use of epidural analgesia.

5. Conclusions

Overall, women who needed oxytocin administration or suffered a caesarean section showed lower flexibility levels. The early identification of pregnant women who fail to meet the suggested standards in the Back-scratch test can assist in better pregnancy monitoring and might help to identify relevant birth-related complications easily, quickly, and cheaply and then initiate preventive strategies (for instance, focused on improving flexibility levels within their exercise program).

The Back-scratch test should be proposed as a discriminative tool for predicting the need for oxytocin administration during labour and the odds of caesarean section. A Back-scratch test score <3.6 cm was associated with a ~5 times greater increased odds ratio of requiring exogenous oxytocin administration to induce or stimulate labour. A Back-scratch test score <4.1 cm was associated with a ~4 times greater increased odds ratio of having a caesarean section. Therefore, optimal flexibility levels during pregnancy might prevent these labour-related complications.

Supplementary Materials: The following supporting information can be downloaded at https://www.mdpi.com/article/10.3390/jcm13175245/s1, Table S1: Study inclusion and exclusion criteria.

Author Contributions: Conceptualization, V.A.A. and L.B.-G.; methodology, V.A.A.; formal analysis, V.A.A. and L.B.-G.; investigation, V.A.A.; writing—original draft preparation, V.A.A.; writing—review and editing, N.M.-J., J.C.-P., M.F.-A., I.C.-R. and L.B.-G.; supervision, L.B.-G.; project administration, V.A.A.; funding acquisition, V.A.A. All authors have read and agreed to the published version of the manuscript.

Funding: This study was funded by the Regional Ministry of Health of the Junta de Andalucía (PI-0395-2016), the Research and Knowledge Transfer Fund (PPIT) 2016, Excellence Actions Programme: Scientific Units of Excellence (UCEES), and the Regional Ministry of Economy, Knowledge, Enterprises and University, European Regional Development Funds (SOMM17/6107/UGR) of the University of Granada. This study is included in the thesis of N.M.J., who is enrolled in the Doctoral Programme in Biomedicine at the University of Granada.

Institutional Review Board Statement: This study was conducted according to the guidelines of the Declaration of Helsinki and approved by the Ethics Committee on Clinical Research (CEIC) of Granada, Regional Government of Andalusia, Spain (protocol code: GESFIT-0448-N-15, 25 May 2015).

Informed Consent Statement: Informed consent was obtained from all subjects involved in this study.

Data Availability Statement: The data that support the findings of this study are available from the corresponding author, M.F.A., upon reasonable request.

Acknowledgments: We are grateful to the staff of the GESTAFIT project for recruiting participants and their teamwork in obtaining the assessments. We are also grateful for the cooperation and participation of all the pregnant women recruited in this study.

Conflicts of Interest: The authors declare no conflicts of interest.

References

1. Boutsikou, T.; Malamitsi-Puchner, A. Caesarean section: Impact on mother and child. *Acta Paediatr.* **2011**, *100*, 1518–1522. [CrossRef] [PubMed]
2. Oishi, A.; Tagashira, H.; Verho, A.; Holden, J.; Brimdyr, K.; Cadwell, K.; Widström, A.M.; Svensson, K.; Phillips, R. The effect of labor medications on normal newborn behavior in the first hour after birth: A prospective cohort study. *BMJ Open* **2019**, *132*, 30–36. [CrossRef]
3. Hobbs, A.J.; Mannion, C.A.; McDonald, S.W.; Brockway, M.; Tough, S.C. The impact of caesarean section on breastfeeding initiation, duration and difficulties in the first four months postpartum. *BMC Pregnancy Childbirth* **2016**, *16*, 90. [CrossRef]
4. Olza Fernández, I.; Marín Gabriel, M.; Malalana Martínez, A.; Fernández-Cañadas Morillo, A.; López Sánchez, F.; Costarelli, V. Newborn feeding behaviour depressed by intrapartum oxytocin: A pilot study. *Acta Paediatr.* **2012**, *101*, 749–754. [CrossRef] [PubMed]
5. Rousseau, A.; Burguet, A. Oxytocin administration during spontaneous labor: Guidelines for clinical practice. Chapter 5: Maternal risk and adverse effects of using oxytocin augmentation during spontaneous labor. *J. Gynecol. Obstet. Hum. Reprod.* **2017**, *46*, 509–521. [CrossRef]
6. Burguet, A.; Rousseau, A. Oxytocin administration during spontaneous labor: Guidelines for clinical practice. Chapter 6: Fetal, neonatal and pediatric risks and adverse effects of using oxytocin augmentation during spontaneous labor. *J. Gynecol. Obstet. Hum. Reprod.* **2017**, *46*, 523–530. [CrossRef]
7. Lothian, J.A. Healthy Birth Practice #4: Avoid Interventions Unless They Are Medically Necessary. *J. Perinat. Educ.* **2019**, *28*, 94–103. [CrossRef]
8. Baena-García, L.; Marín-Jiménez, N. Association of Self-Reported Physical Fitness during Late Pregnancy with Birth Outcomes and Oxytocin Administration during Labour-The GESTAFIT Project. *Int. J. Environ. Res. Public Health* **2021**, *18*, 8201. [CrossRef]
9. Baena-García, L.; Coll-Risco, I. Association of objectively measured physical fitness during pregnancy with maternal and neonatal outcomes. The GESTAFIT Project. *PLoS ONE* **2020**, *15*, e0229079. [CrossRef]
10. Kongkaew, C.; Lertsinthai, P.; Jampachaisri, K.; Mongkhon, P.; Meesomperm, P.; Kornkaew, K.; Malaiwong, P. The Effects of Thai Yoga on Physical Fitness: A Meta-Analysis of Randomized Control Trials. *J. Altern. Complement. Med.* **2018**, *24*, 541–551. [CrossRef]
11. Kawanishi, Y.; Hanley, S.J.; Tabata, K.; Nakagi, Y.; Ito, T.; Yoshioka, E.; Yoshida, T.; Saijo, Y. Effects of prenatal yoga: A systematic review of randomized controlled trials. *Jpn. J. Public Health* **2015**, *62*, 221–231. [CrossRef]
12. Jahdi, F.; Sheikhan, F.; Haghani, H.; Sharifi, B.; Ghaseminejad, A.; Khodarahmian, M.; Rouhana, N. Yoga during pregnancy: The effects on labor pain and delivery outcomes (A randomized controlled trial). *Complement. Ther. Clin. Pract.* **2017**, *27*, 1–4. [CrossRef]
13. Irving, G.; Neves, A.L.; Dambha-Miller, H. International variations in primary care physician consultation time: A systematic review of 67 countries. *BMJ Open* **2017**, *7*, e017902. [CrossRef] [PubMed]
14. Acosta-Manzano, P.; Segura-Jiménez, V.; Coll-Risco, I.; Borges-Cosic, M.; Castro-Piñero, J.; Delgado-Fernández, M.; Aparicio, V.A. Association of sedentary time and physical fitness with ideal cardiovascular health in perimenopausal women: The FLAMENCO project. *Maturitas* **2019**, *120*, 53–60. [CrossRef]
15. Chang, K.V.; Hung, C.Y.; Li, C.M.; Lin, Y.H.; Wang, T.G.; Tsai, K.S.; Han, D.S. Reduced flexibility associated with metabolic syndrome in community-dwelling elders. *PLoS ONE* **2015**, *10*, e0117167. [CrossRef]
16. Aparicio, V.A.; Segura-Jiménez, V.; Álvarez-Gallardo, I.C.; Soriano-Maldonado, A.; Castro-Piñero, J.; Delgado-Fernández, M.; Carbonell-Baeza, A. Fitness testing in the fibromyalgia diagnosis: The al-Ándalus project. *Med. Sci. Sports Exerc.* **2015**, *47*, 451–459. [CrossRef]

17. Aparicio, V.A.; Ocon, O.; Padilla-Vinuesa, C.; Soriano-Maldonado, A.; Romero-Gallardo, L.; Borges-Cosic, M.; Coll-Risco, I.; Ruiz-Cabello, P.; Acosta-Manzano, P.; Estevez-Lopez, F.; et al. Effects of supervised aerobic and strength training in overweight and grade I obese pregnant women on maternal and foetal health markers: The GESTAFIT randomized controlled trial. *BMC Pregnancy Childbirth* **2016**, *16*, 290. [CrossRef] [PubMed]
18. Rikli, R.E.; Jones, J. Development and validation of a functional fitness test for community residing older adults. *J. Aging Phys. Act.* **1999**, *7*, 129–161. [CrossRef]
19. Zweig, M.H.; Campbell, G. Receiver-operating characteristic (ROC) plots: A fundamental evaluation tool in clinical medicine. *Clin. Chem.* **1993**, *39*, 561–577. [CrossRef]
20. World Health Organization. WHO Statement on Cesarean Rate. Available online: http://www.paho.org/hq/index.php?option=com_content&view=article&id=10646:2015-la-cesarea-solo-deberia-realizarse-cuando-es-medicamente-necesaria&Itemid=1926&lang=es (accessed on 16 July 2024).
21. Ministry of Health and Social Policy and Equality. Strategy for Assistance at Normal Childbirth in the National Health System 2007. Available online: https://www.sanidad.gob.es/areas/calidadAsistencial/estrategias/atencionPartoNormal/docs/estrategiaPartoNormalEnglish.pdf (accessed on 30 July 2024).
22. Penfield, C.A.; Wing, D.A. Labor Induction Techniques: Which Is the Best? *Obstet. Gynecol. Clin. N. Am.* **2017**, *44*, 567–582. [CrossRef]
23. Dupont, C.; Carayol, M.; Le Ray, C.; Deneux-Tharaux, C.; Riethmuller, D. Oxytocin administration during spontaneous labor: Guidelines for clinical practice. Guidelines short text. *J. Gynecol. Obstet. Hum. Reprod.* **2017**, *46*, 539–543. [CrossRef] [PubMed]
24. Petersen, L.K.; Vogel, I.; Agger, A.O.; Westergård, J.; Nils, M.; Uldbjerg, N. Variations in serum relaxin (hRLX-2) concentrations during human pregnancy. *Acta Obstet. Gynecol. Scand.* **1995**, *74*, 251–256. [CrossRef] [PubMed]
25. Dehghan, F.; Haerian, B.S.; Muniandy, S.; Yusof, A.; Dragoo, J.L.; Salleh, N. The effect of relaxin on the musculoskeletal system. *Scand. J. Med. Sci. Sports* **2014**, *24*, e220–e229. [CrossRef] [PubMed]
26. Vodstrcil, L.A.; Tare, M.; Novak, J.; Dragomir, N.; Ramirez, R.J.; Wlodek, M.E.; Conrad, K.P.; Parry, L.J. Relaxin mediates uterine artery compliance during pregnancy and increases uterine blood flow. *FASEB J. Off. Publ. Fed. Am. Soc. Exp. Biol.* **2012**, *26*, 4035–4044. [CrossRef]
27. Pantelis, A.; Sotiriadis, A. Serum relaxin and cervical length for prediction of spontaneous preterm birth in second-trimester symptomatic women. *Ultrasound Obstet. Gynecol.* **2018**, *52*, 763–768. [CrossRef]
28. Pupula, M.; MacLennan, A.H. Effect of porcine relaxin on spontaneous, oxytocin-driven and prostaglandin-driven pig myometrial activity in vitro. *J. Reprod. Med.* **1989**, *34*, 819–823.
29. Lee, I.M.; Blair, S.N.; Tashiro, M.; Horikawa, C.; Matsubayashi, Y.; Yamada, T.; Fujihara, K.; Kato, K.; Sone, H.; Earnest, C.P.; et al. Maximal estimated cardiorespiratory fitness, cardiometabolic risk factors, and metabolic syndrome in the aerobics center longitudinal study. *Scand. J. Med. Sci. Sports* **2013**, *88*, 259–270. [CrossRef]
30. Ebrahimzadeh, S.; Golmakani, N.; Kabirian, M.; Shakeri, M.T. Study of correlation between maternal fatigue and uterine contraction pattern in the active phase of labour. *J. Clin. Nurs.* **2012**, *21*, 1563–1569. [CrossRef]
31. Baena-García, L.; Ocón-Hernández, O. Association of sedentary time and physical activity during pregnancy with maternal and neonatal birth outcomes. The GESTAFIT Project. *Menopause* **2019**, *29*, 407–414. [CrossRef]

Disclaimer/Publisher's Note: The statements, opinions and data contained in all publications are solely those of the individual author(s) and contributor(s) and not of MDPI and/or the editor(s). MDPI and/or the editor(s) disclaim responsibility for any injury to people or property resulting from any ideas, methods, instructions or products referred to in the content.

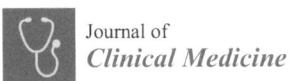

Journal of
Clinical Medicine

Review

Investigating Menstruation and Adverse Pregnancy Outcomes: Oxymoron or New Frontier? A Narrative Review

Kirstin Tindal [1,2,3,*], Fiona L. Cousins [1,2], Stacey J. Ellery [1,2], Kirsten R. Palmer [2,4], Adrienne Gordon [3,5], Caitlin E. Filby [2], Caroline E. Gargett [1,2], Beverley Vollenhoven [2,4] and Miranda L. Davies-Tuck [1,2,3]

1. The Ritchie Centre, Hudson Institute of Medical Research, Clayton, VIC 3168, Australia; caroline.gargett@monash.edu (C.E.G.); miranda.davies@hudson.org.au (M.L.D.-T.)
2. Department of Obstetrics and Gynaecology, Monash University, Clayton, VIC 3168, Australia; kirsten.palmer@monash.edu (K.R.P.); beverley.vollenhoven@monash.edu (B.V.)
3. NHMRC Centre for Research Excellence (CRE) in Stillbirth, Brisbane, QLD 4101, Australia; adrienne.gordon@sydney.edu.au
4. Women's and Newborn Program, Monash Health, Clayton, VIC 3168, Australia
5. Central Clinical School, Faculty of Medicine and Health, University of Sydney, Sydney, NSW 2006, Australia
* Correspondence: kirstin.street@monash.edu

Abstract: Not discounting the important foetal or placental contribution, the endometrium is a key determinant of pregnancy outcomes. Given the inherently linked processes of menstruation, pregnancy and parturition with the endometrium, further understanding of menstruation will help to elucidate the maternal contribution to pregnancy. Endometrial health can be assessed via menstrual history and menstrual fluid, a cyclically shed, easily and non-invasively accessible biological sample that represents the distinct, heterogeneous composition of the endometrial environment. Menstrual fluid has been applied to the study of endometriosis, unexplained infertility and early pregnancy loss; however, it is yet to be examined regarding adverse pregnancy outcomes. These adverse outcomes, including preeclampsia, foetal growth restriction (FGR), spontaneous preterm birth and perinatal death (stillbirth and neonatal death), lay on a spectrum of severity and are often attributed to placental dysfunction. The source of this placental dysfunction is largely unknown and may be due to underlying endometrial abnormalities or endometrial interactions during placentation. We present existing evidence for the endometrial contribution to adverse pregnancy outcomes and propose that a more comprehensive understanding of menstruation can provide insight into the endometrial environment, offering great potential value as a diagnostic tool to assess pregnancy risk. As yet, this concept has hardly been explored.

Keywords: menstruation; endometrium; pregnancy; menstrual fluid; adverse pregnancy outcomes; stillbirth; placenta

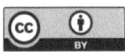

1. Introduction

The death of a baby before its life even begins is a devasting outcome of pregnancy. Globally, more than 4 million babies die in the perinatal period (as a stillbirth or neonatal death (NND)) every year [1,2]. In high-income countries, current approaches to reduce perinatal death focus predominantly on care at the end of pregnancy. While gains are being made in reducing late gestation stillbirth [3,4], 85% of perinatal deaths occur in the preterm period (<37 weeks' completed gestation), with the most common classified causes (excluding congenital anomalies) being spontaneous preterm birth (e.g., preterm premature rupture of membranes (pPROM); 11.5% stillbirths and 38% NND), foetal growth restriction (FGR; 9% stillbirths, where the baby fails to reach its growth potential), or unexplained antepartum deaths, with no cause found (14% stillbirths) [5]. Preeclampsia, a hypertensive disorder of pregnancy, is also a leading cause of maternal morbidity and mortality worldwide [6]. The underlying biological pathways that lead to this continuum of adverse pregnancy outcomes, including preeclampsia and FGR, spontaneous preterm birth and perinatal death, are not fully understood. Even though these outcomes manifest in different ways, 'placental insufficiency' is commonly attributed as the driver of adverse outcomes. The causes of poor placental function, however, remain largely unknown.

The evidence demonstrates that the endometrial environment into which the embryo implants is crucial in the establishment and progression of pregnancy, including placental development [7–10]. Defective decidualisation of the endometrium has been linked with recurrent pregnancy loss, spontaneous preterm birth and preeclampsia [11–14]. Abnormal menstruation, such as irregular periods or early onset of menarche, has also been associated with the development of preeclampsia and FGR [15] and preterm birth [16]. Despite these correlations, the role of the endometrium and menstruation in contributing to adverse pregnancy outcomes has been entirely understudied. The lack of research in this space to date may be attributed to the difficulty in performing non-invasive assessments of the endometrial environment. With the advent of menstrual fluid research, however, it is now possible to non-invasively collect and measure the components of menstrual fluid that reflect the endometrium around the time of embryo implantation [17–19], thus providing a window into this dynamic environment.

In this review, we reiterate that the endometrial environment into which the embryo implants is an integral component in establishing the trajectory of pregnancy. Abnormal placentation likely stems from impaired decidualisation and inflammation, leading to reduced endometrial receptivity and, therefore, aberrant implantation [20,21]. Just as these are thought to be factors leading to infertility and recurrent pregnancy loss, we emphasise that they can lead to a spectrum of adverse outcomes throughout pregnancy (Figure 1). We highlight several studies of placental insufficiency biomarkers detected in peripheral blood or placental tissues, which are not necessarily representative of the endometrial environment, making it difficult to draw inferences from these associations. We also provide detailed evidence from endometrial biopsy and in vitro studies, including differences in cellular and protein pathways and gene expression, demonstrating the contribution of the endometrium to adverse pregnancy outcomes.

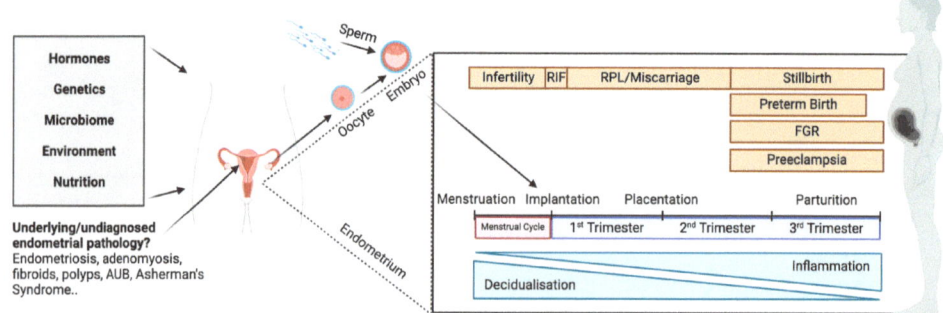

Figure 1. The potential contribution of factors that contribute to the resultant spectrum of adverse pregnancy outcomes. AUB: abnormal uterine bleeding; RIF: recurrent implantation failure; RPL: recurrent pregnancy loss; FGR: foetal growth restriction.

Studying menstruation and menstrual fluid has unrealised potential to better understand the origins of poor placental function. Specifically, there is the prospect for menstrual fluid biomarker screening to be used during preconception care or after adverse events have occurred to guide future pregnancy care. There is also an opportunity to inform the development or repurposing of therapeutics to target specific cellular pathways that underpin poor pregnancy outcomes. Whilst it might seem contradictory to use menstruation, a biological process that signals the very absence of pregnancy, to research obstetric complications and adverse pregnancy outcomes, it provides the perfect window into the endometrial environment of the uterus prior to implantation.

2. The Endometrial Environment

2.1. Endometrial Composition Changes over the Menstrual Cycle

The endometrium is a heterogeneous tissue comprising epithelial, stromal, stem/progenitor and immune cells. Throughout the menstrual cycle and during pregnancy, the composition of the endometrium changes dynamically in response to circulating ovarian hormones. During menstruation, the functional layer of endometrial tissue sheds, and the endometrial 'wound' begins to repair concurrently [22,23]. Following repair and under the influence of rising oestrogen levels during the proliferative phase, endometrial regeneration is likely mediated by stem/progenitor cells to regenerate the glands and vascularised stroma of the functional layer of the endometrium. Regeneration involves the endometrium more than doubling in thickness, growing up to 1 cm of mucosal tissue [23]. After ovulation, the secretory phase involves the differentiation of glandular epithelium into secretory cells that produce mucin-rich secretions for nourishing a future embryo; and stromal cells, which undergo distinct differentiation to become highly secretory epithelioid cells in preparation for embryo implantation. Endometrial glandular epithelium and stroma differentially express proteins throughout the varying phases of the menstrual cycle, and endometrial receptivity is influenced by a suite of molecules [24,25].

The proportion of immune cells in the endometrium also fluctuates dramatically throughout the phases of the menstrual cycle. Previous research shows that the proportion of CD45+ endometrial leukocytes doubles between the late proliferative and late secretory phases and represents up to 90% of all endometrial cells towards the end of the menstrual cycle [17,26]. Of note is the influx of uterine natural killer (uNK) cells, neutrophils and monocytes, which differentiate into macrophages, particularly in the decidualising endometrial stroma [27]. Throughout the menstrual cycle, uNK cells become the dominant immune cell population (>70%) to promote trophoblast invasion and spiral arteriole remodelling [28,29].

2.2. Endometrial Composition Changes during Pregnancy Establishment

The endometrial environment is fundamental for the establishment of pregnancy. After fertilisation and the journey down the oviduct to the uterine cavity, the blastocyst adheres to the endometrial luminal epithelium. This epithelium is crucial in mediating crosstalk between the implanting blastocyst and the endometrium [30,31]. Following implantation, the human embryo is completely enveloped within the endometrial lining by post-conception day 10 [32]. Extravillous trophoblastic cells (EVTs) rapidly proliferate and migrate into the decidua basalis. EVTs invade the underlying endometrial glands to anchor the conceptus to the uterine wall [31] and the spiral arterioles within the endometrium to remodel them into a low resistance, high flow system to allow for gas and nutrient exchange. The invasion and subsequent lining of the spiral arterioles by EVTs is crucial to the establishment of a well-functioning placenta. Paracrine signalling and histotroph secretions from the endometrial glands promote this process and provide nutrition to the conceptus until placentation is well established [33]. Whilst the placenta is critical to the maintenance of pregnancy, it is becoming clearer that the endometrial environment and maternal contribution have a huge influence on implantation and subsequent placentation to establish pregnancy.

3. The Origins of Adverse Pregnancy Outcomes

3.1. Parturition and Pregnancy Outcomes: Is Decidualisation the Determining Factor?

During the mid-secretory phase of each menstrual cycle, endometrial stromal cells commence a terminal morphological and functional differentiation termed decidualisation [34]. Elongated fibroblast-like cells transform into enlarged, round-shaped, highly secretory decidual cells, characterised by the release of insulin-like growth factor binding protein-1 (IGFBP-1) and prolactin (PRL) in preparation for pregnancy [35]. In response to elevated progesterone levels [36], decidualised stromal cells promote angiogenesis, activate matrix metalloproteinases (MMPs) and generate prostaglandins to facilitate trophoblast invasion and prevent immune rejection by recruiting uNK cells to the decidua [34].

Most non-menstruating eutherian mammals undergo decidualisation induced by the arrival of an implanting blastocyst; however, in humans, decidualisation occurs spontaneously [36,37]. The evolution of spontaneous decidualisation and menstruation is thought to coincide with invasive placentation, as decidual cells promote endometrial homeostasis during placentation [38,39]. Thus, in non-conception cycles, it is the terminally differentiated decidualised endometrium of the functionalis layer that is shed during menstruation in humans. The proliferative and differentiation capacity of decidual cells, which are a key determinant of menstrual health and pregnancy outcomes [14,40,41], can be assessed via endometrial and menstrual fluid samples in vitro [42].

There is abundant evidence that impaired decidualisation affects endometrial receptivity regarding early pregnancy loss and infertility [43], and this has also been proposed as a contributing factor to later adverse pregnancy outcomes [44]. Aberrations in the endometrial environment due to impaired decidualisation have been termed 'decidualisation resistance' [9] or maternal immune intolerance. Decidualisation resistance impacts trophoblast invasion, histotroph secretions and spiral artery remodelling, which can cause recurrent implantation failure, underlying infertility, or miscarriage [9,45,46]. Likely, decidual resistance is also involved in the pathogenesis of later pregnancy complications through several mechanisms [11,13,14,47,48], though the specific contribution of the endometrial environment to these adverse pregnancy outcomes remains largely unknown. Well-established hypotheses include decidual resistance impeding spiral arteriole remodelling, contributing to placental insufficiency in preeclampsia and FGR, and downstream effects on progesterone receptor expression leading to spontaneous preterm birth [11,14,48,49]. Most knowledge of endometrial associations with adverse pregnancy outcomes comes from circulating biomarkers present in peripheral blood [50–53] or retrospective analysis of placental tissue [54], and there is limited research using endometrial biospecimens themselves.

Many of the mediators involved in menstruation are also activated during labour, such as prostaglandins, pro-inflammatory cytokines and MMPs, which breakdown the endometrium for menstruation or degrade the extracellular matrix to weaken foetal membranes for rupture during labour [55–59]. While the exact mechanisms for initiating labour, both at term and preterm, are yet to be fully elucidated, it has been hypothesised that a 'decidual clock' is responsible for parturition, and as such, the decidua is vital in determining the onset of labour [60]. When decidual support is withdrawn, separation of the chorioamniotic membranes is initiated. Paracrine signalling by interleukins (IL) and prostaglandins between the endometrium and myometrium causes the switch between anti-inflammatory and pro-inflammatory states, which indicates the transition from a quiescent to a contractile phase. Cervical ripening in preparation for dilation is also mediated by changes in MMPs and inflammatory cytokines [61]. In the instance of spontaneous preterm birth, activation of inflammatory pathways likely signals a premature stimulation of the cascade of hormones responsible for parturition, though it remains unknown why this occurs (in cases that do not involve infection).

3.2. Evidence for the Endometrial Contribution to Adverse Pregnancy Outcomes

Later gestation pregnancy complications, including preeclampsia, FGR, spontaneous preterm birth and perinatal death, represent a continuum of adverse outcomes. These are often attributed to 'placental insufficiency' and share common pathways. Below, we provide detailed evidence of endometrial factors hypothesised to be involved in the development of adverse pregnancy outcomes. These factors are indicative of an altered endometrial environment and could be further explored by investigating menstrual health.

3.2.1. Preeclampsia

Preeclampsia is a progressive hypertensive disorder that worsens as pregnancy continues [62] and is estimated to affect approximately 5% of all pregnancies [63]. Preeclampsia is largely considered to be a placental disorder, and as such, most preeclampsia research has been conducted on the placenta itself [63]. It is believed to stem from shallow trophoblast invasion and inadequate spiral arteriole remodelling, which subsequently leads to narrow maternal vessels and vascular resistance, eventually resulting in placental insufficiency. The contribution of the endometrium to this process, however, has not been fully explored, but there is evidence to suggest that decidualisation plays a crucial role.

Decidualisation assays on cultured human endometrial stromal cells derived from endometrial biopsies have shown reduced decidualisation marker expression (PRL and IGFBP1) and a failure to decidualise in vitro in women with a history of preeclampsia [11]. These findings were replicated in sections of decidua basalis and parietalis collected at the time of delivery from women with preeclampsia and showed a functional reduction in cytotrophoblast invasion [11]. Further transcriptional analyses of both endometrial stromal cells and the decidua basalis in cases of preeclampsia have demonstrated over a hundred differentially expressed genes, demonstrating impaired decidualisation and revealing the maternal contribution to preeclampsia [48,64]. Another study analysing the gene expression of chorionic villous samples showed that the genes dysregulated in preeclamptic cases were of decidual origin [48] and showed concordance with nine genes identified in the previous study [11]. Both studies also demonstrated differential gene expression of maternal immune cells, NK and T-cell receptors [11,48].

Several inflammatory cytokines, secreted by endometrial macrophages, have also been implicated in the pathogenesis of preeclampsia. The overexpression of circulating IL-6, IL-8, IL-1β and tumour necrosis factor-alpha (TNF-α) in cases of preeclampsia maintain a chronic pro-inflammatory state [51]. There is evidence that the source of excess circulating interleukins is the decidua, not the placenta, in preeclamptic cases compared to gestational age-matched controls [65]. Overexpression of these factors may act through varying mechanisms; for example, TNF-α impacts the ability of uNK cells to regulate the level of trophoblast migration and invasion [66]. Overexpressed TNF-α can also promote increased oestrogen biosynthesis in endometrial glandular epithelial cells. This is associated with the development of endometrial disorders such as endometriosis [67], which has an increased risk of preeclampsia [68].

This highlights the crucial importance of considering the endometrium in cases of preeclampsia. Even though the placenta retains some endometrial epithelial cells [69], very little research has been conducted on the pre-placental origins of preeclampsia. Further research into endometrial biomarkers for preeclampsia may provide novel insights into the pathogenesis of preeclampsia.

3.2.2. Foetal Growth Restriction

FGR is defined as the inability of a foetus to reach its intrauterine growth and development potential due to placental compromise [70] and remains a leading cause of perinatal mortality worldwide. More than half of FGR cases remain idiopathic [71], as current clinical detection and diagnosis of FGR remains poor, with as many as four out of five growth-restricted babies remaining undetected in utero [72]. FGR is generally defined as a foetus weighing below the 10th percentile; however, not all foetuses that are small for gestational age have FGR. Incorrectly identified FGR can result in unnecessary harmful interventions, including iatrogenic preterm birth [73]. This can carry significant neonatal comorbidities such as cognitive deficits and cardiovascular disease later in life [74,75].

In the absence of genetic or structural defects in the foetus, placental insufficiency accounts for the majority of FGR cases [76]. A spectrum of placental pathologies contributes to uteroplacental insufficiency, ranging from impaired villous development to deficient vascular remodelling, resulting in inadequate nutrient transfer and foetal hypoxia [77]. There is emerging evidence that FGR and preeclampsia share common pathways, with a pro-inflammatory bias of increased levels of IL-6, IL-8 and TNF-α; however, FGR has been associated with decreased levels of the anti-inflammatory cytokine IL-10 in peripheral blood [53,78]. IL-10 suppresses natural killer-like cells at the uteroplacental interface, and cases of FGR demonstrate a reduced proportion of uNK cells in the decidua basalis compared to controls [79]. Interestingly, this association was significant with FGR, regardless of preeclampsia status; however, the reduction was not significant in isolated cases of preeclampsia without FGR [79]. The balanced composition of decidual leukocytes is crucial for the maintenance of pregnancy, and dysregulation of the decidua may be a prominent early event of pregnancy that affects the regulation of inflammation and spiral artery remodelling. It is unknown what causes this initial dysregulation and subsequent inflammatory responses in the endometrial environment and why this manifests differently in some cases of preeclampsia and FGR.

3.2.3. Spontaneous Preterm Birth

Spontaneous preterm birth remains one of the leading causes of perinatal mortality in high-income countries [5,80]. Some of the top risk factors for spontaneous preterm birth include prior preterm birth [81] and preeclampsia [82]. As many as two-thirds of preterm births may occur in the absence of any evident risk factors [83], and the underlying mechanisms leading to spontaneous preterm birth are largely unknown.

It has been previously proposed that the four following interrelated pathogenic mechanisms cause spontaneous preterm birth [84]:

1. Activation of the maternal or foetal hypothalamic-pituitary-adrenal (HPA) axis;
2. Decidual-chorioamniotic or systemic inflammation;
3. Decidual haemorrhage (abruption);
4. Pathological distention of the uterus [84].

Similar to the spectrum of adverse pregnancy outcomes, it is likely that the origins and severity of spontaneous preterm births also lay on a continuum dependent on the initial endometrial environment and may stem from underlying endometrial abnormalities. This hypothesis is supported in a review by Ng et al. [9], which postulates that these processes are interrelated, as evidenced by overlapping biomarkers and risk factors for other adverse pregnancy outcomes with preterm birth (Figure 1).

Many of the molecular mechanisms implicated in the pathogenesis of preeclampsia and FGR discussed above are also dysregulated in cases of spontaneous preterm birth, and identifying biomarkers for spontaneous preterm birth remains challenging. A cross-sectional study of urine and plasma collected from women who experienced spontaneous preterm birth demonstrated that TNF-α, IL-6, IL-10 and IL-1β were all positively associated with an increased risk for spontaneous preterm birth; however, only IL-10 was found to be statistically significant [50]. IL-10 is specifically elevated among cases of preterm birth with aberrant placentation [85,86]. Whilst of interest, it is unlikely that plasma and urine samples are exclusively representative of the endometrial environment, and as highlighted above, the source of these circulating factors and whether differential expression of these mediators is implicated in endometrial cells requires further investigation.

This could be achieved with a focus on studying menstrual fluid composition in women with pregnancies previously impacted by spontaneous preterm labour. For instance, the expression of MMP-1 and MMP-9 is higher in the placental tissue of preterm [54] compared with term births. The very nature of placental investigations, however, is retrospective, and it can be difficult to separate the foetal and maternal contributions. These factors can be detected in endometrial tissue derived from menstrual fluid, and MMP-1 has been shown to be significantly upregulated in the menstrual fluid of infertility cases [87]. Further research comparing placental tissue with endometrial tissues would determine whether these factors can be used as biomarkers in preconception care to predict an increased risk for spontaneous preterm birth.

3.2.4. Perinatal Death

Perinatal death can occur as a result of the aforementioned pregnancy complications. Regardless of the gestation or cause, perinatal death is a traumatic experience that has a profound impact on all of those affected. Due to the logistical considerations of obtaining endometrial samples from women impacted by pregnancy and infant loss, there has been very little research into the exact endometrial contribution. However, both uterine maturity [88–91] and decidualisation capacity [92] have been implicated in pregnancy loss, highlighting the importance of exploring this concept further.

As progesterone is essential to maintaining the menstrual cycle, there is a theory that cyclic menstruation 'preconditions' the uterus for pregnancy by protecting the uterus from inflammatory and oxidative stress associated with placentation [88]. This may explain why adolescent pregnancies (<20 years old) have a higher risk of perinatal death and adverse pregnancy outcomes [89,90]. This has often been attributed to socioeconomic disadvantage and insufficient reproductive education associated with teenage pregnancy [91]. Uterine immaturity due to progesterone resistance, however, has also been indicated as a potential underlying factor that impacts endocrine pathways and decidualisation capacity [92]. This is evident when we consider that neonates have inactive endometrium, and females transition to a state of cyclic ovarian oestrogen and progesterone production, followed by progesterone responsiveness during puberty. This then triggers the onset of regular menstruation and decidual gene expression [92]. Inadequate vascular remodelling in adolescent pregnancies may be a result of incomplete cyclic programming of uNK cells. The higher rate of stillbirth among adolescent pregnancies may be an indication of insufficient menstrual cycles to precondition the uterus for adaptation to pregnancy [88]. This highlights the significance of the functional decidua for both a healthy menstrual cycle and pregnancy.

Conversely, advanced maternal age (>35 years old) is also a risk factor for perinatal deaths [93]. This is often attributed to declining oocyte quality and increased rates of embryonic chromosomal abnormalities. Emerging evidence from preclinical models, however, indicates that most pregnancies with later adverse outcomes occur in the absence of a chromosomal abnormality, indicating a role for the uterine environment [94]. Age-related inflammation occurs in the endometrium [95], and it has been demonstrated in mice models that advanced maternal age interferes with the progesterone response of stromal cells, resulting in a reduced capacity to decidualise [94]. This has downstream implications for placental establishment and function, which has been shown to gradually decrease in a maternal age-dependent manner via reduced concentration of pro-inflammatory cytokines IL-1β and TNF-α [96]. Placentas from advanced-aged mothers also weigh significantly more even though there is an increased incidence of FGR [96,97], which may be indicative of a response to compensate for poor placental function. This evidence emphasises the complexity of elucidating the molecular mechanisms underpinning pregnancy complications but reiterates that a healthy endometrium is key to maintaining pregnancy.

4. Is Menstrual Assessment the New Frontier in Understanding the Endometrial Contribution to Adverse Pregnancy Outcomes?

The complexities of menstruation, conception, decidualisation, implantation, placentation and parturition are inevitably difficult to replicate and study in vivo in humans. As detailed in the previous sections, understanding of these processes and the errors that occur in these pathways have largely come from animal models, placental examinations and in vitro studies using tissue from endometrial biopsies. Given the copious molecular mechanisms that are spatiotemporally regulated during implantation and placentation, retrospective placental examination is inadequate to gain the critical insights required to understand the aetiology of these adverse pregnancy outcomes. Many of these approaches are also time-consuming and invasive, and sample sizes for studies are often small due to difficulty recruiting relevant populations to prospective clinical studies. The potential to uncover the endometrium's contribution to adverse pregnancy outcomes via menstrual history taking, clinical assessments and biological evaluation of menstrual fluid can overcome these challenges, paving the way to drive this important research field forward.

4.1. The Potential for Investigating Menstrual Characteristics Associated with Adverse Pregnancy Outcomes

Menstrual characteristics, including age at menarche, cycle length, period regularity, length and heaviness, period pain and associated menstrual symptoms, are all indications of menstrual health.

There is some evidence for the association between certain menstrual characteristics and adverse pregnancy outcomes. Early studies in the 1980s indicated that there may be a higher risk of miscarriage [98], spontaneous abortion [99] and ectopic pregnancy [100] in women who experience early menarche, traditionally defined as the onset of menstruation before 12 years old. Early menarche has since been associated with a higher risk of preeclampsia [101–104], preterm birth [16] and the likelihood of a low birth weight baby [102]. Interestingly, self-reported heavy or irregular periods prior to a second or subsequent birth in multiparous women were also associated with an increased risk of preterm birth in the subsequent pregnancy, demonstrating that new menstrual symptoms may arise after pregnancy [105]. There is also evidence of an increased risk for preterm birth when there is prolonged menstruation before conception [106], likely due to an extended proliferative phase. This implies that pregnancy, where implantation occurs outside of the critical fertile window, may still progress but have consequences that manifest later in pregnancy. Despite this, most antenatal assessments only obtain clinical information about the date of the last menstrual period to determine an estimated birth due date, with no consideration of previous menstrual health. This could be a critically missed opportunity to gather more information about the endometrial environment.

Abnormal menstruation and adverse pregnancy outcomes may have common causes that effect the endometrium. For example, both increased and decreased body mass index (BMI) is known to impact the menstrual cycle and is often attributed to hormonal factors. Increased BMI is associated with heavy menstrual bleeding and increased risk of premenstrual disorders [107], whereas decreased BMI is associated with irregular menstruation or amenorrhea (the absence of menstruation), and both report painful periods more frequently than those with an average BMI [108]. Maternal pre-pregnancy BMI also increases the risk of preeclampsia [101,109]. This is thought to be caused by influencing the length of the menstrual cycle, and thus, differential expression of endometrial receptors throughout the menstrual cycle may result in inadequate trophoblast invasion and subsequent placental insufficiency [101,109]. Rather than implicating a direct cause-and-effect model, we emphasise that the association between menstrual characteristics and pregnancy outcomes can be used as a proxy measure of endometrial health to warrant further investigation.

4.2. The Potential for Analysing Menstrual Fluid Regarding Adverse Pregnancy Outcomes

Menstrual fluid can be collected non-invasively and used to assess the composition of the endometrial environment (reviewed in [110]). Menstrual fluid demonstrates a reproducible profile with minimal variation between menstrual cycles, indicating that it is an appropriate biospecimen representative of an individual's endometrial environment [17]. Whilst menstrual fluid has recently been adopted to study endometriosis [18,19,111–118] and unexplained infertility [45,98,99,119], there is no evidence of its use in investigating adverse pregnancy outcomes. We are currently conducting a case–control study, where participants who have experienced adverse pregnancy outcomes in the second and third trimesters donate menstrual fluid samples for molecular analyses [100]. In this study, women who have experienced a preterm stillbirth or livebirth (20–36 + 6 weeks' gestation), FGR (birth weight <3rd centile by population charts [101]) or second-trimester miscarriage in the past 3 years (cases) and those who have not (healthy term birth matched for maternal age, BMI and gravidity) (controls) are being recruited [100]. Differences in cellular and immune cell composition, secreted proteins and menstrual cycle characteristics are being compared [100]. The potential for this research is just emerging, and modern techniques, such as endometrial organoids derived from menstrual fluid, provide a particularly exciting opportunity to understand the endometrial contribution to adverse pregnancy outcomes better than ever through in vitro experimentation [19,102]. Placental organoids can also be co-cultured with paired endometrial samples to elucidate these mechanisms further.

4.3. Limitations and Opportunities for Assessing the Associations between Menstruation and Pregnancy Outcomes

We acknowledge the limitations that are inherent in a narrative review; however, this methodology was appropriate given the sparse current evidence connecting menstruation and pregnancy outcomes. The aim of this review was to collate evidence for the endometrial contribution to adverse pregnancy outcomes, understand the landscape of menstrual associations with pregnancy outcomes, and provide a novel hypothesis as further rationale to address this as a research question.

Menstruation is a unique biological process, observed in only 1.6% of all eutherian species [103], making it difficult to study in preclinical settings. Even though approximately half of the human population menstruate throughout their reproductive life, menstruation remains a taboo topic in public discourse. Menstrual fluid has been referred to as 'one of nature's most stigmatized fluids' [104]. For example, it was not until 2023 that real blood was used to measure the absorbability of menstrual sanitary products to assess heavy menstrual bleeding [109]. Menstrual blood, or menstrual fluid, itself has still never been utilised for this purpose.

There are many advantages to using menstrual fluid samples for research, including ease and non-invasiveness of collection and the fact that it is readily obtainable from reproductive-aged women. Up to 80% of women are willing to donate menstrual fluid for medical research [105,106], indicating that it is a feasible collection method. When surveyed about their perspectives on donating menstrual fluid, some women had hygiene concerns, but most responded positively. Reasons to donate menstrual fluid included current use of a menstrual cup, which is environmentally friendly, and it being an empowering, easy and "excellent use of a waste product" [105]. If advertised correctly and sensitively, such research may also give women a sense of purpose for their menses, with one woman stating, "If I felt I could help in any way to improve the lives of others in such a simple way it can only be a good thing" [105].

Sampling shed endometrium using menstrual fluid mitigates the risk of cycle bias, which is often not accounted for with endometrial biopsies. Due to the cyclical nature of menstruation, though, menstrual fluid may not accurately reflect the endometrium during earlier phases of the menstrual cycle and should be considered in the context of the late-secretory phase. For example, drawing inferences from immune cell proportions at one time-point may not be indicative of an abnormality throughout the menstrual cycle or pregnancy. Findings may still require comparison with endometrial tissue during other menstrual cycle phases or gestational-age-matched placental tissue samples to investigate if this phenotype persists.

Gathering a menstrual history over time and in the preconception phase provides valuable insight into endometrial health and potential future pregnancies. While concerns of recall bias have been expressed when taking menstrual histories, most women recall their menstrual history accurately [120], and for those who do not, the ever-changing nature of menstruation throughout reproductive life may be the reason. With the emergence of modern period-tracking apps and enhanced reproductive education, menstrual tracking is simple, valid and easier than ever.

Pregnancy loss and infertility also remain highly stigmatised topics [121,122]. Collecting menstrual fluid samples from women who have experienced traumatic pregnancy outcomes may make participating in such studies emotionally challenging and should be treated sensitively [123]. There is an underwhelming amount of research connecting these two areas, and the associated taboos have engrained social and systemic barriers to conducting such research. For such research to prevail, successful participant recruitment relies on addressing the taboos that underlie these barriers.

As highlighted in Figure 1, numerous other factors contribute to establishing and progressing pregnancy. Various confounders include nutrition, the environment, maternal and paternal conditions and anomalies of the foetus itself. We also acknowledge that with advancements in assisted reproductive technologies, menstruation is not necessitated to achieve pregnancy. Women who are postmenopausal or do not menstruate following a uterine transplant can now become pregnant. We emphasise here, though, that the endometrial contribution to pregnancy success has been underestimated and under-researched to date and that a better understanding of menstruation can aid further progress.

4.4. Elucidating the Endometrial Environment via Menstrual Assessment: What's Next?

For this research to progress, several things must be addressed. Firstly, standardised definitions for what constitutes 'abnormal' menstruation should be updated and implemented. A classification system for symptoms and causes of abnormal uterine bleeding was established in 2011 and revised in 2018 [124]; however, it is still not routinely used in clinical practice. It is essential that we can delineate between idiopathic abnormal menstruation and endometrial pathologies. Abnormal menstruation may be more prevalent than previously realised, and updated criteria will aid pathways for those that warrant further investigation regarding potential pregnancy outcomes. Large datasets from period-tracking apps may challenge current definitions of abnormal menstruation and reveal which menstrual characteristics are most helpful for assessing pregnancy risk.

If the menstrual fluid is to be pursued as a legitimate sample for biochemical analyses, further characterisation of menstrual fluid composition and normal parameters should also be determined. For this to occur, a standardised protocol for the optimal collection, processing, storage and experimentation of menstrual fluid must be established. In our recent review of menstrual fluid, we detail how this can be achieved [110].

Furthermore, during this review, we identified crucial knowledge gaps regarding the endometrial contribution to adverse pregnancy outcomes. A recent systematic review revealed that of 74 endometrial transcriptome studies, all were conducted regarding menstrual cycle differences, endometrial and fertility-related pathologies and response to hormone treatment [125]. None of these studies investigated adverse pregnancy outcomes. We emphasise the need for further scientific discovery, particularly investigating genetic and epigenetic differences in endometrial tissue related to adverse pregnancy outcomes, to explicate upstream mechanisms of observations at the functional level.

5. Conclusions

Menstrual health and women's health are finally being drawn into focus, and now is the time for advanced investigations into the links between menstruation, the endometrium and pregnancy [126]. As detailed here, there is increasing data regarding the endometrial contribution to adverse pregnancy outcomes; however, most evidence is derived from invasive endometrial biopsies, peripheral blood biomarkers, preclinical models, or retrospective placental examinations. We and others hypothesise that understanding menstrual history and menstrual fluid collection is a non-invasive and novel approach for better understanding the endometrial environment regarding adverse pregnancy outcomes [9,38,103,127]; however, this call to action has not yet been answered. Exploring this avenue of research will lead to identifying completely new and undiscovered drivers of poor placentation, unravelling the potential for preconception biomarkers and therapies to mitigate some of the greatest causes of death, disability and heartbreak that is seen in obstetrics, including preeclampsia, FGR, preterm birth and perinatal death.

Author Contributions: Conceptualisation, K.T., M.L.D.-T., C.E.G., F.L.C. and C.E.F.; methodology, K.T.; investigation, K.T.; resources, K.T.; data curation, K.T.; writing—original draft preparation, K.T.; writing—review and editing, K.T., F.L.C., S.J.E.; K.R.P., A.G., C.E.G., C.E.F., B.V. and M.L.D.-T.; visualisation, K.T.; supervision, M.L.D.-T., C.E.G., F.L.C. and C.E.F.; project administration, K.T., M.L.D.-T., C.E.G., F.L.C. and C.E.F.; funding acquisition, M.L.D.-T., C.E.G., F.L.C. and C.E.F.; All authors have read and agreed to the published version of the manuscript.

Funding: This research was funded by Stillbirth Foundation Australia. K.T. receives support through an Australian Government Research Training Program (RTP) Scholarship and the Stillbirth Centre of Research Excellence (CRE). K.R.P. and C.E.G. are supported by the National Health and Medical Research Council (NHMRC, Australia) Investigator Grants (2009765 and 1173882, respectively). M.D.T. is supported by an NHMRC Ideas Grant (2023288).

Institutional Review Board Statement: Not applicable.

Conflicts of Interest: The authors declare no conflicts of interest.

References

1. UNICEF; WHO; World Bank Group; United Nations. *A Neglected Tragedy: The Global Burden of Stillbirths*; The United Nations Inter-Agency Group for Child Mortality Estimation: New York, NY, USA, 2020; Available online: https://www.unicef.org/reports/neglected-tragedy-global-burden-of-stillbirths-2020 (accessed on 8 April 2024).
2. UNICEF. Neonatal Deaths. 2024. Available online: https://data.unicef.org/topic/child-survival/neonatal-mortality/ (accessed on 8 April 2024).
3. Flenady, V.; Ellwood, D. Making real progress with stillbirth prevention. *Aust. N. Z. J. Obstet. Gynaecol.* **2020**, *60*, 495–497. [CrossRef] [PubMed]
4. Australian Institute of Health and Welfare (AIHW). Australia's Mothers and Babies. 2023. Available online: https://www.aihw.gov.au/reports/mothers-babies/stillbirths-and-neonatal-deaths (accessed on 8 April 2024).
5. Tindal, K.; Bimal, G.; Flenady, V.; Gordon, A.; Farrell, T.; Davies-Tuck, M. Causes of perinatal deaths in Australia: Slow progress in the preterm period. *Aust. N. Z. J. Obstet. Gynaecol.* **2022**, *62*, 511–517. [CrossRef]
6. Rana, S.; Lemoine, E.; Granger, J.P.; Karumanchi, S.A. Preeclampsia. *Circ. Res.* **2019**, *124*, 1094–1112. [CrossRef]
7. Su, R.-W.; Fazleabas, A.T. Implantation and Establishment of Pregnancy in Human and Nonhuman Primates. In *Regulation of Implantation and Establishment of Pregnancy in Mammals: Tribute to 45 Year Anniversary of Roger V. Short's "Maternal Recognition of Pregnancy"*; Geisert, R.D., Bazer, F.W., Eds.; Springer International Publishing: Cham, Switzerland, 2015; pp. 189–213.
8. Cha, J.; Sun, X.; Dey, S.K. Mechanisms of implantation: Strategies for successful pregnancy. *Nat. Med.* **2012**, *18*, 1754–1767. [CrossRef] [PubMed]
9. Ng, S.-W.; Norwitz, G.A.; Pavlicev, M.; Tilburgs, T.; Simón, C.; Norwitz, E.R. Endometrial Decidualization: The Primary Driver of Pregnancy Health. *Int. J. Mol. Sci.* **2020**, *21*, 4092. [CrossRef]
10. Burton, G.J.; Jauniaux, E.; Charnock-Jones, D.S. Human early placental development: Potential roles of the endometrial glands. *Placenta* **2007**, *28* (Suppl. A), S64–S69. [CrossRef]
11. Garrido-Gomez, T.; Dominguez, F.; Quiñonero, A.; Diaz-Gimeno, P.; Kapidzic, M.; Gormley, M.; Ona, K.; Padilla-Iserte, P.; McMaster, M.; Genbacev, O.; et al. Defective decidualization during and after severe preeclampsia reveals a possible maternal contribution to the etiology. *Proc. Natl. Acad. Sci. USA* **2017**, *114*, E8468–E8477. [CrossRef] [PubMed]
12. Lucas, E.S.; Dyer, N.P.; Murakami, K.; Lee, Y.H.; Chan, Y.-W.; Grimaldi, G.; Muter, J.; Brighton, P.J.; Moore, J.D.; Patel, G.; et al. Loss of Endometrial Plasticity in Recurrent Pregnancy Loss. *Stem Cells* **2016**, *34*, 346–356. [CrossRef]
13. Romero, R.; Dey, S.K.; Fisher, S.J. Preterm labor: One syndrome, many causes. *Science* **2014**, *345*, 760–765. [CrossRef]
14. Schatz, F.; Guzeloglu-Kayisli, O.; Arlier, S.; Kayisli, U.A.; Lockwood, C.J. The role of decidual cells in uterine hemostasis, menstruation, inflammation, adverse pregnancy outcomes and abnormal uterine bleeding. *Hum. Reprod. Update* **2016**, *22*, 497–515. [CrossRef]
15. Bonnesen, B.; Oddgeirsdóttir, H.L.; Naver, K.V.; Jørgensen, F.S.; Nilas, L. Women with minor menstrual irregularities have increased risk of preeclampsia and low birthweight in spontaneous pregnancies. *Acta Obstet. Gynecol. Scand.* **2016**, *95*, 88–92. [CrossRef] [PubMed]
16. Li, H.; Song, L.; Shen, L.; Liu, B.; Zheng, X.; Zhang, L.; Li, Y.; Xia, W.; Lu, B.; Zhang, B.; et al. Age at menarche and prevalence of preterm birth: Results from the Healthy Baby Cohort study. *Sci. Rep.* **2017**, *7*, 12594. [CrossRef] [PubMed]
17. Wyatt, K.A.; Filby, C.E.; Davies-Tuck, M.L.; Suke, S.G.; Evans, J.; Gargett, C.E. Menstrual fluid endometrial stem/progenitor cell and supernatant protein content: Cyclical variation and indicative range. *Hum. Reprod.* **2021**, *36*, 2215–2229. [CrossRef] [PubMed]
18. Masuda, H.; Schwab, K.E.; Filby, C.E.; Tan, C.S.C.; Tsaltas, J.; Weston, G.C.; Gargett, C.E. Endometrial stem/progenitor cells in menstrual blood and peritoneal fluid of women with and without endometriosis. *Reprod. Biomed. Online* **2021**, *43*, 3–13. [CrossRef] [PubMed]
19. Filby, C.E.; Wyatt, K.A.; Mortlock, S.; Cousins, F.L.; McKinnon, B.; Tyson, K.E.; Montgomery, G.W.; Gargett, C.E. Comparison of Organoids from Menstrual Fluid and Hormone-Treated Endometrium: Novel Tools for Gynecological Research. *J. Pers. Med.* **2021**, *11*, 1314. [CrossRef] [PubMed]
20. Norwitz, E.R. Defective implantation and placentation: Laying the blueprint for pregnancy complications. *Reprod. Biomed. Online* **2007**, *14*, 101–109. [CrossRef] [PubMed]
21. Tong, J.; Lv, S.; Yang, J.; Li, H.; Li, W.; Zhang, C. Decidualization and Related Pregnancy Complications. *Matern. Fetal Med.* **2022**, *4*, 24–35. [CrossRef]
22. Cousins, F.L.; Filby, C.E.; Gargett, C.E. Endometrial Stem/Progenitor Cells-Their Role in Endometrial Repair and Regeneration. *Front. Reprod. Health* **2021**, *3*, 811537. [CrossRef] [PubMed]

23. Salamonsen, L.A.; Hutchison, J.C.; Gargett, C.E. Cyclical endometrial repair and regeneration. *Development* **2021**, *148*, 199577. [CrossRef]
24. Desouza, L.; Diehl, G.; Yang, E.C.C.; Guo, J.; Rodrigues, M.J.; Romaschin, A.D.; Colgan, T.J.; Siu, K.W.M. Proteomic analysis of the proliferative and secretory phases of the human endometrium: Protein identification and differential protein expression. *Proteomics* **2005**, *5*, 270–281. [CrossRef]
25. Hood, B.L.; Liu, B.; Alkhas, A.; Shoji, Y.; Challa, R.; Wang, G.; Ferguson, S.; Oliver, J.; Mitchell, D.; Bateman, N.W.; et al. Proteomics of the Human Endometrial Glandular Epithelium and Stroma from the Proliferative and Secretory Phases of the Menstrual Cycle1. *Biol. Reprod.* **2015**, *92*, 106. [CrossRef] [PubMed]
26. Flynn, L.; Byrne, B.; Carton, J.; O'Farrelly, C.; Kelehan, P.; O'Herlihy, C. Menstrual Cycle Dependent Fluctuations in NK and T-Lymphocyte Subsets from Non-Pregnant Human Endometrium. *Am. J. Reprod. Immunol.* **2000**, *43*, 209–217. [CrossRef] [PubMed]
27. Yang, F.; Zheng, Q.; Jin, L. Dynamic Function and Composition Changes of Immune Cells During Normal and Pathological Pregnancy at the Maternal-Fetal Interface. *Front. Immunol.* **2019**, *10*, 2317. [CrossRef] [PubMed]
28. Radović Janošević, D.; Trandafilović, M.; Krtinić, D.; Čolović, H.; Stevanović, J.M.; Dinić, S.P.-T. Endometrial immunocompetent cells in proliferative and secretory phase of normal menstrual cycle. *Folia Morphol.* **2020**, *79*, 296–302. [CrossRef] [PubMed]
29. Hanna, J.; Goldman-Wohl, D.; Hamani, Y.; Avraham, I.; Greenfield, C.; Natanson-Yaron, S.; Prus, D.; Cohen-Daniel, L.; Arnon, T.I.; Manaster, I.; et al. Decidual NK cells regulate key developmental processes at the human fetal-maternal interface. *Nat. Med.* **2006**, *12*, 1065–1074. [CrossRef] [PubMed]
30. Denker, H.-W. Cell Biology of Endometrial Receptivity and of Trophoblast-Endometrial Interactions. In *Endocrinology of Embryo-Endometrium Interactions*; Glasser, S.R., Mulholland, J., Psychoyos, A., Eds.; Springer: Boston, MA, USA, 1994; pp. 17–32.
31. Enders, A.C. Trophoblast-Uterine Interactions in the First Days of Implantation: Models for the Study of Implantation Events in the Human. *Semin. Reprod. Med.* **2000**, *18*, 255–264. [CrossRef] [PubMed]
32. Garrido-Gómez, T.; Castillo-Marco, N.; Cordero, T.; Simón, C. Decidualization resistance in the origin of preeclampsia. *Am. J. Obstet. Gynecol.* **2022**, *226*, S886–S894. [CrossRef] [PubMed]
33. Burton, G.J.; Watson, A.L.; Hempstock, J.; Skepper, J.N.; Jauniaux, E. Uterine Glands Provide Histiotrophic Nutrition for the Human Fetus during the First Trimester of Pregnancy. *J. Clin. Endocrinol. Metab.* **2002**, *87*, 2954–2959. [CrossRef] [PubMed]
34. Okada, H.; Tsuzuki, T.; Murata, H. Decidualization of the human endometrium. *Reprod. Med. Biol.* **2018**, *17*, 220–227. [CrossRef]
35. Dunn, C.L.; Kelly, R.W.; Critchley, H.O.D. Decidualization of the human endometrial stromal cell: An enigmatic transformation. *Reprod. Biomed. Online* **2003**, *7*, 151–161. [CrossRef]
36. Diessler, M.E.; Hernández, R.; Castro, G.G.; Barbeito, C.G. Decidual cells and decidualization in the carnivoran endotheliochorial placenta. *Front. Cell Dev. Biol.* **2023**, *11*, 1134874. [CrossRef] [PubMed]
37. Wagner, G.; Kin, K.; Muglia, L.; Pavličev, M. Evolution of mammalian pregnancy and the origin of the decidual stromal cell. *Int. J. Dev. Biol.* **2014**, *58*, 117–126. [CrossRef] [PubMed]
38. Pavlicev, M.; Norwitz, E.R. Human Parturition: Nothing More Than a Delayed Menstruation. *Reprod. Sci.* **2018**, *25*, 166–173. [CrossRef] [PubMed]
39. Emera, D.; Romero, R.; Wagner, G. The evolution of menstruation: A new model for genetic assimilation. *Bioessays* **2012**, *34*, 26–35. [CrossRef] [PubMed]
40. Salker, M.; Teklenburg, G.; Molokhia, M.; Lavery, S.; Trew, G.; Aojanepong, T.; Mardon, H.J.; Lokugamage, A.U.; Rai, R.; Landles, C.; et al. Natural selection of human embryos: Impaired decidualization of endometrium disables embryo-maternal interactions and causes recurrent pregnancy loss. *PLoS ONE* **2010**, *5*, e10287. [CrossRef] [PubMed]
41. Rawlings, T.M.; Makwana, K.; Taylor, D.M.; Molè, M.A.; Fishwick, K.J.; Tryfonos, M.; Odendaal, J.; Hawkes, A.; Zernicka-Goetz, M.; Hartshorne, G.M.; et al. Modelling the impact of decidual senescence on embryo implantation in human endometrial assembloids. *elife* **2021**, *10*, 69603. [CrossRef]
42. Domnina, A.P.; Novikova, P.V.; Fridlyanskaya, I.I.; Shilina, M.A.; Zenin, V.V.; Nikolsky, N.N. Induction of decidual differentiation in endometrial mesenchymal stem cells. *Cell Tissue Biol.* **2016**, *10*, 95–99. [CrossRef]
43. Teklenburg, G.; Salker, M.; Heijnen, C.; Macklon, N.S.; Brosens, J.J. The molecular basis of recurrent pregnancy loss: Impaired natural embryo selection. *Mol. Hum. Reprod.* **2010**, *16*, 886–895. [CrossRef]
44. Dunk, C.; Kwan, M.; Hazan, A.; Walker, S.; Wright, J.K.; Harris, L.K.; Jones, R.L.; Keating, S.; Kingdom, J.C.P.; Whittle, W.; et al. Failure of Decidualization and Maternal Immune Tolerance Underlies Uterovascular Resistance in Intra Uterine Growth Restriction. *Front. Endocrinol.* **2019**, *10*, 160. [CrossRef]
45. Hosseini, S.; Shokri, F.; Pour, S.A.; Khoshnoodi, J.; Jeddi-Tehrani, M.; Zarnani, A.-H. Diminished Frequency of Menstrual and Peripheral Blood NKT-Like Cells in Patients With Unexplained Recurrent Spontaneous Abortion and Infertile Women. *Reprod. Sci.* **2019**, *26*, 97–108. [CrossRef]
46. Teklenburg, G.; Salker, M.; Molokhia, M.; Lavery, S.; Trew, G.; Aojanepong, T.; Mardon, H.J.; Lokugamage, A.U.; Rai, R.; Landles, C.; et al. Natural selection of human embryos: Decidualizing endometrial stromal cells serve as sensors of embryo quality upon implantation. *PLoS ONE* **2010**, *5*, e10258. [CrossRef] [PubMed]
47. Gellersen, B.; Brosens, J.J. Cyclic Decidualization of the Human Endometrium in Reproductive Health and Failure. *Endocr. Rev.* **2014**, *35*, 851–905. [CrossRef] [PubMed]

48. Rabaglino, M.B.; Uiterweer, E.D.P.; Jeyabalan, A.; Hogge, W.A.; Conrad, K.P. Bioinformatics Approach Reveals Evidence for Impaired Endometrial Maturation Before and During Early Pregnancy in Women Who Developed Preeclampsia. *Hypertension* **2015**, *65*, 421–429. [CrossRef] [PubMed]
49. Blanks, A.M.; Brosens, J.J. Progesterone action in the myometrium and decidua in preterm birth. *Facts Views Vis. Obgyn.* **2012**, *4*, 33–43. [PubMed]
50. Aung, M.T.; Yu, Y.; Ferguson, K.K.; Cantonwine, D.E.; Zeng, L.; McElrath, T.F.; Pennathur, S.; Mukherjee, B.; Meeker, J.D. Prediction and associations of preterm birth and its subtypes with eicosanoid enzymatic pathways and inflammatory markers. *Sci. Rep.* **2019**, *9*, 17049. [CrossRef] [PubMed]
51. Black, K.H. June, Inflammatory Markers and Preeclampsia: A systematic Review. *Nurs. Res.* **2018**, *67*, 242–251. [CrossRef]
52. Szentpéteri, I.; Rab, A.; Kornya, L.; Kovács, P.; Joó, J.G. Gene expression patterns of vascular endothelial growth factor (VEGF-A) in human placenta from pregnancies with intrauterine growth restriction. *J. Matern. Fetal Neonatal Med.* **2013**, *26*, 984–989. [CrossRef] [PubMed]
53. Al-Azemi, M.; Raghupathy, R.; Azizieh, F. Pro-inflammatory and anti-inflammatory cytokine profiles in fetal growth restriction. *Clin. Exp. Obstet. Gynecol.* **2017**, *44*, 98–103. [CrossRef] [PubMed]
54. Sundrani, D.P.; Chavan-Gautam, P.M.; Pisal, H.R.; Mehendale, S.S.; Joshi, S.R. Matrix Metalloproteinase-1 and -9 in Human Placenta during Spontaneous Vaginal Delivery and Caesarean Sectioning in Preterm Pregnancy. *PLoS ONE* **2012**, *7*, e29855. [CrossRef]
55. Vannuccini, S.; Bocchi, C.; Severi, F.M.; Challis, J.R.; Petraglia, F. Endocrinology of human parturition. *Ann. Endocrinol.* **2016**, *77*, 105–113. [CrossRef]
56. Fuentes, A.; Spaziani, E.P.; O'Brien, W.F. The expression of cyclooxygenase-2 (COX-2) in amnion and decidua following spontaneous labor. *Prostaglandins* **1996**, *52*, 261–267. [CrossRef] [PubMed]
57. Gao, L.; Lu, C.; Xu, C.; Tao, Y.; Cong, B.; Ni, X. Differential Regulation of Prostaglandin Production Mediated by Corticotropin-Releasing Hormone Receptor Type 1 and Type 2 in Cultured Human Placental Trophoblasts. *Endocrinology* **2008**, *149*, 2866–2876. [CrossRef] [PubMed]
58. Kota, S.K.; Gayatri, K.; Jammula, S.; Kota, S.K.; Krishna, S.V.; Meher, L.K.; Modi, K.D. Endocrinology of parturition. *Indian J. Endocrinol. Metab.* **2013**, *17*, 50–59. [CrossRef] [PubMed]
59. Vincent, Z.L.; Mitchell, M.D.; Ponnampalam, A.P. Regulation of TIMP-1 in Human Placenta and Fetal Membranes by lipopolysaccharide and demethylating agent 5-aza-2′-deoxycytidine. *Reprod. Biol. Endocrinol.* **2015**, *13*, 136. [CrossRef] [PubMed]
60. Norwitz, E.R.; Bonney, E.A.; Snegovskikh, V.V.; Williams, M.A.; Phillippe, M.; Park, J.S.; Abrahams, V.M. Molecular Regulation of Parturition: The Role of the Decidual Clock. *Cold Spring Harb. Perspect. Med.* **2015**, *5*, a023143. [CrossRef] [PubMed]
61. Tosto, V.; Giardina, I.; Tsibizova, V.; Renzo, G.C.D. Preterm Birth, From the Biological Knowledges to the Prevention: An Overview. *Matern. Fetal Med.* **2020**, *2*, 162–171. [CrossRef]
62. Lowe, S.A.; Bowyer, L.; Lust, K.; McMahon, L.P.; Morton, M.; North, R.A.; Paech, M.; Said, J.M. SOMANZ guidelines for the management of hypertensive disorders of pregnancy 2014. *Aust. N. Z. J. Obstet. Gynaecol.* **2015**, *55*, e1–e29. [CrossRef]
63. Fox, R.; Kitt, J.; Leeson, P.; Aye, C.Y.L.; Lewandowski, A.J. Preeclampsia: Risk Factors, Diagnosis, Management, and the Cardiovascular Impact on the Offspring. *J. Clin. Med.* **2019**, *8*, 1625. [CrossRef]
64. Løset, M.; Mundal, S.B.; Johnson, M.P.; Fenstad, M.H.; Freed, K.A.; Lian, I.A.; Eide, I.P.; Bjørge, L.; Blangero, J.; Moses, E.K. A transcriptional profile of the decidua in preeclampsia. *Am. J. Obstet. Gynecol.* **2011**, *204*, 84.e1–84.e27. [CrossRef]
65. Lockwood, C.J.; Yen, C.-F.; Basar, M.; Kayisli, U.A.; Martel, M.; Buhimschi, I.; Buhimschi, C.; Huang, S.J.; Krikun, G.; Schatz, F. Preeclampsia-Related Inflammatory Cytokines Regulate Interleukin-6 Expression in Human Decidual Cells. *Am. J. Pathol.* **2008**, *172*, 1571–1579. [CrossRef]
66. Wallace, A.E.; Host, A.J.; Whitley, G.S.; Cartwright, J.E. Decidual natural killer cell interactions with trophoblasts are impaired in pregnancies at increased risk of preeclampsia. *Am. J. Pathol.* **2013**, *183*, 1853–1861. [CrossRef] [PubMed]
67. Salama, S.A.; Kamel, M.W.; Diaz-Arrastia, C.R.; Xu, X.; Veenstra, T.D.; Salih, S.; Botting, S.K.; Kumar, R. Effect of tumor necrosis factor-alpha on estrogen metabolism and endometrial cells: Potential physiological and pathological relevance. *J. Clin. Endocrinol. Metab.* **2009**, *94*, 285–293. [CrossRef] [PubMed]
68. Drummond, K.; Danesh, N.M.; Arseneault, S.; Rodrigues, J.; Tulandi, T.; Raina, J.; Suarthana, E. Association between Endometriosis and Risk of Preeclampsia in Women Who Conceived Spontaneously: A Systematic Review and Meta-analysis. *J. Minim. Invasive Gynecol.* **2023**, *30*, 91–99. [CrossRef] [PubMed]
69. Cheung, V.C.; Peng, C.Y.; Marinić, M.; Sakabe, N.J.; Aneas, I.; Lynch, V.J.; Ober, C.; Nobrega, M.A.; Kessler, J.A. Pluripotent stem cell-derived endometrial stromal fibroblasts in a cyclic, hormone-responsive coculture model of human decidua. *Cell Rep.* **2021**, *35*, 109138. [CrossRef] [PubMed]
70. Resnik, R. Intrauterine growth restriction. *Obstet. Gynecol.* **2002**, *99*, 490–496. [CrossRef] [PubMed]
71. Ghidini, A. Idiopathic fetal growth restriction: A pathophysiologic approach. *Obstet. Gynecol. Surv.* **1996**, *51*, 376–382. [CrossRef] [PubMed]
72. Sparks, T.N.; Cheng, Y.W.; McLaughlin, B.; Esakoff, T.F.; Caughey, A.B. Fundal height: A useful screening tool for fetal growth? *J. Matern. Fetal Neonatal Med.* **2011**, *24*, 708–712. [CrossRef]
73. Selvaratnam, R.; Davey, M.A.; Anil, S.; McDonald, S.; Farrell, T.; Wallace, E. Does public reporting of the detection of fetal growth restriction improve clinical outcomes: A retrospective cohort study. *BJOG* **2020**, *127*, 581–589. [CrossRef] [PubMed]

74. Crispi, F.; Miranda, J.; Gratacós, E. Long-term cardiovascular consequences of fetal growth restriction: Biology, clinical implications, and opportunities for prevention of adult disease. *Am. J. Obstet. Gynecol.* **2018**, *218*, S869–S879. [CrossRef]
75. Pels, A.; Beune, I.M.; Van Wassenaer-Leemhuis, A.G.; Limpens, J.; Ganzevoort, W. Early-onset fetal growth restriction: A systematic review on mortality and morbidity. *Acta Obstet. Gynecol. Scand.* **2020**, *99*, 153–166. [CrossRef]
76. Tang, L.; He, G.; Liu, X.; Xu, W. Progress in the understanding of the etiology and predictability of fetal growth restriction. *Reproduction* **2017**, *153*, R227–R240. [CrossRef]
77. Hendrix, N.; Berghella, V. Non-Placental Causes of Intrauterine Growth Restriction. *Semin. Perinatol.* **2008**, *32*, 161–165. [CrossRef]
78. Raghupathy, R.; Al-Azemi, M.; Azizieh, F. Intrauterine growth restriction: Cytokine profiles of trophoblast antigen-stimulated maternal lymphocytes. *Clin. Dev. Immunol.* **2012**, *2012*, 734865. [CrossRef]
79. Eide, I.P.; Rolfseng, T.; Isaksen, C.V.; Mecsei, R.; Roald, B.; Lydersen, S.; Salvesen, K.Å.; Harsem, N.K.; Austgulen, R. Serious foetal growth restriction is associated with reduced proportions of natural killer cells in decidua basalis. *Virchows Arch.* **2006**, *448*, 269–276. [CrossRef]
80. Gravett, M.G.; Rubens, C.E.; Nunes, T.M. Global report on preterm birth and stillbirth (2 of 7): Discovery science. *BMC Pregnancy Childbirth* **2010**, *10*, S2. [CrossRef]
81. Phillips, C.; Velji, Z.; Hanly, C.; Metcalfe, A. Risk of recurrent spontaneous preterm birth: A systematic review and meta-analysis. *BMJ Open* **2017**, *7*, e015402. [CrossRef]
82. Connealy, B.D.; Carreno, C.A.; Kase, B.A.; Hart, L.A.; Blackwell, S.C.; Sibai, B.M. A history of prior preeclampsia as a risk factor for preterm birth. *Am. J. Perinatol.* **2014**, *31*, 483–488. [CrossRef]
83. Vogel, J.P.; Chawanpaiboon, S.; Moller, A.-B.; Watananirun, K.; Bonet, M.; Lumbiganon, P. The global epidemiology of preterm birth. *Best Pract. Res. Clin. Obstet. Gynaecol.* **2018**, *52*, 3–12. [CrossRef] [PubMed]
84. Lockwood, C.J.; Kuczynski, E. Risk stratification and pathological mechanisms in preterm delivery. *Paediatr. Perinat. Epidemiol.* **2001**, *15*, 78–89. [CrossRef] [PubMed]
85. Institute of Medicine (US). *Committee on Understanding Premature Birth and Assuring Healthy Outcomes*; Behrman, R.E., Butler, A.S., Eds.; Preterm Birth: Causes, Consequences, and Prevention; National Academies Press: Washington, DC, USA, 2007.
86. Ferguson, K.K.; McElrath, T.F.; Chen, Y.H.; Mukherjee, B.; Meeker, J.D. Longitudinal profiling of inflammatory cytokines and C-reactive protein during uncomplicated and preterm pregnancy. *Am. J. Reprod. Immunol.* **2014**, *72*, 326–336. [CrossRef] [PubMed]
87. Skliutė, G.; Baušytė, R.; Borutinskaitė, V.; Valiulienė, G.; Kaupinis, A.; Valius, M.; Ramašauskaitė, D.; Navakauskienė, R. Menstrual Blood-Derived Endometrial Stem Cells' Impact for the Treatment Perspective of Female Infertility. *Int. J. Mol. Sci.* **2021**, *22*, 6774. [CrossRef] [PubMed]
88. Brosens, J.J.; Parker, M.G.; McIndoe, A.; Pijnenborg, R.; Brosens, I.A. A role for menstruation in preconditioning the uterus for successful pregnancy. *Am. J. Obstet. Gynecol.* **2009**, *200*, e1–e615. [CrossRef] [PubMed]
89. Zhang, T.; Wang, H.; Wang, X.; Yang, Y.; Zhang, Y.; Tang, Z.; Wang, L. The adverse maternal and perinatal outcomes of adolescent pregnancy: A cross sectional study in Hebei, China. *BMC Pregnancy Childbirth* **2020**, *20*, 339. [CrossRef] [PubMed]
90. Ganchimeg, T.; Ota, E.; Morisaki, N.; Laopaiboon, M.; Lumbiganon, P.; Zhang, J.; Yamdamsuren, B.; Temmerman, M.; Say, L.; Tunçalp, Ö.; et al. Network, Pregnancy and childbirth outcomes among adolescent mothers: A World Health Organization multicountry study. *BJOG* **2014**, *121*, 40–48. [CrossRef] [PubMed]
91. Amjad, S.; MacDonald, I.; Chambers, T.; Osornio-Vargas, A.; Chandra, S.; Voaklander, D.; Ospina, M.B. Social determinants of health and adverse maternal and birth outcomes in adolescent pregnancies: A systematic review and meta-analysis. *Paediatr. Perinat. Epidemiol.* **2019**, *33*, 88–99. [CrossRef] [PubMed]
92. Brosens, I.; Muter, J.; Gargett, C.E.; Puttemans, P.; Benagiano, G.; Brosens, J.J. The impact of uterine immaturity on obstetrical syndromes during adolescence. *Am. J. Obstet. Gynecol.* **2017**, *217*, 546–555. [CrossRef]
93. Saccone, G.; Gragnano, E.; Ilardi, B.; Marrone, V.; Strina, I.; Venturella, R.; Berghella, V.; Zullo, F. Maternal and perinatal complications according to maternal age: A systematic review and meta-analysis. *Int. J. Gynaecol. Obstet.* **2022**, *159*, 43–55. [CrossRef]
94. Woods, L.; Perez-Garcia, V.; Kieckbusch, J.; Wang, X.; DeMayo, F.; Colucci, F.; Hemberger, M. Decidualisation and placentation defects are a major cause of age-related reproductive decline. *Nat. Commun.* **2017**, *8*, 352. [CrossRef] [PubMed]
95. Tanikawa, N.; Ohtsu, A.; Kawahara-Miki, R.; Kimura, K.; Matsuyama, S.; Iwata, H.; Kuwayama, T.; Shirasuna, K. Age-associated mRNA expression changes in bovine endometrial cells in vitro. *Reprod. Biol. Endocrinol.* **2017**, *15*, 63. [CrossRef]
96. Hirata, Y.; Katsukura, Y.; Henmi, Y.; Ozawa, R.; Shimazaki, S.; Kurosawa, A.; Torii, Y.; Takahashi, H.; Iwata, H.; Kuwayama, T.; et al. Advanced maternal age induces fetal growth restriction through decreased placental inflammatory cytokine expression and immune cell accumulation in mice. *J. Reprod. Dev.* **2021**, *67*, 257–264. [CrossRef]
97. Lean, S.C.; Heazell, A.E.P.; Dilworth, M.R.; Mills, T.A.; Jones, R.L. Placental Dysfunction Underlies Increased Risk of Fetal Growth Restriction and Stillbirth in Advanced Maternal Age Women. *Sci. Rep.* **2017**, *7*, 9677. [CrossRef] [PubMed]
98. Hosseini, S.; Shokri, F.; Tokhmechy, R.; Savadi-Shiraz, E.; Jeddi-Tehrani, M.; Rahbari, M.; Zarnani, A.-H. Menstrual blood contains immune cells with inflammatory and anti-inflammatory properties. *J. Obstet. Gynaecol. Res.* **2015**, *41*, 1803–1812. [CrossRef]
99. Hosseini, S.; Zarnani, A.-H.; Asgarian-Omran, H.; Vahedian-Dargahi, Z.; Eshraghian, M.R.; Akbarzadeh-Pasha, Z.; Arefi, S.; Jeddi-Tehrani, M.; Shokri, F. Comparative analysis of NK cell subsets in menstrual and peripheral blood of patients with unexplained recurrent spontaneous abortion and fertile subjects. *J. Reprod. Immunol.* **2014**, *103*, 9–17. [CrossRef]

100. Tindal, K.; Filby, C.E.; Gargett, C.E.; Cousins, F.; Palmer, K.R.; Vollenhoven, B.; Davies-Tuck, M. Endometrial Origins of Stillbirth (EOS), a case–control study of menstrual fluid to understand and prevent preterm stillbirth and associated adverse pregnancy outcomes: Study protocol. *BMJ Open* **2023**, *13*, e068919. [CrossRef] [PubMed]
101. Joseph, F.A.; Hyett, J.A.; Schluter, P.J.; McLennan, A.; Gordon, A.; Chambers, G.M.; Hilder, L.; Choi, S.K.; Vries, B. New Australian birthweight centiles. *Med. J. Aust.* **2020**, *213*, 79–85. [CrossRef] [PubMed]
102. Cindrova-Davies, T.; Zhao, X.; Elder, K.; Jones, C.J.P.; Moffett, A.; Burton, G.J.; Turco, M.Y. Menstrual flow as a non-invasive source of endometrial organoids. *Commun. Biol.* **2021**, *4*, 651. [CrossRef]
103. Critchley, H.O.D.; Babayev, E.; Bulun, S.E.; Clark, S.; Garcia-Grau, I.; Gregersen, P.K.; Kilcoyne, A.; Kim, J.-Y.J.; Lavender, M.; Marsh, E.E.; et al. Menstruation: Science and society. *Am. J. Obstet. Gynecol.* **2020**, *223*, 624–664. [CrossRef]
104. Johnston-Robledo, I.; Chrisler, J.C. The Menstrual Mark: Menstruation as Social Stigma. In *The Palgrave Handbook of Critical Menstruation Studies*; Bobel, C., Ed.; Palgrave Macmillan: Singapore, 2020; pp. 181–199.
105. Manley, H.; Sprinks, J.; Breedon, P. Menstrual Blood-Derived Mesenchymal Stem Cells: Women's Attitudes, Willingness, and Barriers to Donation of Menstrual Blood. *J. Womens Health* **2019**, *28*, 1688–1697. [CrossRef]
106. Bouzid, K.; Bourdon, M.; Bartkowski, R.; Verbanck, M.; Chapron, C.; Marcellin, L.; Batteux, F.; Santulli, P.; Doridot, L. Menstrual Blood Donation for Endometriosis Research: A Cross-Sectional Survey on Women's Willingness and Potential Barriers. *Reprod. Sci.* **2024**, *31*, 1617–1625. [CrossRef]
107. Itriyeva, K. The effects of obesity on the menstrual cycle. *Curr. Probl. Pediatr. Adolesc. Health Care* **2022**, *52*, 101241. [CrossRef]
108. Aladashvili-Chikvaidze, N.; Kristesashvili, J.; Gegechkori, M. Types of reproductive disorders in underweight and overweight young females and correlations of respective hormonal changes with BMI. *Iran J. Reprod. Med.* **2015**, *13*, 135–140. [PubMed]
109. DeLoughery, E.; Colwill, A.C.; Edelman, A.; Bannow, B.S. Red blood cell capacity of modern menstrual products: Considerations for assessing heavy menstrual bleeding. *BMJ Sex. Reprod. Health* **2023**, *50*, 201895. [CrossRef]
110. Tindal, K.; Filby, C.E.; Cousins, F.L.; Ellery, S.J.; Vollenhoven, B.; Palmer, K.; Gordon, A.; Gargett, C.E.; Davies-Tuck, M. The composition of menstrual fluid, its applications, and recent advances to understand the endometrial environment: A narrative review. *FS Rev.* **2024**, *5*, 100075. [CrossRef]
111. Nikoo, S.; Ebtekar, M.; Jeddi-Tehrani, M.; Shervin, A.; Bozorgmehr, M.; Vafaei, S.; Kazemnejad, S.; Zarnani, A.H. Menstrual blood-derived stromal stem cells from women with and without endometriosis reveal different phenotypic and functional characteristics. *Mol. Hum. Reprod.* **2014**, *20*, 905–918. [CrossRef]
112. Da Silva, C.M.; Belo, A.V.; Andrade, S.P.; Campos, P.P.; Ferreira, M.C.F.; Da Silva-Filho, A.L.; Carneiro, M.M. Identification of local angiogenic and inflammatory markers in the menstrual blood of women with endometriosis. *Biomed. Pharmacother.* **2014**, *68*, 899–904. [CrossRef]
113. Warren, L.A.; Shih, A.; Renteira, S.M.; Seckin, T.; Blau, B.; Simpfendorfer, K.; Lee, A.; Metz, C.N.; Gregersen, P.K. Analysis of menstrual effluent: Diagnostic potential for endometriosis. *Mol. Med.* **2018**, *24*, 1. [CrossRef]
114. Madjid, T.H.; Ardiansyah, D.F.; Permadi, W.; Hernowo, B. Expression of Matrix Metalloproteinase-9 and Tissue Inhibitor of Metalloproteinase-1 in Endometriosis Menstrual Blood. *Diagnostics* **2020**, *10*, 364. [CrossRef]
115. Nayyar, A.; Saleem, M.I.; Yilmaz, M.; DeFranco, M.; Klein, G.; Elmaliki, K.M.; Kowalsky, E.; Chatterjee, P.K.; Xue, X.; Viswanathan, R.; et al. Menstrual Effluent Provides a Novel Diagnostic Window on the Pathogenesis of Endometriosis. *Front. Reprod. Health* **2020**, *2*, 3. [CrossRef] [PubMed]
116. Shih, A.J.; Adelson, R.P.; Vashistha, H.; Khalili, H.; Nayyar, A.; Puran, R.; Herrera, R.; Chatterjee, P.K.; Lee, A.T.; Truskinovsky, A.M.; et al. Single-cell analysis of menstrual endometrial tissues defines phenotypes associated with endometriosis. *BMC Med.* **2022**, *20*, 315. [CrossRef]
117. Sahraei, S.S.; Asl, F.D.; Kalhor, N.; Sheykhhasan, M.; Fazaeli, H.; Moud, S.S.; Sheikholeslami, A. A Comparative Study of Gene Expression in Menstrual Blood-Derived Stromal Cells between Endometriosis and Healthy Women. *Biomed Res. Int.* **2022**, *2022*, 7053521. [CrossRef]
118. Ji, S.; Liu, Y.; Yan, L.; Zhang, Y.; Li, Y.; Zhu, Q.; Xia, W.; Ge, S.; Zhang, J. DIA-based analysis of the menstrual blood proteome identifies association between CXCL5 and IL1RN and endometriosis. *J. Proteom.* **2023**, *289*, 104995. [CrossRef]
119. Hosseini, S.; Shokri, F.; Pour, S.A.; Jeddi-Tehrani, M.; Nikoo, S.; Yousefi, M.; Zarnani, A.-H. A shift in the balance of T17 and Treg cells in menstrual blood of women with unexplained recurrent spontaneous abortion. *J. Reprod. Immunol.* **2016**, *116*, 13–22. [CrossRef]
120. Jukic, A.M.Z.; Weinberg, C.R.; Wilcox, A.J.; McConnaughey, D.R.; Hornsby, P.; Baird, D.D. Accuracy of Reporting of Menstrual Cycle Length. *Am. J. Epidemiol.* **2007**, *167*, 25–33. [CrossRef]
121. Burden, C.; Bradley, S.; Storey, C.; Ellis, A.; Heazell, A.E.P.; Downe, S.; Cacciatore, J.; Siassakos, D. From grief, guilt pain and stigma to hope and pride—A systematic review and meta-analysis of mixed-method research of the psychosocial impact of stillbirth. *BMC Pregnancy Childbirth* **2016**, *16*, 9. [CrossRef]
122. Pollock, D.D.; Pearson, D.E.; Cooper, D.M.; Ziaian, A.P.T.; Foord, C.; Warland, A.P.J. Breaking the silence: Determining Prevalence and Understanding Stillbirth Stigma. *Midwifery* **2021**, *93*, 102884. [CrossRef]
123. Wojcieszek, A.M.; Shepherd, E.; Middleton, P.; Gardener, G.; Ellwood, D.A.; McClure, E.M.; Gold, K.J.; Khong, T.Y.; Silver, R.M.; Erwich, J.J.H.; et al. Interventions for investigating and identifying the causes of stillbirth. *Cochrane Database Syst. Rev.* **2018**, *4*, CD012504. [CrossRef]

124. Munro, M.G.; Critchley, H.O.D.; Fraser, I.S. The two FIGO systems for normal and abnormal uterine bleeding symptoms and classification of causes of abnormal uterine bleeding in the reproductive years: 2018 revisions. *Int. J. Gynecol. Obstet.* **2018**, *143*, 393–408. [CrossRef]
125. Walker, E.R.; McGrane, M.; Aplin, J.D.; Brison, D.R.; Ruane, P.T. A systematic review of transcriptomic studies of the human endometrium reveals inconsistently reported differentially expressed genes. *Reprod. Fertil.* **2023**, *4*, e220115. [CrossRef]
126. Hennegan, J.; Winkler, I.T.; Bobel, C.; Keiser, D.; Hampton, J.; Larsson, G.; Chandra-Mouli, V.; Plesons, M.; Mahon, T. Menstrual health: A definition for policy, practice, and research. *Sex. Reprod. Health Matters* **2021**, *29*, 1911618. [CrossRef]
127. Khoury, M.; Alcayaga-Miranda, F.; Illanes, S.E.; Figueroa, F.E. The Promising Potential of Menstrual Stem Cells for Antenatal Diagnosis and Cell Therapy. *Front. Immunol.* **2014**, *5*, 205. [CrossRef]

Disclaimer/Publisher's Note: The statements, opinions and data contained in all publications are solely those of the individual author(s) and contributor(s) and not of MDPI and/or the editor(s). MDPI and/or the editor(s) disclaim responsibility for any injury to people or property resulting from any ideas, methods, instructions or products referred to in the content.

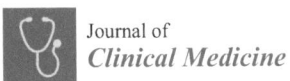

Article

Predelivery Haemostatic Biomarkers in Women with Non-Severe Postpartum Haemorrhage

Claire de Moreuil [1,2,3,*], Brigitte Pan-Petesch [1,4], Dino Mehic [3], Daniel Kraemmer [3], Theresa Schramm [3], Casilda Albert [5], Christophe Trémouilhac [6], Sandy Lucier [7], Hubert Galinat [8], Liana Le Roux [9], Johanna Gebhart [3], Francis Couturaud [1,2], Alisa S. Wolberg [10], Cihan Ay [3] and Ingrid Pabinger [3]

1. UMR 1304 GETBO, INSERM, University of Brest, 29200 Brest, France
2. Internal Medicine, Vascular Medicine and Pneumology Department, Centre Hospitalier Universitaire de Brest, 29200 Brest, France
3. Department of Medicine I, Clinical Division of Haematology and Haemostaseology, Medical University of Vienna, 1090 Vienna, Austria
4. Center for Haemophilia Treatment, Haematology, Centre Hospitalier Universitaire de Brest, 29200 Brest, France
5. Gynecology and Obstetrics Department, Centre Hospitalier Universitaire de Brest, 29200 Brest, France
6. Gynecology and Obstetrics Department, Morlaix Hospital, 29672 Morlaix, France
7. CIC1412, INSERM, Centre Hospitalier Universitaire de Brest, 29200 Brest, France
8. Haemostasis Laboratory, Centre Hospitalier Universitaire de Brest, 29200 Brest, France
9. CIC-RB Ressources Biologiques (UF 0827), Centre Hospitalier Universitaire de Brest, 29200 Brest, France
10. Department of Pathology and Laboratory Medicine, UNC Blood Research Center, University of North Carolina at Chapel Hill, NC 27514, USA
* Correspondence: claire.demoreuil@chu-brest.fr

Abstract: Background: Postpartum haemorrhage (PPH) is a frequent complication of childbirth that is difficult to predict. Predelivery coagulation biomarkers may help to guide preventive strategies. Our objective was to evaluate the association of predelivery haemostatic biomarkers with non-severe PPH. **Methods**: A nested case-control study was conducted within the « Study of Biological Determinants of Bleeding Postpartum » in order to compare different haemostatic biomarkers in plasma from pregnant women with non-severe PPH (cases) and controls without PPH matched for age, body mass index, term, and mode of delivery. Blood was collected at entry in the delivery room. Global haemostatic assays (thrombin generation assay (TGA) and plasmin generation assay (PGA)) were then performed on freshly thawed aliquots of platelet-poor plasma. **Results**: A total of 370 pregnant women (185 cases and 185 controls) were included. Median [interquartile range] predelivery platelet count was lower in PPH cases than in controls (217 [181–259] versus 242 [196–280] G/L). TGA and PGA parameters were similar between cases and controls. In a subset analysis of vaginal deliveries (n = 144), median predelivery TGA thrombin peak was lower, and median predelivery PGA lag phase was longer in cases compared to controls. In multivariable analysis, only predelivery platelet count was independently associated with non-severe PPH. **Conclusions**: Predelivery platelet count is associated with non-severe PPH. Differences in other haemostatic parameters are tenuous, questioning their usefulness in predicting non-severe PPH.

Keywords: coagulation; plasmin generation; postpartum haemorrhage; predelivery; thrombin generation

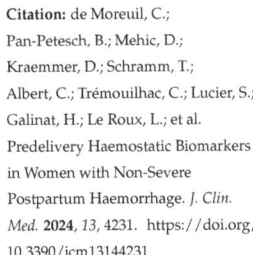

Citation: de Moreuil, C.; Pan-Petesch, B.; Mehic, D.; Kraemmer, D.; Schramm, T.; Albert, C.; Trémouilhac, C.; Lucier, S.; Galinat, H.; Le Roux, L.; et al. Predelivery Haemostatic Biomarkers in Women with Non-Severe Postpartum Haemorrhage. *J. Clin. Med.* **2024**, *13*, 4231. https://doi.org/10.3390/jcm13144231

Academic Editors: Apostolos Mamopoulos and Ioannis Tsakiridis

Received: 21 May 2024
Revised: 17 July 2024
Accepted: 18 July 2024
Published: 19 July 2024

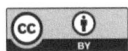

Copyright: © 2024 by the authors. Licensee MDPI, Basel, Switzerland. This article is an open access article distributed under the terms and conditions of the Creative Commons Attribution (CC BY) license (https://creativecommons.org/licenses/by/4.0/).

1. Introduction

Postpartum haemorrhage (PPH) is a frequent complication of childbirth that can affect pregnant women worldwide [1–3]. The prevalence of PPH is estimated to range from 7 to 25% of deliveries, depending on the definition of PPH, on the mode of evaluation of blood loss, and on the country [4]. Despite the identification of a number of obstetric risk factors for PPH, this complication is still difficult to predict in the general population of delivering women, and targeted preventive strategies are still not uniformly implemented in the maternity wards [5,6]. Most PPH cases are attributed to uterine atony, and the coagulation state of pregnant women prior to delivery has not been extensively investigated as a potential co-factor for bleeding. Most studies have focused on haemostatic biomarkers measured at PPH diagnosis after delivery to guide transfusion procedures or administration of factor concentrates, e.g., fibrinogen [7,8]. In this context, viscoelastic haemostatic assays can be useful to monitor and treat PPH-associated coagulopathy [9,10]. Moreover, the usefulness in preventing PPH would avoid the need for blood product transfusion, emergency surgery, and the negative psychological impact on women experiencing such a complication. That is why we focused our research on the exploration of predelivery haemostatic biomarkers in the context of PPH.

In a previous work within the "Study of Biological Determinants of Bleeding Postpartum" (HPP-IPF), a French cohort study, we found that predelivery endogenous thrombin potential (ETP) measured with the thrombin generation assay (TGA) was lower in women with severe PPH compared to matched pregnant controls, despite similar results in conventional coagulation tests [11].

While severe PPH is defined by a blood loss higher or equal to 1 L (L) at delivery and has a prevalence of around 2% of deliveries, non-severe PPH has a milder clinical phenotype but is much more frequent [4]. As such, the question arises whether predelivery haemostatic biomarkers could therefore help with predicting and possibly preventing this frequent complication of childbirth.

In this nested case-control study within the HPP-IPF cohort study, we aimed to investigate the association of predelivery haemostatic biomarkers with non-severe PPH. For this purpose, we performed global haemostatic assays (thrombin generation assay (TGA) and plasmin generation assay (PGA)) using plasma samples collected at entry in the delivery room in women who went on to have non-severe PPH and in matched pregnant controls, and evaluated associations of haemostatic biomarkers with non-severe PPH. Since the impact of the haemostatic system might be a more important determinant of bleeding following vaginal delivery versus Caesarean section (C-section), we also evaluated women with vaginal delivery separately in a subset analysis.

2. Materials and Methods

2.1. Recruitment of Participants, Blood and Data Collection

The HPP-IPF "Study of Biological Determinants of Bleeding Postpartum" is a French prospective single-centre cohort study designed to evaluate the biomarkers associated with PPH among various biological and clinical parameters collected before delivery [12]. All pregnant women entering Brest University Hospital for a delivery between 1 April 2013 and 29 May 2015 were included in the study if they had given their oral consent for the study (Clinicaltrials.gov identifier: NCT02884804). Around 1862 deliveries per year took place at Brest University Hospital during the study period.

Biological data were measured from a blood sample routinely collected before delivery at entry in the delivery room for blood group determination, complete blood count, and conventional haemostatic tests. The following biomarkers were measured directly in fresh blood samples: haemoglobin, haematocrit, platelet count, immature platelet fraction (IPF) (XE 5000, Sysmex, Villepinte, France), prothrombin rate (STAGO Néoplastine CI + 10, STA-R, Stago, Asnières sur Seine, France), activated partial thromboplastin time (aPTT) ratio (Triniclot Automated APTT, STA-R, Stago, Asnières sur Seine, France), fibrinogen (STAGO STA Fibrinogen 5, STA-R, Stago, Asnières sur Seine, France), D-dimer (STAGO STA Liatest D-Di, STA-R, Stago, Asnières sur Seine, France), and fibrin monomers (STAGO STA Liatest MOFB, STA-R, Stago, Asnières sur Seine, France).

Platelet-poor plasma was prepared after centrifugation ($2500 \times g$, 15 min), aliquoted, and immediately stored at $-80\ °C$.

Clinical data on women and their pregnancies were collected by midwives and obstetricians in the medical files during each antenatal care visit, from the end of first trimester of pregnancy until delivery, and then in the delivery room, and finally during the maternity stay until discharge. These data were then recorded by trained research assistants in a standardised electronic case report form. Abnormal placental insertion comprised low-lying placentas, placenta previa, placenta percreta, placenta accreta, and placenta bipartita. Antepartum haemorrhage comprised all episodes of uterine haemorrhage occurring at any time during pregnancy, before delivery. The definition of pre-eclampsia was the one provided by the American College of Obstetricians and Gynecologists and published in 2013 [13]. Macrosomia corresponded to a weight of the newborn $\geq$4000 g.

2.2. Definition of Non-Severe PPH

Blood loss at delivery was measured systematically with a graduated collector bag.

Non-severe PPH diagnosis was based on the World Health Organization's (WHO) definitions of PPH and severe PPH, i.e., a blood loss between 500 and 999 mL in the 24 h following delivery [14].

For each PPH case, the aetiology of PPH was diagnosed by the midwife or the obstetrician in charge of the delivery, according to the "4T" rule [15]. The main aetiology of PPH was recorded if the PPH case was multifactorial. All cases were reviewed and adjudicated by two obstetricians (CaA and CT) in order to confirm the main aetiology of PPH.

2.3. Selection of Cases and Controls

Cases were women included in the HPP-IPF cohort study and diagnosed with non-severe PPH based on the volume of blood loss at delivery. Women for whom the volume of blood loss had not been objectively measured were excluded from the study, as were women delivering before 21 weeks of gestation (WG). Women who had no available frozen plasma sample were also excluded from the study.

Finally, each case was matched with one pregnant woman from the HPP-IPF cohort study as a control with no PPH (i.e., a volume of blood loss < 500 mL at delivery), a delivery at a term $\geq$21WG, and a stored plasma sample. This matching was performed with the support of an experienced data manager (SL) who created a list of potential controls for each case, matched for age at delivery (<35 years versus $\geq$35 years), pre-pregnancy body mass index (BMI) (<25.0 kg/m^2 versus [25.0–29.9] kg/m^2 and $\geq$30.0 kg/m^2), term at delivery (<37 WG versus $\geq$37 WG), and delivery mode (vaginal versus C-section). Then, for each case, CDM selected the pregnant woman without PPH who matched best the PPH case for the four clinical parameters described above. Thus, each non-severe PPH case was matched with the pregnant control woman included in the study who had not presented PPH at delivery and who had the closest clinical characteristics regarding the four matching criteria (age at delivery, pre-pregnancy BMI, term at delivery, and delivery mode). If more than one woman could match one case according to these four matching criteria, CDM chose the control that was the most similar to the case regarding age, BMI, and term at delivery.

The matching of the PPH cases and controls for the main clinical parameters which could represent confounding biases ensures a good reliability of the comparison between non-severe PPH cases and controls, and compensates for the reduced number of controls. This design was also chosen in order to reduce the overall cost of the study and in order to make the measurements feasible by one unique researcher in a period of six months.

2.4. Thrombin Generation Assay (TGA)

TGA was performed in plasma using a commercially available kit (Technothrombin, Technoclone, Vienna, Austria) and a low concentration of tissue factor (TF) (PPP Low Reagent, <3 pM final, Stago, Asnières sur Seine, France), as previously described [16]. The following parameters were analysed, using a specifically adapted software (Technothrombin TGA® evaluation software, Biotek KC4, Technoclone, Vienna, Austria, www.technoclone.com): lag phase (minutes), maximum thrombin concentration generated (thrombin peak, nmol/L), time to peak (minutes), velocity index (nmol/L/min), and endogenous thrombin potential (ETP, nmol/L $\times$ min).

2.5. Plasmin Generation Assay (PGA)

PGA was performed as described [17]. Briefly, two measurements were collected for each plasma sample: one in which endogenous plasmin generation was triggered with a 10 μL solution containing TF, phospholipids, and recombinant tissue plasminogen activator (rtPA), and one in which 10 μL α2M-Pm (calibrator) was added. Plasma was diluted (40 μL of 1:2 dilution in HBS) and added to each well, and the plate was incubated for 10 min at 37 °C. $CaCl_2$ and fluorogenic substrate were then dispensed into each well. Final concentrations of reagents were the following: TF (0.5 pmol/L), phospholipids (4 μmol/L), rtPA (0.31 μg/mL), $CaCl_2$ (16.6 mmol/L), and fluorogenic substrate (0.5 mmol/L). Measurements were performed with the Calibrated Automated Thrombogram (Stago, Vienna, Austria). Data were analysed as previously described [17].

All experiments were performed in a blinded fashion.

2.6. Statistical Analysis

To describe the study population, continuous variables are displayed as medians with interquartile ranges (IQR) and categorical variables as counts with percentages. Parameters were compared between non-severe PPH and matched controls without PPH using the Wilcoxon rank sum test for quantitative parameters and Pearson's chi-squared test for qualitative parameters. They were also compared in a subgroup analysis restricting the cohort to those with vaginal delivery and C-section, respectively. Correlations between quantitative parameters were measured with Spearman's rank correlation coefficient (ρ).

The association of haemostatic biomarkers with non-severe PPH was investigated in a logistic regression model, adjusting for clinical parameters described in the literature associated with PPH, and presenting odds ratios (OR) with their 95% confidence intervals (95% CI) [1,2]. We ranked included biomarkers for importance by their "fraction of new information", that is, the proportion of total predictive information in the full model that was added by the respective biomarker, as described by Harrell [18]. Due to the large number of parameters of interest given the number of events, we conducted principal component analyses of the PGA and TGA parameters, respectively, which were a priori judged to be highly correlated, representing them in the model by their respective first principal component. To further account for the limited number of events per included covariate, we calculated 95% percentile bootstrap confidence intervals running a bootstrap, clustered for matched pairs, for 10,000 iterations. The ability of the final model to discriminate between non-severe PPH and controls was quantified by c-index and Nagelkerke's R^2. Additionally, we visualised the correlation between all biomarkers in a heatmap of their pairwise absolute Spearman's ρ and using hierarchical clustering of the absolute values of their Spearman's ρ with a complete agglomeration method.

Missing data were not imputed. All statistical analyses were conducted in R version 4.3.2 using the rms package version 6.7-1 [19,20].

2.7. Ethics Approval

Pregnant women were informed by midwives and/or obstetricians of Brest University Hospital about the study, and gave their oral consent to participate in the study. The protocol of the study was approved by our institutional review board on 23 August 2011 (Protocol RB 11.080; ID RCB: 2011-A00802-39).

3. Results

3.1. Characteristics of the Pregnant Women

In this nested case-control study within the HPP-IPF cohort study, 370 pregnant women were investigated: 185 cases who went on to have non-severe PPH and 185 matched pregnant controls (Figure 1). The median [IQR] volume of blood loss in non-severe PPH cases and controls was 600 mL [500–750] and 200 mL [100–300], respectively.

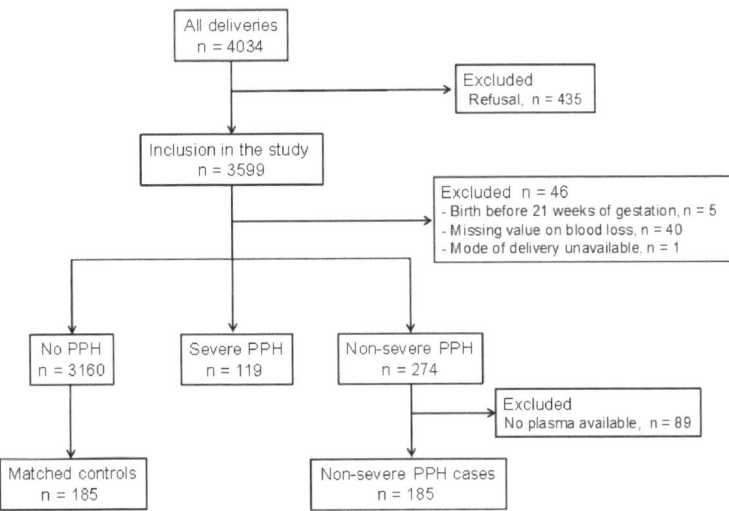

Figure 1. Flow chart of the case-control study. PPH = postpartum haemorrhage.

Table 1 illustrates the clinical characteristics of the pregnant women included in this case-control study.

Table 1. Clinical characteristics of the 370 pregnant women.

Characteristics	Non-Severe PPH (n = 185)	Controls (n = 185)	p
Women's characteristics			
Age *, years, median (IQR)	30 (26–34)	30 (26–33)	0.54
BMI *, kg/m^2, median (IQR)	23 (21–27)	23 (21–28)	0.77
25–29.9 kg/m^2, n (%)	44 (23.8%)	44 (23.8%)	
≥30 kg/m^2, n (%)	24 (13.0%)	24 (13.0%)	
Smokers, n (%)	51 (27.6%)	58 (31.4%)	0.42
Blood group			
O group, n (%)	82 (44.3%)	86 (46.5%)	0.68
Nulliparous, n (%)	97 (52.4%)	89 (48.1%)	0.41
Pregnancy characteristics			
Conception by ART, n (%)	21 (11.4%)	15 (8.1%)	0.29
Gemellar pregnancy, n (%)	17 (9.2%)	9 (4.9%)	0.10
Gestational diabetes, n (%)	20 (10.8%)	19 (10.3%)	1.0
Gestational weight gain, kg, median (IQR)	13 (8–18)	13 (9–17)	0.85
Pre-eclampsia, n (%)	12 (6.5%)	9 (4.9%)	0.50
IUGR, n (%)	6 (3.2%)	3 (1.6%)	0.51
Placental abruption, n (%)	2 (1.1%)	1 (0.5%)	0.50
Abnormal placental insertion, n (%)	17 (9.2%)	4 (2.2%)	0.003
Antepartum haemorrhage, n (%)	25 (13.5%)	14 (7.6%)	0.01
Delivery characteristics			
Term * at delivery, WG, median (IQR)	39 (37–40)	39 (37–40)	0.77
Induced labour, n (%)	69 (37.3%)	67 (36.2%)	0.83
Vaginal * delivery, n (%)	72 (38.9%)	72 (38.9%)	1.0
Instrumental delivery, n (%)	27 (14.6%)	17 (9.2%)	0.11
C-section *, n (%)	113 (61.1%)	113 (61.1%)	1.0
Emergency C-section, n (%)	77 (41.6%)	91 (49.2%)	0.14
Episiotomy, n (%)	42 (22.7%)	19 (10.3%)	0.001
Perineal tears, n (%)	48 (25.9%)	40 (21.6%)	0.33
Macrosomia, n (%)	17 (9.2%)	16 (8.6%)	0.86

* Matching criteria. ART = Assisted reproductive technology; BMI = body mass index; C-section = Caesarean section; IQR = interquartile range; IUGR = intrauterine growth restriction; PPH = postpartum haemorrhage; WG = weeks of gestation.

The characteristics of the women and pregnancies between both groups were similar, except for abnormal placental insertion, antepartum haemorrhage, and episiotomy, which were more frequently observed in the non-severe PPH cases compared to controls.

No pregnant women received anticoagulants the day before delivery, but three pregnant women in the control group were on low-dose aspirin in the days preceding delivery.

Among the 185 non-severe PPH cases, the three main aetiologies of PPH were uterine atony (n = 56, 30.3%), traumatic (n = 54, 29.2%), or placental causes (n = 38, 20.5%). In 39 pregnant women, two PPH aetiologies were combined; and in four, three PPH aetiologies were noted. In 33 (17.8%) PPH cases, no aetiology of PPH could be identified.

3.2. Predelivery Haemostatic Biomarkers and Their Association with Non-Severe PPH

Table 2 displays the median values of biomarkers of interest with interquartile ranges, stratified by group.

Table 2. Predelivery haemostatic biomarkers of the 370 pregnant women.

Haemostatic Biomarkers	Non-Severe PPH (n = 185)	Controls (n = 185)	p
Blood count parameters			
Haemoglobin, g/dL, median (IQR)	12.1 (11.4–12.8)	12.3 (11.4–12.9)	0.35
Platelets, G/L, median (IQR)	217 (181–259)	242 (196–280)	0.003
IPF, ratio, median (IQR)	5.1 (3.3–7.9)	4.9 (3.1–7.7)	0.63
Conventional haemostatic tests			
Prothrombin rate, %, median (IQR)	100 (94–100)	99 (94–100)	0.73
aPTT, ratio, median (IQR)	1.01 (0.95–1.06)	0.99 (0.94–1.06)	0.12
Fibrinogen, g/L, median (IQR)	4.85 (4.35–5.63)	5.09 (4.46–5.56)	0.32
D-dimer, µg/mL, median (IQR)	1.64 (1.24–2.21)	1.54 (1.08–2.06)	0.06
Fibrin monomers, µg/mL, median (IQR)	5.64 (4.39–9.61)	5.32 (3.98–7.08)	0.10
Thrombin generation assay			
Lag phase, min, median (IQR)	14.1 (12.6–15.1)	14.1 (12.1–15.6)	0.89
Thrombin peak, nmol/L, median (IQR)	294.5 (237.5–389.8)	314.9 (239.3–388.1)	0.57
Time to peak, min, median (IQR)	23.6 (20.6–25.6)	23.1 (20.6–25.6)	0.58
Velocity index, nmol/L/min, median (IQR)	32.6 (22.9–48.3)	35.1 (24.2–49.0)	0.50
ETP, nmol/L × min, median (IQR)	5 419 (4 978–5 919)	5 349 (5 038–5 876)	0.78
Plasmin generation assay			
Lag phase, min, median (IQR)	2.7 (2.6–3.0)	2.7 (2.3–3.0)	0.10
Plasmin peak, nmol/L, median (IQR)	66.8 (52.9–78.0)	67.9 (56.3–78.0)	0.46
Time to peak, min, median (IQR)	7.3 (7.0–8.0)	7.3 (7.0–8.0)	0.67
Velocity index, nmol/L/min, median (IQR)	14.2 (11.9–17.1)	13.8 (11.4–17.0)	0.65
EPP, nmol/L × min, median (IQR)	840.8 (540.6–1 111.8)	844.4 (537.1–1 070.4)	0.87

aPTT = activated partial thromboplastin time; EPP = endogenous plasmin potential; ETP = endogenous thrombin potential; IQR = interquartile range; IPF = immature platelet fraction; PPH = postpartum haemorrhage.

Pregnant women with non-severe PPH had a lower median [IQR] predelivery platelet count (217 [181–259] versus 242 [196–280] G/L, p = 0.003) compared to their matched pregnant controls. Two pregnant women (one case and one control) had a predelivery platelet count below 50 G/L. No significant difference was observed in conventional haemostatic tests. In the subset of women delivering vaginally, we found only weak evidence for lower median [IQR] predelivery platelet count (213 [170–256] versus 234 [192–279] G/L, p = 0.06) and median D-dimer levels (1.68 [1.31–2.13] versus 1.56 [1.15–1.86] µg/mL, p = 0.05) in non-severe PPH compared to matched controls (Table S1).

3.3. Thrombin Generation Assay (TGA)

We found no evidence for a difference in predelivery TGA parameters between non-severe PPH cases and pregnant controls in the full population (n = 370, Table 2). In women delivering vaginally (n = 144, 72 in each group), a decrease in median [IQR] thrombin peak was observed in non-severe PPH cases compared to matched pregnant controls (277.5 [228.6–355.0] versus 317.1 [258.9–410.8] nmol/L, $p = 0.047$) (Figure S1, Table S1).

Over the full population, a weak correlation between blood loss and predelivery TGA time to peak was observed ($\rho = 0.11$; 95% CI 0.01, 0.21) (Table S2), as it was the case in the subset of women delivering vaginally ($\rho = 0.22$; 95% CI 0.05, 0.37). In women delivering vaginally, blood loss was also weakly inversely correlated with predelivery TGA thrombin peak ($\rho = -0.20$; 95% CI -0.36, -0.04) and TGA velocity index ($\rho = -0.21$; 95% CI -0.36, -0.05).

3.4. Plasmin Generation Assay (PGA)

We found no evidence for a difference in predelivery PGA parameters between non-severe PPH cases and matched pregnant controls in the full population. However, in women delivering vaginally (n = 144), median [IQR] predelivery PGA lag phase was longer in non-severe PPH cases compared to matched controls (2.9 [2.7–3.2] versus 2.7 [2.3–3.0] min, $p = 0.008$) (Figure S2, Table S1).

3.5. Logistic Regression Analysis for Parameters Associated with Non-Severe PPH

The linear association of haemostatic biomarkers with non-severe PPH was investigated in a logistic regression model, adjusting for clinical parameters described in the literature associated with PPH.

To reduce the number of biomarkers, we conducted principal component analyses of the PGA and TGA parameters, respectively, representing them in the model with their respective first principal component.

Figure 2 depicts a hierarchical cluster analysis of all biomarkers of interest and a heatmap of their pairwise absolute Spearman's correlation coefficients. Expectedly, TGA parameters formed a separate cluster, showing high correlation between the curve parameters, albeit less so for ETP. With the exception of the PGA lag phase, which showed barely any correlation with the other curve parameters, PGA presented as a separate cluster with fibrinogen but only modest pairwise correlations, except for PGA plasmin peak and velocity index.

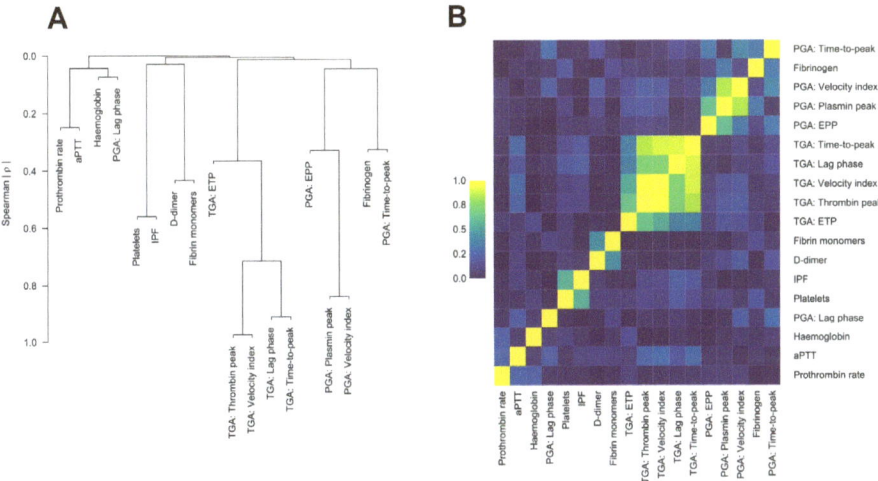

Figure 2. (**A**) Hierarchical cluster analysis of biomarkers of interest using the absolute values of the Spearman correlation coefficients to compute pairwise similarities. (**B**) Heatmap of the absolute values of pairwise Spearman correlation coefficients between biomarkers of interest.

In the logistic regression model presented in Table 3, only two parameters were significantly associated with non-severe PPH: abnormal placental insertion (OR = 3.37; 95%

CI 1.06–25.06) and predelivery platelet count. For each decrease in 10 G/L and 50 G/L of predelivery platelet count, the OR of predelivery platelet count for non-severe PPH was 1.06 (95% CI 1.02–1.12) and 1.35 (95% CI 1.10–1.80), respectively. Accordingly, the fraction of new information added to the model was highest for platelets (0.252), which was higher by a factor of 2.7 compared to the second-ranked biomarker, immature platelet fraction (0.094). The concordance index for the model was 0.66 and the Nagelkerke R2 0.11.

Table 3. Logistic regression analysis for biological and clinical parameters associated with non-severe PPH.

Biomarker	25th Percentile	75th Percentile	Difference	OR	95% CI	Fraction of New Information
Platelets (G/L)	187.50	271.50	84.00	0.61	0.37–0.86	0.252
Immature platelet fraction (%)	3.25	7.95	4.70	0.76	0.51–1.05	0.094
aPTT ratio (%)	0.94	1.06	0.12	1.31	0.98–2.02	0.093
Prothrombin time (%)	94.00	100.00	6.00	1.15	0.90–1.51	0.066
D-dimer (µg/mL)	1.16	2.12	0.96	1.10	0.88–1.96	0.024
Haemoglobin (g/dL)	11.40	12.90	1.50	0.92	0.65–1.30	0.009
PC1 plasmin generation assay	−0.92	0.96	1.88	0.93	0.63–1.25	0.007
Fibrinogen (g/L)	4.41	5.58	1.17	0.96	0.65–1.38	0.002
Fibrin monomers (µg/mL)	4.20	8.23	4.04	1.00	0.94–1.05	<0.001
PC1 thrombin generation assay	−0.75	1.12	1.87	0.99	0.72–1.30	<0.001
Adjusted for clinical covariates:						
Age (years)—matched	26.00	33.00	7.00	0.99	0.78–1.24	
BMI (kg/m^2)—matched	20.70	27.50	6.80	1.08	0.88–1.34	
Nulliparous (yes/no)	No	Yes		1.18	0.73–2.04	
Gemellar pregnancy (yes/no)	No	Yes		2.01	0.62–7.56	
Abnormal placental insertion (yes/no)	No	Yes		3.37	1.06–25.06	
Antepartum haemorrhage (yes/no)	No	Yes		1.51	0.67–3.65	
Pre-eclampsia (yes/no)	No	Yes		0.77	0.14–3.42	
Macrosomia (yes/no)	No	Yes		1.39	0.58–3.58	
Induced labour (yes/no)	No	Yes		1.09	0.67–1.84	
Term at delivery (WG)—matched	37.00	40.00	3.00	1.04	0.80–1.34	
Type of delivery—matched (elective/emergency C-section)				1.67	0.78–3.97	
(vaginal/emergency C-section)				1.23	0.91–1.66	

BMI = body mass index; CI = confidence interval; C-section = Caesarean section; OR = odds ratio; WG = weeks of gestation.

4. Discussion

In this nested case-control study derived from the French HPP-IPF cohort study, we aimed at evaluating the association of predelivery haemostatic biomarkers with non-severe PPH. Among the parameters that were measured in the study population, only one was significantly different between non-severe PPH cases and matched pregnant controls: the predelivery platelet count. We found no evidence for a difference in predelivery TGA and PGA parameters between non-severe PPH cases and matched controls. However, in pregnant women delivering vaginally, median predelivery TGA thrombin peak was lower and median predelivery PGA lag phase was longer in non-severe PPH cases compared to matched controls. Finally, when incorporating all the haemostatic parameters of interest in a logistic regression model adjusting for established clinical risk factors, predelivery platelet count remained independently associated with non-severe PPH, suggesting a potential role as a predictive biomarker for the assessment of PPH risk at entry in the delivery room.

The platelet count was the sole parameter that remained associated with non-severe PPH among a battery of haemostatic tests in our study. The association of predelivery platelet count with PPH is a consistent and important finding [11,12,21]. The platelet count as part of the blood count analysis is easy to perform and globally widely available. Recently, we published a systematic review and meta-analyses on predelivery haemostatic biomarkers associated with PPH [21]. That review included a total of 81 articles, of which 17 articles were included in the final quantitative synthesis, and various haemostatic parameters. We did not focus on non-severe PPH, but for severe PPH, predelivery platelet count was associated with the clinical outcome [21]. The results of this review are in line with the findings of the present study.

We did not find any significant difference in predelivery TGA parameters between non-severe PPH cases and controls in the study population. However, in the subgroup of women delivering vaginally, those with non-severe PPH had a slightly but significantly lower thrombin peak compared to matched controls. In a small case-control study focusing on severe PPH, within the same HPP-IPF cohort study, we observed lower predelivery ETP values measured with TGA in pregnant women who developed severe PPH, compared with matched controls [11]. Thus, reduced thrombin generation potential might promote PPH under certain circumstances. We hypothesise that changes in the coagulation profile observed before delivery could be more pronounced in pregnant women who later develop severe PPH than in women who develop non-severe PPH.

To the best of our knowledge, this is the first study exploring the association of predelivery PGA parameters with non-severe PPH. While we noted no significant difference in predelivery PGA parameters between non-severe PPH cases and matched controls, we detected a difference in predelivery PGA lag phase between cases and controls in the subgroup of pregnant women delivering vaginally. The longer predelivery PGA lag phase observed in non-severe PPH cases delivering vaginally could be interpreted not as a hypofibrinolytic tendency, but as a reflection of the lower predelivery thrombin generation potential, as suggested by their concomitant lower predelivery TGA thrombin peak.

PPH is a frequent complication of childbirth with many short-term and long-term consequences on women health [22]. Identifying pregnant women at risk for PPH is a key element in preventing this complication, but it remains a challenge. Our study suggests a potential role for predelivery platelet count in predicting PPH. Predelivery platelet count is already used in the USA to assess the risk of PPH at entry in the delivery room [23]. Other countries do not recommend performing a complete blood count prior to delivery. For example, in France, a complete blood count is recommended only at the sixth month of pregnancy, but it is not repeated before delivery in case of physiological pregnancy [24].

However, the role of coagulation in the occurrence of non-severe PPH could also be minor, compared with the role of other factors such as uterine atony. Indeed, uterine atony is the main aetiology of PPH, accounting for approximately 70% of PPH cases [25]. Risk factors for uterine atony are well known, such as obesity, excessive gestational weight gain, multiple pregnancy, macrosomia, labour induction or a prolonged duration of labour [25]. Efforts have been made in the past decade to reduce the occurrence of uterine atony worldwide by the systematic administration of uterotonics after delivery, as recommended by the WHO and the FIGO, but without significant reduction in the incidence of PPH [26,27]. Future research should focus on tools to identify pregnant women at risk for uterine atony and on efficient strategies to manage them appropriately during childbirth in order to avoid the occurrence of PPH. An American case-control study recently published in AJOG by Reitsma et al. performed mass spectrometry on predelivery plasma samples from pregnant women diagnosed with PPH and pregnant controls without PPH matched for age and delivery mode [28]. The authors identified differentially abundant plasma proteins, in particular prostaglandin D2 synthase (PTGDS), which was higher in PPH cases compared with controls [28]. As PTGDS is involved in smooth muscle relaxation and in the inhibition of platelet aggregation, this could be a missing link explaining the association between uterine atony, platelets, and PPH. The authors suggested that the biomarkers they identified as differentially expressed could be incorporated into a score predictive for PPH, which was also our objective in performing this exploratory study.

Our study has some limitations. The monocentric design of the study induced a selection bias, making our results not easily generalizable to other populations of pregnant women. The large number of biomarkers we looked at and the many univariable formal tests and subset analysis we performed led to a highly inflated alpha error and multiple testing issues. However, our study was exploratory and, thus, we refrained from any multiple-testing adjustments; nevertheless, we presented all formal testing that we conducted. The large number of tests thus weakens the evidence for differences found between study cohorts and needs to be acknowledged when interpreting the results. The logistic regression model further includes a large number of biomarkers and clinical covariates. As such, PGA and TGA were represented by their respective first principal component. Moreover, while we did model biomarkers continuously, we did not allow for non-linearity due to sample size limitations, which would be another important research question to investigate. Considering the study design and matching, we further only modelled associations and could not evaluate the predictive performance of the model or biomarkers.

The main strength of our study is the time of blood collection, i.e., at entry in the delivery room, before the clinical bleeding. This prospective design allowed us to investigate the predelivery coagulation profile of pregnant women who later developed non-severe PPH and test for haemostatic biomarkers potentially predictive for non-severe PPH. Second, we collected numerous clinical and biological data on each pregnant woman included in the study, which enabled us to consider a large number of parameters in the risk assessment of non-severe PPH. This study is one of the most comprehensive dealing with haemostatic parameters and the basis for further clinical research in that most important field.

5. Conclusions

In this case-control study of pregnant women from a large prospective cohort, predelivery platelet count was associated with non-severe PPH. Changes in other haemostatic parameters were tenuous in pregnant women later diagnosed with non-severe PPH and may not help for the prediction of PPH. Further prospective observational studies are needed to help with improving the prediction of PPH, what could result in efficient and tailored preventive strategies to avoid PPH events and their consequences on women's health.

Supplementary Materials: The following supporting information can be downloaded at https://www.mdpi.com/article/10.3390/jcm13144231/s1, Figure S1. Comparison of predelivery TGA thrombin peak in non-severe PPH cases and matched pregnant controls delivering vaginally. The superimposed box plot displays quartiles with whiskers extending to data points 1.5 times the interquartile range; Figure S2. Comparison of predelivery PGA lag phase in non-severe PPH cases and matched pregnant controls delivering vaginally. The superimposed box plot displays quartiles with whiskers extending to data points 1.5 times the interquartile range; Table S1. Predelivery biological characteristics of the 144 pregnant women with a vaginal delivery; Table S2. Correlation between blood loss in mL at delivery and predelivery biomarkers.

Author Contributions: C.d.M., I.P. and B.P.-P. designed the study. C.A. (Casilda Albert) and C.T. advocated the aetiology of PPH for each non-severe PPH case. C.d.M. and S.L. identified the women included in this study within the database of the HPP-IPF cohort study. C.d.M. and D.M. performed the biological measurements. A.S.W. provided the protocol for PGA. D.K. performed the statistical analyses. C.d.M. wrote the manuscript. C.d.M., I.P., D.K., B.P.-P., F.C., C.T., C.A. (Casilda Albert), H.G., D.M., A.S.W., J.G., T.S., L.L.R. and C.A. (Cihan Ay) interpreted the results. All authors have read and agreed to the published version of the manuscript.

Funding: This research received no external funding. The study was conducted in agreement and with the institutional support of Brest University Hospital, France, and the Medical University of Vienna, Austria, but without a specific grant.

Institutional Review Board Statement: The study was conducted in accordance with the Declaration of Helsinki, and approved by the Institutional Review Board of Brest University Hospital (Protocol RB 11.080; ID RCB: 2011-A00802-39) on 23 August 2011.

Informed Consent Statement: Informed consent was obtained from all the pregnant women included in the study.

Data Availability Statement: The data that support the findings of this study are available from the corresponding author (C.d.M.), upon reasonable request.

Acknowledgments: The authors thank the CIC 1412 CRB Santé BB-0033-00037 of Brest for providing high-quality and annotated samples. The authors thank in particular Sylvain Rosec, CIC-RB

Ressources Biologiques (UF 0827), Brest University Hospital, Brest, France, for his help in the identification of plasma samples. The authors also thank Birgit Fortsner and Marietta Kollars, Department of Medicine I, Clinical Division of Haematology and Haemostaseology, Medical University of Vienna, Vienna, Austria, for their technical support. Last, the authors thank all obstetricians, midwives, anaesthetists, and research assistants involved in the recruitment and inclusion of participants in Brest University Hospital, Brest, France.

Conflicts of Interest: The authors declare no conflict of interest.

References

1. Patek, K.; Friedman, P. Postpartum Hemorrhage—Epidemiology, Risk Factors, and Causes. *Clin. Obstet. Gynecol.* **2023**, *66*, 344–356. [CrossRef] [PubMed]
2. Oyelese, Y.; Ananth, C.V. Postpartum Hemorrhage: Epidemiology, Risk Factors, and Causes. *Clin. Obstet. Gynecol.* **2010**, *53*, 147–156. [CrossRef] [PubMed]
3. McLintock, C. Prevention and treatment of postpartum hemorrhage: Focus on hematological aspects of management. *Hematology 2020*, **2020**, 542–546. [CrossRef] [PubMed]
4. Calvert, C.; Thomas, S.L.; Ronsmans, C.; Wagner, K.S.; Adler, A.J.; Filippi, V. Identifying Regional Variation in the Prevalence of Postpartum Haemorrhage: A Systematic Review and Meta-Analysis. *PLoS ONE* **2012**, *7*, e41114. [CrossRef] [PubMed]
5. Dahlke, J.D.; Mendez-Figueroa, H.; Maggio, L.; Hauspurg, A.K.; Sperling, J.D.; Chauhan, S.P.; Rouse, D.J. Prevention and management of postpartum hemorrhage: A comparison of 4 national guidelines. *Am. J. Obstet. Gynecol.* **2015**, *213*, 76.e1–76.e10. [CrossRef] [PubMed]
6. Neary, C.; Naheed, S.; McLernon, D.J.; Blac, M. Predicting risk of postpartum haemorrhage: A systematic review. *BJOG Int. J. Obstet. Gynaecol.* **2021**, *128*, 46–53. [CrossRef] [PubMed]
7. Charbit, B.; Mandelbrot, L.; Samain, E.; Baron, G.; Haddaoui, B.; Keita, H.; Sibony, O.; Mahieu-Caputo, D.; Hurtaud-Roux, M.F.; Huisse, M.G.; et al. The decrease of fibrinogen is an early predictor of the severity of postpartum hemorrhage. *J. Thromb. Haemost.* **2007**, *5*, 266–273. [CrossRef] [PubMed]
8. Cortet, M.; Deneux-Tharaux, C.; Dupont, C.; Colin, C.; Rudigoz, R.-C.; Bouvier-Colle, M.-H.; Huissoud, C. Association between fibrinogen level and severity of postpartum hemorrhage: Secondary analysis of a prospective trial. *Br. J. Anaesth.* **2012**, *108*, 984–989. [CrossRef] [PubMed]
9. Huissoud, C.; Carrabin, N.; Audibert, F.; Levrat, A.; Massignon, D.; Berland, M.; Rudigoz, R. Bedside assessment of fibrinogen level in postpartum haemorrhage by thrombelastometry. *BJOG Int. J. Obstet. Gynaecol.* **2009**, *116*, 1097–1102. [CrossRef]
10. Collins, P.; Cannings-John, R.; Bruynseels, D.; Mallaiah, S.; Dick, J.; Elton, C.; Weeks, A.; Sanders, J.; Aawar, N.; Townson, J.; et al. Viscoelastometric-guided early fibrinogen concentrate replacement during postpartum haemorrhage: OBS2, a double-blind randomized controlled trial. *Br. J. Anaesth.* **2017**, *119*, 411–421. [CrossRef]
11. De Moreuil, C.; Dargaud, Y.; Nougier, C.; Dupré, P.-F.; Trémouilhac, C.; Le Joliff, D.; Rosec, S.; Lucier, S.; Pabinger, I.; Ay, C.; et al. Women with severe postpartum hemorrhage have a decreased endogenous thrombin potential before delivery. *J. Thromb. Haemost.* **2023**, *21*, 3099–3108. [CrossRef] [PubMed]
12. Salomon, C.; De Moreuil, C.; Hannigsberg, J.; Trémouilhac, C.; Drugmanne, G.; Gatineau, F.; Nowak, E.; Anouilh, F.; Briend, D.; Le Moigne, E.; et al. Haematological parameters associated with postpartum haemorrhage after vaginal delivery: Results from a French cohort study. *J. Gynecol. Obstet. Hum. Reprod.* **2021**, *50*, 102168. [CrossRef] [PubMed]
13. American College of Obstetricians and Gynecologists. Hypertension in pregnancy: Report of the American College of Obstetricians and Gynecologists' Task Force on Hypertension in Pregnancy. *Obstet. Gynecol.* **2013**, *122*, 1122–1131. [CrossRef]
14. World Health Organisation. WHO Recommendations for the Prevention and Treatment of Postpartum Haemorrhage. 2012. Available online: http://apps.who.int/iris/bitstream/handle/10665/75411/9789241548502_eng.pdf;jsessionid=8F11A00EB1C7BD4C058948030FBD1D77?sequence=1 (accessed on 14 January 2024).
15. Solomon, C.; Collis, R.; Collins, P. Haemostatic monitoring during postpartum haemorrhage and implications for management. *Br. J. Anaesth.* **2012**, *109*, 851–863. [CrossRef] [PubMed]
16. Hofer, S.; Ay, C.; Rejtö, J.; Wolberg, A.S.; Haslacher, H.; Koder, S.; Pabinger, I.; Gebhart, J. Thrombin-generating potential, plasma clot formation, and clot lysis are impaired in patients with bleeding of unknown cause. *J. Thromb. Haemost.* **2019**, *17*, 1478–1488. [CrossRef] [PubMed]
17. Miszta, A.; Ahmadzia, H.K.; Luban, N.L.C.; Li, S.; Guo, D.; Holle, L.A.; Berger, J.S.; James, A.H.; Gobburu, J.V.S.; Anker, J.v.D.; et al. Application of a plasmin generation assay to define pharmacodynamic effects of tranexamic acid in women undergoing cesarean delivery. *J. Thromb. Haemost.* **2021**, *19*, 221–232. [CrossRef] [PubMed]
18. Statistically Efficient Ways to Quantify Added Predictive Value of New Measurements. Available online: https://www.fharrell.com/post/addvalue/ (accessed on 14 January 2024).
19. R Core Team. *R: A Language and Environment for Statistical Computing*; R Foundation for Statistical Computing: Vienna, Austria, 2023. Available online: https://www.R-project.org/ (accessed on 14 January 2024).
20. Harrell, F.E., Jr. rms: Regression Modeling Strategies. R Package Version 6.7-1. 2023. Available online: https://CRAN.R-project.org/package=rms (accessed on 14 January 2024).

21. De Moreuil, C.; Mehic, D.; Nopp, S.; Kraemmer, D.; Gebhart, J.; Schramm, T.; Couturaud, F.; Ay, C.; Pabinger, I. Hemostatic biomarkers associated with postpartum hemorrhage: A systematic review and meta-analysis. *Blood Adv.* **2023**, *7*, 5954–5967. [CrossRef] [PubMed]
22. Eckerdal, P.; Kollia, N.; Löfblad, J.; Hellgren, C.; Karlsson, L.; Högberg, U.; Wikström, A.-K.; Skalkidou, A. Delineating the Association between Heavy Postpartum Haemorrhage and Postpartum Depression. *PLoS ONE* **2016**, *11*, e0144274. [CrossRef] [PubMed]
23. Kawakita, T.; Mokhtari, N.; Huang, J.C.; Landy, H.J. Evaluation of Risk-Assessment Tools for Severe Postpartum Hemorrhage in Women Undergoing Cesarean Delivery. *Obstet. Gynecol.* **2019**, *134*, 1308–1316. [CrossRef]
24. Collège National des Gynécologues et Obstétriciens Français (CNGOF). Guidelines for postpartum hemorrhage. *J. Gynecol. Obstet. Biol. Reprod.* **2004**, *33*, 4S130–134S136.
25. Bienstock, J.L.; Eke, A.C.; Hueppchen, N.A. Postpartum Hemorrhage. *N. Engl. J. Med.* **2021**, *384*, 1635–1645. [CrossRef] [PubMed]
26. World Health Organization. WHO Reommendations: Uterotonics for the Prevention of Postpartum Haemorrhage. Available online: https://www.who.int/publications/i/item/9789241550420 (accessed on 13 June 2024).
27. Escobar, M.F.; Nassar, A.H.; Theron, G.; Barnea, E.R.; Nicholson, W.; Ramasauskaite, D.; Lloyd, I.; Chandraharan, E.; Miller, S.; Burke, T.; et al. FIGO recommendations on the management of postpartum hemorrhage 2022. *Int. J. Gynecol. Obstet.* **2022**, *157* (Suppl. S1), 3–50. [CrossRef] [PubMed]
28. Reitsma, S.E.; Barsoum, J.R.; Hansen, K.C.; Sassin, A.M.; Dzieciatkowska, M.; James, A.H.; Aagaard, K.M.; Ahmadzia, H.K.; Wolberg, A.S. Agnostic identification of plasma biomarkers for postpartum hemorrhage risk. *Am. J. Obstet. Gynecol.* **2024**, in press. [CrossRef] [PubMed]

Disclaimer/Publisher's Note: The statements, opinions and data contained in all publications are solely those of the individual author(s) and contributor(s) and not of MDPI and/or the editor(s). MDPI and/or the editor(s) disclaim responsibility for any injury to people or property resulting from any ideas, methods, instructions or products referred to in the content.

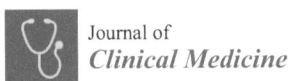

Article

Comparative Analysis of Therapeutic Showers and Bathtubs for Pain Management and Labor Outcomes—A Retrospective Cohort Study

Elena Mellado-García [1], Lourdes Díaz-Rodríguez [1], Jonathan Cortés-Martín [1], Juan Carlos Sánchez-García [1,*], Beatriz Piqueras-Sola [2], Juan Carlos Higuero Macías [3], Francisco Rivas Ruiz [3] and Raquel Rodríguez-Blanque [1,4]

1. Department of Nursing, Faculty of Health Sciences, University of Granada, 18016 Granada, Spain; e.elenamellado@go.ugr.es (E.M.-G.); cldiaz@ugr.es (L.D.-R.); jcortesmartin@ugr.es (J.C.-M.); rarobladoc@ugr.es (R.R.-B.)
2. Virgen de las Nieves University Hospital, 18014 Granada, Spain; beatriz.piqueras.sspa@juntadeandalucia.es
3. Costa del Sol University Hospital, 29603 Marbella, Spain; juancarlos.higueromacas@gmail.com (J.C.H.M.); francisco.rivas.ruiz.sspa@juntadeandalucia.es (F.R.R.)
4. San Cecilio University Hospital, 18016 Granada, Spain
* Correspondence: jsangar@ugr.es

Abstract: Hydrotherapy, including the use of therapeutic showers and bathtubs, has been studied for its potential benefits in labor pain management. Previous research has indicated that hydrotherapy can alleviate pain, but comparative studies between therapeutic showers and bathtubs are scarce. **Objective**: This study aims to compare the effects of therapeutic showers and bathtubs on pain perception, labor duration, use of epidural analgesia, and maternal and neonatal outcomes during labor. **Methods**: A total of 124 pregnant women were included in this study. Participants were divided into two groups: those who used a therapeutic shower and those who used a bathtub during labor. Pain levels were measured using a visual analog scale (VAS). Labor duration, use of epidural analgesia, types of delivery, maternal outcomes (postpartum hemorrhage, perineal status, maternal hypotension, fever, and breastfeeding), and neonatal outcomes (APGAR scores, fetal heart rate, complications, and neonatal unit admissions) were recorded and analyzed. **Results**: Both the therapeutic shower and the bathtub effectively reduced pain perception, with the bathtub showing a greater reduction in VAS scores. The therapeutic shower group experienced a significantly shorter labor duration compared to the bathtub group. The majority of participants in both groups did not require epidural analgesia, with no significant differences between the groups. There were no significant differences in the types of delivery. Maternal outcomes indicated a lower incidence of perineal tears and episiotomies in the therapeutic shower group. Neonatal outcomes, including APGAR scores and fetal heart rate, were similar between the groups, with no significant differences in complications or neonatal unit admissions. **Conclusions**: Both therapeutic showers and bathtubs are effective for pain relief during labor, with the bathtub showing a higher reduction in pain intensity. The therapeutic shower is associated with a shorter labor duration and a lower incidence of perineal tears and episiotomies. Both methods are safe for neonatal well-being, making hydrotherapy a viable non-pharmacological option for pain management in labor. However, the therapeutic shower may offer additional benefits in terms of labor duration and maternal outcomes.

Keywords: hydrotherapy; waterbirth; immersion; first labor stage; maternal health

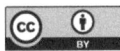

1. Introduction

Hydrotherapy as a method for managing pain during childbirth has been used for thousands of years, and its exact origin is unknown [1]. Currently, many women seek non-pharmacological methods for pain relief during labor. The use of hydrotherapy can provide natural pain relief because warm water helps relax muscles and can reduce the sensation of pain, allowing women to better manage contractions [1,2].

The use of warm water can help reduce anxiety and stress, promoting a state of calm that facilitates the birthing process. The option to choose hydrotherapy for pain management during labor can give women a sense of control and empowerment over their birthing experience [3]. It allows them to actively participate in their care and make informed decisions about pain management. It is important to consider that each woman has her own preferences and needs during labor, and the decision to use hydrotherapy should be individualized [4].

In 2022, the Health Technology Assessment Service of the Basque Country (OSTEBA), supported by the Spanish Ministry of Health, published a comprehensive report on water immersion during labor. This study focused on two main aspects: evaluating the efficacy, effectiveness, and safety of water immersion during labor, and understanding the values and preferences of women who had experienced this birthing method. Given existing concerns, particularly regarding the safety of the newborn, the report aimed to analyze the available evidence to determine the safety and efficacy of water immersion during labor for both the mother and the neonate [5].

According to the literature review, various studies have been conducted to demonstrate the efficacy of therapeutic showers during labor for pain relief, compared to women who do not use water during the birthing process [6,7]. However, as of our review, we have not found specific studies that directly compare therapeutic showers and bathtubs in this context. Nevertheless, there are articles that compare therapeutic showers with other non-pharmacological methods, such as the use of perineal exercises with a Swiss ball during the dilation phase. These studies have yielded equally interesting results, demonstrating that the combination of therapeutic showers with these exercises is associated with reduced pain during labor and greater comfort for the mother [8].

In a pretest-posttest design study with a single group of 24 women who used the therapeutic shower for 30 min, numerical pain rating scales were evaluated before and after use. A significant decrease in both pain perception and levels of tension and anxiety was observed after the intervention [9].

Currently, in Spain, maternity units are incorporating bathtubs in their delivery rooms, but not all hospitals in the country can offer these services due to a lack of necessary infrastructure, specifically bathtubs for water immersion use by pregnant women during labor. Some delivery rooms have therapeutic showers available, but these do not provide full water immersion. The purpose of the present study was to compare whether therapeutic showers can be as effective as bathtubs regarding labor duration, use of analgesia, pain relief, and maternal and fetal outcomes.

Objectives

To evaluate and compare the effects of using a bathtub and a therapeutic shower during labor on pain perception, the use of epidural analgesia, labor duration, and maternal and fetal outcomes.

2. Materials and Methods

2.1. Study Design

This is a retrospective cohort study of women who chose to use hydrotherapy during their labor. The report of this research follows the STROBE guidelines for observational studies. The study was conducted in accordance with the Declaration of Helsinki for research involving humans and was approved by the Ethics Committee of Hospital Costa del Sol (002_oct18_PI-hydrotherapy in labor) in November 2018.

2.2. Setting

These are secondary outcomes from a study that evaluated the use of hydrotherapy during labor. The initial study included women who gave birth at Hospital Costa del Sol,

Málaga (Spain), during the period between January 2010, when hydrotherapy began to be offered during labor at the hospital, and December 2020. In this hospital, the use of hydrotherapy is indicated in the first stage of labor, either through a therapeutic shower or by immersion in a bathtub. Data were collected from each woman's partogram as well as from the medical records of both the mother and the newborn.

2.3. Participants

Our study included women with low-risk pregnancies and labors, which means they had a healthy singleton pregnancy, a body mass index of 30 kg/m^2 or less, cephalic presentation, spontaneous onset of labor, a gestational age between 37 + 0 and 41 + 6 weeks, and a normal cardiotocographic record upon admission. Women with multiple pregnancies and those who gave birth before 37 weeks or after 42 weeks were excluded. According to the protocol of our Labor Unit, all admitted women were offered the option to use hydrotherapy during the labor process. The participants in this study had no history of opioid medication use.

2.4. Variables and Data Sources

The study meticulously planned data coding in advance, extracting data directly from medical records into a structured database. It analyzes a variety of variables related to labor and hydrotherapy. Regarding pain relief during labor, pain perception was assessed using the visual analogue scale (VAS) in both the therapeutic shower group and the bathtub group, as well as comparing the median pain scores before and after the use of each method. Regarding labor duration, dilation times and overall labor time were examined in both groups. The use of epidural analgesia during labor was also recorded. In terms of delivery types, the proportion of spontaneous and operative deliveries in each group was observed. Additionally, various maternal outcomes were explored, including the incidence of postpartum hemorrhage, perineal status, presence of hypotension, maternal fever, and breastfeeding. As for neonatal outcomes, APGAR scores, fetal heart rate, fetal complications, and neonatal unit admission were analyzed.

2.5. Bias

To mitigate potential biases, the study established precise inclusion and exclusion criteria for participants, ensured data anonymity, and conducted meticulous data coding. Additionally, confounding variables were controlled through multivariable statistical analysis. These measures ensured the validity and reliability of the findings obtained in this retrospective cohort study.

2.6. Study Size

The sample size for this study was determined using the same parameters and methodology as the previously published initial study [10]. For the primary objective of comparing the duration of the first stage of labor between the hydrotherapy group and the non-hydrotherapy group, a statistically significant difference of 16 min between the groups was considered. Based on the study by Torkamani, Kangani, and Janani (2010) [11], a standard deviation of 48 min was used for each group. With a type I error (alpha) of 0.05 and a type II error (beta) of 0.20, it was determined that 111 patients per group were required. Considering a 10% loss rate in the evaluation of medical records, the total sample size was adjusted to 248 patients, evenly distributed as 124 patients per group.

To ensure the robustness of the results and to study additional data of interest, the sample was expanded to a total of 377 women, with 253 individuals in the control group and 124 in the hydrotherapy experimental group. This approach allowed us to further explore various relevant clinical and demographic aspects while maintaining consistency with the originally calculated sample size from the initial study.

2.7. Statistical Methods

Descriptive analysis was performed using measures of central tendency, dispersion, and position (median and interquartile range (P75–P25)) for quantitative variables and frequency distribution for qualitative variables. To assess differences between study groups (bath vs. shower), the chi-squared test (or Fisher's exact test if expected frequencies were less than 5) was used for qualitative variables, while Student's t-test (or Mann–Whitney U test if the distribution was non-normal) was used for quantitative variables. Using pain as the outcome variable, a multivariate linear regression model was employed, including unbalanced independent variables from previous bivariate analysis, selecting variables with a criterion of $p < 0.05$, and describing the Beta coefficient (β) with respective 95% confidence intervals (CI95%). This involved checking for normality, homoscedasticity, and multicollinearity.

For all analyses, the level of statistical significance was set at $p < 0.05$. The analysis was performed using SPSS vs. 28.0 program for Windows (IBM Corporation, Armonk, NY, USA) statistical software.

2.8. Ethics Statement

This study was conducted in accordance with the Declaration of Helsinki for research involving human subjects. The Ethics Committee of the Costa del Sol Hospital approved the study in November 2018 under reference number 002_oct18_PI-hydrotherapy birth, ensuring the ethical compliance of the research.

No personal or identifying information was collected. Anonymity was guaranteed by the research service of Hospital Costa del Sol, which anonymized the personal or identifying data of the women involved in the study. Additionally, the data were stored on a password-protected personal computer.

3. Results

The results examined the effect of hydrotherapy, both in the form of a bathtub and a therapeutic shower, in relation to pain relief during labor, its duration, the use of pharmacological analgesia, and delivery types. Additionally, maternal and fetal outcomes were analyzed based on whether water immersion in a bathtub or the use of water in a therapeutic shower was performed.

For this study, a sample of 124 laboring women was recruited using a systematic sampling approach. This included 44 women (35.5%) who utilized the therapeutic shower and 80 women (64.5%) who immersed themselves in a bathtub with water immersion (Figure 1).

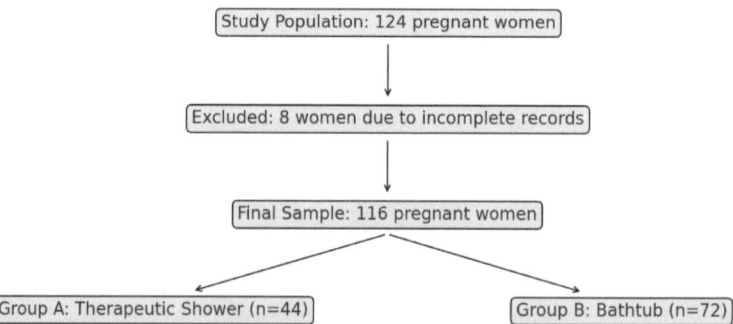

Figure 1. Flow diagram.

To determine if there were significant differences between the groups, the obstetric characteristics of the sample were evaluated, which are presented in Table 1:

Table 1. Baseline characteristics of the sample.

Variables		Therapeutic Shower	Bathtub	Total	p-Value
Age; Mean ± SD		30.70 ± 5.083	32.25 ± 5.784		0.140
Gestation grouped; n (%)	1	19 (43.2%)	43 (53.8%)	62 (50%)	0.549
	2	17 (38.6%)	21 (26.3%)	38 (30.6%)	
	3 or more	8 (18.2%)	16 (20%)	24 (19.4%)	
Abortions; n (%)	Absence	36 (81.8%)	59 (73.8%)	95 (76.6%)	0.427
	Presence	8 (18.2%)	21 (26.3%)	29 (23.4%)	
Previous Children	0	23 (52.3%)	54 (67.5%)	77 (62.1%)	0.139
	1 or more	21 (47.7%)	26 (32.5%)	47 (37.9%)	

These results demonstrate the distribution of key obstetric characteristics between women who used a therapeutic shower and those who used a bathtub during labor. No statistically significant differences were found between the groups in terms of age, grouped gestation, history of abortions, or the number of previous children.

As shown in Table 2, the primary and secondary outcomes of our study indicate significant differences in the total labor time and intact perineal state between the groups using the therapeutic shower and the bathtub. However, no significant differences were found in the use of epidural analgesia, types of delivery, or the incidence of maternal fever and breastfeeding.

Table 2. Summary of Primary and Secondary Outcomes.

Outcomes	Therapeutic Shower Group	Bathtub Group	p-Value
Primary Outcomes			
Total labor time (minutes)	155 (96.25–242.5)	227.5 (141.25–403.75)	0.004
Use of epidural analgesia	7 (15.9%)	18 (22.5%)	0.521
Types of delivery (% spontaneous)	97.7%	97.5%	>0.05
Pain perception before (VAS)	8 (7–9)	7 (7–8)	-
Pain perception after (VAS)	7.5 (6.25–8.75)	5 (4–7)	-
Secondary Outcomes			
Postpartum hemorrhage	2 (4.5%)	4 (5.0%)	>0.05
Intact perineal state	45.5%	23.8%	0.022
Maternal hypotension	9.1%	3.8%	0.244
Maternal fever	0%	1 (1.3%)	>0.05
Breastfeeding	95.5%	96.3%	1.000
APGAR score at 1 min (median, IQR)	Not specified	Not specified	Not specified
APGAR score at 5 min (median, IQR)	Not specified	Not specified	Not specified
Fetal heart rate	No specified complications	No specified complications	>0.05

3.1. Pain Relief

The initial findings of this study revealed statistically significant differences between the use of hydrotherapy during labor compared to non-use, regardless of whether a therapeutic shower or bathtub was utilized during labor [10]. At this juncture, we scrutinized the sensation of pain in the bathtub versus the therapeutic shower.

Our sample, comprised of 124 pregnant women, furnishes comparative data on perceived pain during the use of therapeutic showers and bathtubs. In the therapeutic shower group, eight cases were lost, while in the bathtub group, five cases were lost due to lack of recording.

According to the results presented, both the use of therapeutic showers and bathtubs show a reduction in pain perception compared to the sensation of pain prior to their use. However, this decrease is more pronounced in the bathtub group, with the difference in the pain perception scale before and after use being statistically significant ($p = 0.003$). In contrast, in the therapeutic shower group, although there is a noticeable reduction in pain perception, this difference does not reach statistical significance ($p = 0.083$) (Figures 2 and 3).

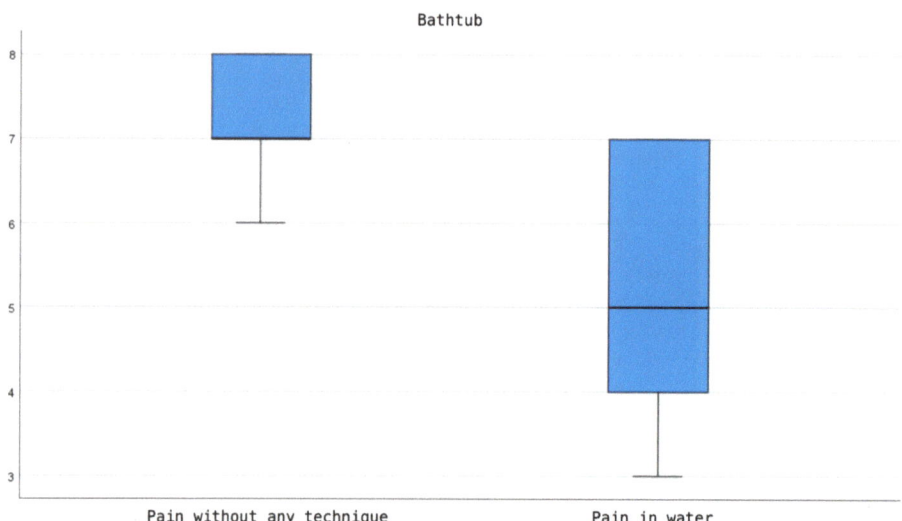

Figure 2. Comparison of Pain Intensity in the Bathtub, Before and After Use.

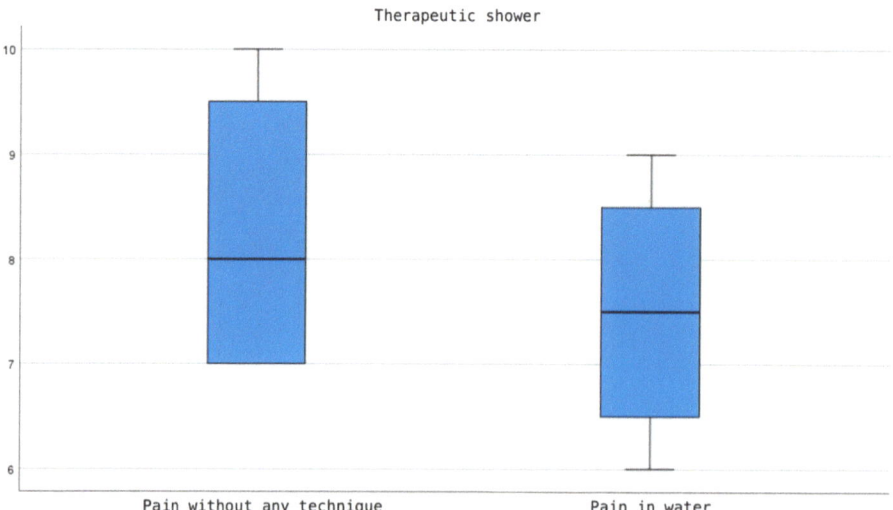

Figure 3. Comparison of Pain Intensity in the Therapeutic Shower, Before and After Use.

3.2. Duration of Labor

Upon examining the results between the group using the therapeutic shower and the group using the bathtub, it was found that dilation times and overall labor duration showed significant differences between the two groups, favoring the group that used the therapeutic shower (Table 3).

Table 3. Results of Labor Duration by Stages in the Use of Bathtub and Therapeutic Shower.

Therapeutic Shower vs. Bathtub			Dilation Time	Expulsive Time	Placental Expulsion Time	Total Labor Time
Therapeutic shower	n	Valid	44	44	44	44
		Missing	0	0	0	0
	Median		90	31	10	155
	Percentile	25	56.25	16.25	10	96.25
		75	133.75	53.75	16.75	242.5
Bathtub	n	Valid	80	80	80	80
		Missing	0	0	0	0
	Median		150	44	10	227.5
	Percentile	25	93.75	15	10	141.25
		75	240	90	15	403.75
p valor			0.002	0.167	0.865	0.004

3.3. Use of Analgesia

A total of 99 pregnant women did not use epidural analgesia, representing 79.8% of the 124 women in our study. The comparison between groups yielded a non-significant result, indicating no association between epidural use and the bathing method, whether therapeutic shower or bathtub.

3.4. Types of Delivery

The data comparing the therapeutic shower group and the bathtub group, as well as the types of delivery, are very similar. According to the *p*-values obtained, none of the statistical tests performed indicate a statistically significant association between the type of delivery and the bathing method. All *p*-values are well above the 0.05 threshold. Therefore, no significant differences were found between the use of the bathtub and the therapeutic shower concerning the types of delivery. The analysis indicates that in the therapeutic shower group, 2.3% of deliveries were operative vaginal and operative cesarean, while 97.7% were spontaneous vaginal. In the bathtub group, 2.5% of deliveries were operative vaginal and operative cesarean, and 97.5% were spontaneous vaginal.

3.5. Maternal Outcomes

The effect of the therapeutic shower and bathtub on various maternal parameters has been investigated:

3.5.1. Postpartum Hemorrhage

There were two cases of postpartum hemorrhage in the therapeutic shower group and four cases in the bathtub group, representing 4.5% and 5.0% of the sample, respectively. However, no statistically significant differences were found regarding this variable.

3.5.2. Postpartum Perineal Status

The study results indicate a statistically significant decrease in the frequency of 1st, 2nd, and 3rd-degree tears, as well as episiotomies, in favor of the group that used the therapeutic shower. In the therapeutic shower group, 45.5% of women had an intact perineum after delivery, compared to 23.8% in the bathtub group. The incidence of 1st, 2nd, and 3rd-degree tears and episiotomies was 54.5% and 76.3%, respectively. The *p*-value of 0.022 suggests that the use of the therapeutic shower was associated with a lower incidence of tears and episiotomies compared to the use of the bathtub.

3.5.3. Maternal Hypotension

It was observed that 9.1% of women in the therapeutic shower group experienced hypotension, compared to 3.8% of women who used the bathtub. However, the *p*-value of 0.244 does not show statistically significant differences between the groups.

3.5.4. Maternal Fever

In the therapeutic shower group, no cases of fever were recorded, while in the bathtub group, there was one case with a fever above 38 °C. No significant differences were found between the groups concerning this variable.

3.5.5. Breastfeeding

No statistically significant differences were recorded ($p = 1.000$); both percentages were high, with 95.5% for women who used the therapeutic shower compared to 96.3% for those who used the bathtub.

3.6. Neonatal Outcomes

Regarding fetal parameters, the analysis between the groups revealed no significant differences in APGAR scores at 1 and 5 min, except for one case in the bathtub group with an APGAR score at 1 min below 7. Fetal heart rate (FHR) was normal in 94.4% of cases in both groups. Specifically, in the therapeutic shower group, 6.8% had a non-reassuring fetal cardiotocographic record (FCTG), while in the bathtub group, this percentage was 5%. No significant differences were found in the APGAR and FCTG variables.

Regarding fetal complications and neonatal unit admissions (NICU), 119 newborns did not have complications, and 118 did not require NICU admission, representing 96% and 95.2% of the sample, respectively. Fetal complications occurred in 5% of the newborns in the bathtub group and 2.3% of the newborns in the therapeutic shower group. NICU admission occurred in 5% of the newborns in the bathtub group and 4.5% of the newborns in the therapeutic shower group. No significant differences were found for these two variables, thus no relationship could be established between the method of water use during labor and the presence of fetal complications or NICU admissions.

4. Discussion

We focused on investigating the effect of hydrotherapy during labor, according to the use of a bathtub or therapeutic shower, in relation to perceived pain, labor duration, analgesia use, and maternal and neonatal outcomes. The objective is to contribute to the scientific evidence by comparing these two groups, which is uncommon due to the scarcity of literature addressing this comparison.

Pain management is a fundamental aspect of labor care, which is why it has been the subject of numerous scientific investigations studying its relationship with non-pharmacological methods such as hydrotherapy. Publications analyzing both the therapeutic shower and the bathtub encompassed in hydrotherapy in general emphasize how the sensation of pain can decrease through the use of hydrotherapy. Our study also corroborates these findings: the comparison between the groups shows that the bathtub reduces the sensation of pain by one point more on the visual analog scale (VAS) compared to the therapeutic shower. Other studies, such as the one conducted by Davim et al. [12], have observed that pain relief increases as dilation progresses during labor when using the therapeutic shower. In a clinical trial conducted by Lee et al. [6], it was demonstrated that the therapeutic shower is a cost-effective, comfortable, and easy-to-perform non-pharmacological method for reducing pain, with positive results on a visual analog pain scale. A systematic review by Vargens, Silva, and Progianti [3] compiled 21 articles on the use of hydrotherapy and concluded that both the bathtub and the therapeutic shower effectively reduce pain during labor.

Our study also shows that the therapeutic shower results in a shorter labor duration compared to the use of the bathtub. Numerous studies discuss the use of the bathtub as a pain relief method [13–17], while there are also studies addressing the use of the therapeutic shower [6,7,12,13,18]. A decrease in dilation time and total labor duration has been observed when using the therapeutic shower as a method. Gallo et al. [13] detailed in their randomized trial how a warm shower at more than 7 cm dilation, combined with exercises on a Swiss ball and lumbosacral massage before 7 cm, yielded significant benefits, such as a reduction of 72 min compared to the group that did not use non-pharmacological techniques during labor, as well as differences in faster expulsion times.

Regarding specific research on analgesia use, the systematic review by Cluett et al. [1] revealed discrepancies in the use of epidural analgesia among women who opted for water immersion during the first stage of labor and those who did not. It was observed that in the group of women who experienced water labor, a smaller proportion opted for epidural analgesia compared to the groups that did not use water as a pain relief method. However, no significant differences were found in the use of epidural analgesia or the use of pethidine/narcotics between the different groups. In our study, we found a significant association between the use of epidural and the use of hydrotherapy, either in a bathtub or therapeutic shower, considering that the majority of pregnant women who used the therapeutic shower or bathtub did not use epidural analgesia. Authors like Gallo et al. [13] and Stark [7] describe the therapeutic shower as one of the beneficial non-pharmacological interventions, with few side effects or contraindications, allowing for a reduction in pain perception and even reducing the use of epidural analgesia, although Stark's study [7] found similar use of epidural analgesia in both the therapeutic shower group and the control group.

The randomized trial by Gallo et al. [13] not only studied variables such as pain and labor duration in women who used the therapeutic shower but also examined other parameters similar to those measured in our study. However, it is important to note that Gallo et al.'s study compared the use of the therapeutic shower with exercises on a Swiss ball and lumbosacral massage. Among the results, neonatal effects stood out: the experimental group had a lower risk of respiratory distress and significantly better Apgar scores. However, no significant differences were observed regarding delivery types, perineal status, or obstetric complications. In our study, we also evaluated these parameters and found no significant differences, except in postpartum perineal status, where we observed a decrease in the frequency of tears and episiotomies in the group that used the therapeutic shower.

The main limitation was the lack of exhaustive records in medical histories, leading to a sample of sixteen pregnant women, as previous information was not typically recorded in these histories. Another limitation was the absence of data related to the water temperature of the bathtub or therapeutic shower, information that would have been useful to assess its possible impact on the health of pregnant women and fetal development. Water temperature could influence various physiological factors, such as blood circulation and muscle relaxation, in addition to preventing risks associated with extreme temperatures, such as overheating or thermal shock. Additionally, the retrospective nature of the study conducted at a single institution is a significant limitation, predisposing the results to considerable bias. This characteristic prevents the generalization of the findings to other populations or contexts.

5. Conclusions

The study demonstrates that hydrotherapy, through the use of both bathtubs and therapeutic showers, effectively reduces pain perception during labor. The bathtub, in particular, provides a slightly higher pain relief compared to the therapeutic shower. Moreover, the therapeutic shower is associated with a shorter labor duration. Despite these benefits, it is important to acknowledge the limitations, such as the retrospective nature of the study conducted at a single institution, which may introduce significant bias and limit the generalizability of the results. Further research with larger, multicenter studies is needed to validate these findings.

Author Contributions: Conceptualization, R.R.-B., J.C.-M., E.M.-G. and J.C.S.-G.; data curation, J.C.-M., L.D.-R., J.C.S.-G. and J.C.H.M.; formal analysis, F.R.R. and J.C.S.-G.; investigation, R.R.-B., L.D.-R., E.M.-G. and J.C.S.-G.; methodology, F.R.R., E.M.-G., R.R.-B. and L.D.-R.; project administration, R.R.-B., B.P.-S., J.C.-M. and J.C.S.-G.; resources, E.M.-G., J.C.S.-G., R.R.-B. and L.D.-R.; supervision, L.D.-R. and R.R.-B.; validation, R.R.-B., J.C.-M., L.D.-R., B.P.-S. and E.M.-G.; visualization,

R.R.-B., J.C.-M. and L.D.-R.; writing—original draft preparation, J.C.-M., R.R.-B., E.M.-G. and J.C.S.-G.; writing—review and editing, R.R.-B., J.C.-M., B.P.-S., E.M.-G., L.D.-R. and J.C.S.-G. All authors have read and agreed to the published version of the manuscript.

Funding: This research received no external funding.

Institutional Review Board Statement: The Ethics Committee of the Hospital Costa del Sol approved this study in November 2018 under reference number 002_oct18_PI-hydrotherapy birth, thus ensuring the ethical compliance of the research in question.

Informed Consent Statement: Not applicable.

Data Availability Statement: Data regarding this study are available upon request from the corresponding author.

Acknowledgments: This study was carried out within the framework of the research project "Effects of hydrotherapy during labor in terms of maternal and neonatal health", which is part of the Doctoral Programme in Clinical Medicine and Public Health at the University of Granada. We are grateful to the Official College of Nursing of Granada (CODEGRA) for their help in the research support program, and to the Chair of Research in Nursing Care of the University of Granada and the Official College of Nursing of Granada. We thank the Research and Innovation Unit of the Costa del Sol Universitary Hospital for their help in obtaining the data related to the study. We thank our medical translator Megan Berry for her services and comments that contributed to improving this manuscript for publication.

Conflicts of Interest: The authors declare no conflicts of interest.

References

1. Cluett, E.R.; Burns, E.; Cuthbert, A. Immersion in Water during Labour and Birth. *Cochrane Database Syst. Rev.* **2018**, *5*, CD000111. [CrossRef] [PubMed]
2. Benko A Waterbirth: Is It a Real Choise. *Midwifery Matters* **2009**, *122*, 9–12.
3. Vargens, O.M.C.; Silva, A.C.V.; Progianti, J.M. Non-Invasive Nursing Technologies for Pain Relief during Childbirth—The Brazilian Nurse Midwives' View. *Midwifery* **2013**, *29*, e99–e106. [CrossRef] [PubMed]
4. Fair, C.D.; Crawford, A.; Houpt, B.; Latham, V. "After Having a Waterbirth, I Feel like It's the Only Way People Should Deliver Babies": The Decision Making Process of Women Who Plan a Waterbirth. *Midwifery* **2020**, *82*, 102622. [CrossRef] [PubMed]
5. Reviriego Rodrigo, E.; Ibargoyen-Roteta, N.; Carreguí Vilar, S.; Mediavilla Serrano, L.; Montero Carcaboso, S.; Ares Mateos, G.; Castelló Zamora, B.; Moreno Rodríguez, A.; Hernández Tejada, N.; Koetsenruyter, C. *Inmersión En Agua Durante El Parto. Informes de Evaluación de Tecnologías Sanitarias*, Vitoria-Gasteiz, 2022.
6. Lee, S.; Liu, C.; Lu, Y.; Gau, M. Efficacy of Warm Showers on Labor Pain and Birth Experiences During the First Labor Stage. *J. Obstet. Gynecol. Neonatal Nurs.* **2013**, *42*, 19–28. [CrossRef] [PubMed]
7. Stark, M.A. Testing the Effectiveness of Therapeutic Showering in Labor. *J. Perinat. Neonatal Nurs.* **2017**, *31*, 109–117. [CrossRef] [PubMed]
8. Barbieri, M.; Henrique, A.J.; Chors, F.M.; de Maia, N.L.; Gabrielloni, M.C. Warm Shower Aspersion, Perineal Exercises with Swiss Ball and Pain in Labor. *Acta Paul. Enferm.* **2013**, *26*, 478–484. [CrossRef]
9. Stark, M.A. Therapeutic Showering in Labor. *Clin. Nurs. Res.* **2013**, *22*, 359–374. [CrossRef] [PubMed]
10. Mellado-García, E.; Díaz-Rodríguez, L.; Cortés-Martín, J.; Sánchez-García, J.C.; Piqueras-Sola, B.; Higuero Macías, J.C.; Rodríguez-Blanque, R. Effects of Hydrotherapy on the Management of Childbirth and Its Outcomes—A Retrospective Cohort Study. *Nurs. Rep.* **2024**, *14*, 1251–1259. [CrossRef] [PubMed]
11. Akbari Torkamani, S.; Kangani, F.; Janani, F. The Effects of Delivery in Water on Duration of Delivery and Pain Compared with Normal Delivery. *Pak. J. Med. Sci.* **2010**, *26*, 551–555.
12. Davim, R.M.B.; Torres, G.D.V.; Dantas, J.D.C.; de Melo, E.S.; Paiva, C.P.; Vieira, D.; Costa, I.K.F. Showering as a Non Pharmacological Strategy to Relief the Parturients Pain. *Rev. Eletrônica Enferm.* **2008**, *10*, 600–609. [CrossRef]
13. Gallo, R.B.S.; Santana, L.S.; Marcolin, A.C.; Duarte, G.; Quintana, S.M. Sequential Application of Non-Pharmacological Interventions Reduces the Severity of Labour Pain, Delays Use of Pharmacological Analgesia, and Improves Some Obstetric Outcomes: A Randomised Trial. *J. Physiother.* **2018**, *64*, 33–40. [CrossRef] [PubMed]
14. Ulfsdottir, H.; Saltvedt, S.; Georgsson, S. Women's Experiences of Waterbirth Compared with Conventional Uncomplicated Births. *Midwifery* **2019**, *79*. [CrossRef] [PubMed]
15. Camargo, J.C.S.; Varela, V.; Ferreira, F.M.; Pougy, L.; Ochiai, A.M.; Santos, M.E.; Grande, M.C.L.R. The Waterbirth Project: São Bernardo Hospital Experience. *Women Birth* **2018**, *31*, e325–e333. [CrossRef] [PubMed]
16. Zanetti-Daellenbach, R.A.; Tschudin, S.; Zhong, X.Y.; Holzgreve, W.; Lapaire, O.; Hösli, I. Maternal and Neonatal Infections and Obstetrical Outcome in Water Birth. *Eur. J. Obstet. Gynecol. Reprod. Biol.* **2007**, *134*, 37–43. [CrossRef] [PubMed]

17. Nutter, E.; Meyer, S.; Shaw-Battista, J.; Marowitz, A. Waterbirth: An Integrative Analysis of Peer-Reviewed Literature. *J. Midwifery Womens Health* **2014**, *59*, 286–319. [CrossRef] [PubMed]
18. Benfield, R.; Heitkemper, M.M.; Newton, E.R. Culture, Bathing and Hydrotherapy in Labor: An Exploratory Descriptive Pilot Study. *Midwifery* **2018**, *64*, 110–114. [CrossRef] [PubMed]

Disclaimer/Publisher's Note: The statements, opinions and data contained in all publications are solely those of the individual author(s) and contributor(s) and not of MDPI and/or the editor(s). MDPI and/or the editor(s) disclaim responsibility for any injury to people or property resulting from any ideas, methods, instructions or products referred to in the content.

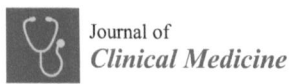

Systematic Review

Hydrotherapy in Pain Management in Pregnant Women: A Meta-Analysis of Randomized Clinical Trials

Elena Mellado-García [1], Lourdes Díaz-Rodríguez [1], Jonathan Cortés-Martín [1], Juan Carlos Sánchez-García [1,*], Beatriz Piqueras-Sola [2], María Montserrat Prieto Franganillo [3] and Raquel Rodríguez-Blanque [1,3]

[1] Department of Nursing, Faculty of Health Sciences, University of Granada, 18016 Granada, Spain; e.elenamellado@go.ugr.es (E.M.-G.); cldiaz@ugr.es (L.D.-R.); jcortesmartin@ugr.es (J.C.-M.); rarobladoc@ugr.es (R.R.-B.)
[2] Virgen de las Nieves University Hospital, 18014 Granada, Spain; beatriz.piqueras.sspa@juntadeandalucia.es
[3] San Cecilio University Clinical Hospital, 18016 Granada, Spain; montseprietof@gmail.com
* Correspondence: jsangar@ugr.es

Abstract: Background: the benefits of water are significant during the birth process. Improved maternal experience of labor, less use of epidurals, better pain management, shorter labor, and a greater sense of control are observed during the birth process. **Objective**: This report aims to determine the benefits of hydrotherapy in clinical childbirth approaches and its applicability in pain control. **Methods:** A meta-analysis of randomized clinical trials selected from various databases with no publication date limits was conducted, comparing groups that did not use hydrotherapy with groups that did during labor. **Results:** Seven articles met the inclusion criteria, with five articles using hot water immersion and two using hot water shower as hydrotherapy treatments. This study identified 840 participants, with the intervention groups including 417 term pregnant women and the control groups including 423 pregnant women. The effect size of hydrotherapy on pain was calculated using the visual analog scale in five articles and analgesic use in the other two articles. Hydrotherapy significantly reduced pain during labor with a mean difference of -0.97 (95% CI: -1.91 to -0.03; $I^2 = 97.32\%$, $p < 0.001$). The duration of the first stage of labor was not significantly affected, with a mean difference of -0.17 h (95% CI: -0.55 to 0.21; $I^2 = 56.75\%$, $p = 0.059$). Additionally, hydrotherapy did not significantly impact the newborns' Apgar scores at 5 min, with a mean difference of 0.18 (95% CI: -0.48 to 0.85; $I^2 = 2.15\%$, $p = 0.939$). **Conclusions:** Hydrotherapy is beneficial for pain control in the first stage of labor and does not increase its duration or negatively affect the Apgar score of newborns.

Keywords: hydrotherapy; waterbirth; immersion; first labor stage; neonatal health; maternal health

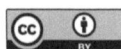

1. Introduction

The use of water as a therapeutic medium has ancient origins, with evidence showing its use in China, Egypt, Japan, Greece, and Rome for treating physical and psychological ailments. In their literature review, Cluett, Burns, and Cuthbert report on the existence of historical references documenting the use of water immersion during childbirth for the purpose of achieving relaxation and pain relief [1]. Hydrotherapy during childbirth focuses on the comfort and support of pregnant women, and many find this method beneficial [2]. Water can be used during the first stage of labor (dilation), the second stage (expulsion), or both. In Spain, the Clinical Practice Guideline on Normal Childbirth recommends warm water immersion as an effective pain relief method during the active first stage of labor [3].

This method has several key features that make it an attractive option. Hydrotherapy is primarily used during the first stage of labor, when contractions are most intense and cervical dilation is in progress. The water temperature is typically maintained around 37.4 °C, which is comfortable for the mother and safe for the newborn. The water helps reduce pain and stress and can accelerate the dilation process. Warm water relaxes the muscles, reduces the perception of pain, and decreases the need for epidural analgesia.

Additionally, the buoyancy of the water allows women to move more freely and adopt more comfortable positions during labor, which can relieve pressure in certain areas of the body. Moreover, the reduced gravity and abdominal pressure facilitate fetal rotation and descent, providing further advantages of hydrotherapy [4,5].

Defining the stages of labor is essential: the first stage (the latent phase from the beginning to 4 cm of cervical dilation and the active phase from 4 cm to 10 cm of cervical dilation), the second stage (expulsion), and the third stage (delivery of the placenta). Proper definition helps differentiate the maternal and neonatal risks and benefits of hydrotherapy [3].

A woman should give birth in a place where she feels secure and receives appropriate care (International Federation of Gynecology and Obstetrics, 1982). Hydrotherapy can enhance the childbirth experience and maternal health, as indicated by a qualitative study involving 23 women [6]. The benefits of water, such as buoyancy, hydrostatic pressure, and temperature, positively affect the dilation process. Studies report reduced epidurals use, better pain management, and shorter labor durations [7–9]. A systematic review and meta-analysis by Burns et al. (2022) [10] indicated a trend favoring water immersion for pain relief since 2009.

A Cochrane review of 15 trials involving 3663 women [1] compared water immersion with non-immersion. Eight studies involved water immersion during the first stage, and four involved it during both stages. The review found physical and emotional benefits [1], including higher pain thresholds, shorter dilation stages, reduced medical intervention, improved relaxation, and greater overall satisfaction with childbirth [11].

A cross-sectional study at São Bernardo Hospital in Portugal evaluated maternal and neonatal outcomes during labor stages. Excellent Apgar scores and pain relief were reported by 98.9% of the 90 women, with immersion time influencing labor duration significantly [12].

Despite these findings, some associations, such as the American College of Obstetricians and Gynecologists (ACOG) and the American Academy of Pediatrics (AAP) [13], discuss neonatal outcomes and safety, emphasizing the need for more high-quality studies.

Contrary to these concerns, Burns et al.'s meta-analysis [10] reported clear benefits for women and newborns from hydrotherapy, with no worse outcomes for water births. Other studies compare births with and without hydrotherapy and do not suggest worse outcomes for babies born through water birth [7,14]. The American College of Nurse-Midwives (ACNM) recommends providing evidence-based information on water birth for uncomplicated pregnancies [7].

A systematic review by Jacoby et al. [15] found varying perinatal outcomes for hydrotherapy, highlighting the need for further research. Meta-analyses and reviews of observational studies, including over 30,000 births, do not demonstrate increased risks for mothers or babies.

This meta-analysis aims to address pain management during the first stage of labor using minimally invasive techniques, enhancing healthcare quality and supporting the use of hydrotherapy for its beneficial impact on labor times and safety.

Objectives

The primary objective is to determine the benefits of hydrotherapy in clinical childbirth approaches and its applicability in pain control. The secondary objectives include assessing its impact on the duration of the first stage of labor and the newborns' physical condition.

2. Materials and Methods

2.1. Review Protocol

This systematic review and meta-analysis followed the PRISMA protocol and was registered with PROSPERO (CRD42023399625).

2.2. Search Strategy and Inclusion Criteria

Studies were selected based on the PICOS criteria (participants, interventions, comparisons, outcomes, and study design). Articles using the RCT methodology and involving pregnant women in the first stage of labor receiving hydrotherapy treatment were included. Two of the investigators (J.C.S.-G. and E.M.-G.) searched the Scopus, PubMed, Cinahl, and WOS databases. A manual search was also performed using the reference lists of studies to find other relevant research.

The structured language used was obtained using MeSH terms and Health Sciences (DeCS) descriptors. The descriptors used were "labor stage, first" and "immersion" along with the corresponding natural language descriptors, using the Boolean operator AND. Supplementary Table S1 shows the search strategy employed for each of the databases consulted, along with the dates on which the searches were conducted. The searches were performed without a year filter to obtain all relevant information related to the objective of the search. The articles were collected between December 2022 and January 2023.

2.3. Data Extraction and Quality Assessment

After carrying out the search strategy, the articles found were transferred to the Mendeley web application using the Mendeley web importer tool. They were then organized into folders according to the database from which they were obtained, and all duplicates were removed. The included studies were RCTs that met the objective of the search. Two reviewers (J.C.S.-G. and E.M.-G.) independently examined the title, abstract, and keywords of each study identified in the search and applied the inclusion and exclusion criteria. The same procedure was applied to potentially eligible full-text articles. Differences between reviewers were resolved by discussion or by a third reviewer (R.R.-B.).

Data on the quality, patient characteristics, interventions, and relevant outcomes were extracted independently by two reviewers (E.M.-G. and J.C.-M.).

Two reviewers (J.C.S.-G. and E.M.-G.) independently extracted the following data from each article: author, country and methodology of the study; intervention characteristics; sample size and sample distribution; weeks of gestation; sample selection criteria; and mean age. Regarding the results of the RCTs, we extracted the type of intervention, start of intervention, and duration of intervention, pain scale; furthermore, relative to the newborn, we assessed their physical condition at 5 min after birth. These data are reported in Table 1. The reviewers also assessed the strengths and weaknesses of each RCT.

Table 1. Characteristics of included trials.

Author	Country	Method	Interventions Characteristics					Outcomes			
			Gestation Weeks (Media)	Sample Size	Distribution of the Sample	Type of Population	Average Age	Type of Intervention	Intervention Time	Pain Scale	Physical Condition of the Newborn
Chaichian, 2009 [16]	Iran	RCT	37–42 weeks	106	EG 53; CG 53	No risks	EG: 26.4 ± 5.9; CG: 27.1 ± 5.9	Warm water pools	On demand	Use of analgesics	Not reported
Cluett et al., 2004 [17]	England	RCT	EG: 284 ± 7 days; CG: 280 ± 8 days	99	EG: 49; CG: 50	Nulliparous women with dystocia and low risk of complications	EG: 26.0 ± 4.8; CG: 24.8 ± 6.0	Warm water pools	Maximum 4 h in the pool	Visual Analog Scale	Apgar 5 min
Eckert, Turnbull and MCallister, 2001 [18]	Australia	RCT	EG: 39.9 ± 1,0; CG: 39.9 ± 1,0	274	EG: 137; CG: 137	Singleton pregnancy. No risks	EG: 28.4 ± 5.4; CG: 27.2 ± 5.1	Warm water pools	On demand during the first stage of labor	Visual Analog Scale	Apgar 5 min
Schorn, McAllister and Blanco, 1993 [19]	USA	RCT	EG: 39.1 ± 1.4; CG: 39.2 ± 1.1	93	EG: 45; CG: 48	Intact membranes and no obstetric risks	EG: 21.4 ± 4.6; CG: 22.6 ± 6.1	Warm water pools	On demand	Use of analgesics	Apgar 5 min
Lee et al., 2013 [20]	Taiwan	RCT	EG: 38.91 ± 1.26; CG: 39.19 ± 1.05	80	EG: 39; CG: 41	Pregnant women with a single foetus with no risk of complications	EG: 31.44 ± 3.85; CG: 31.83 ± 4.62	Warm showers	20 min per shower	Visual Analog Scale for Pain (VASP)	Not reported
Solt and Kanza Gul, 2022 [21]	Turkey	RCT	EG: 39.2 ± 0.8; CG: 39.2 ± 0.8	80	EG: 40; CG: 40	Primiparas between 20 and 40 years old, single foetus.	EG: 28.7 ± 3.1; CG: 28.3 ± 3.2	Warm showers	20 min per shower (18 showers)	Visual Analog Scale	Apgar 5 min
da Silva et al., 2009 [22]	Brazil	RCT	EG: 39.5 ± 0.9; CG: 39.5 ± 1.1	108	EG: 54; CG: 54	Uncomplicated full-term pregnancies	EG: 19.7 ± 3.6; CG: 21.1 ± 4.1	Warm water pools	60 min	Visual Analog Scale	Apgar 5 min

A methodological quality assessment was performed using the PEDro (Physiotherapy Evidence Database) scale, as the methodology corresponded to RCTs. Publication bias was determined by visual inspection of the funnel plots.

2.4. Statistical Analysis

Statistical analysis was performed by analyzing the mean difference between the hydrotherapy and control groups, calculated in each study by subtracting the mean change (post-intervention minus pre-intervention) in the control group from the mean change in the hydrotherapy group.

The effect size of the intervention was studied by analyzing Cohen's d for each of the studies, using random-effects models based on the Sidik–Jonkman method. Cohen's d values below 0.20 indicate no effect; values between 0.21 and 0.49 indicate a small effect; values between 0.50 and 0.70 indicate a moderate effect; and values above 0.80 indicate a large effect [23]. Heterogeneity was assessed with the I^2 statistic, and its values were classified as non-significant (0–40%), moderate (30–60%), substantial (50–90%), or considerable (75–100%) [24]; the corresponding *p*-values were also considered.

Egger's regression asymmetry test was performed to assess publication bias, with $p < 0.10$ being considered statistically significant [25].

Meta-analyses were performed with the free and open-source statistical software Jamovi, Version 2.3.21.0, based on the R programming language.

Based on the information provided by this review, a series of premises are obtained as results that will serve to homogenize concepts about hydrotherapy during labor.

3. Results

Seven potentially eligible studies were identified by searching electronic databases, and none were identified through other sources. Details regarding the inclusion and exclusion of studies at each stage are provided in the flow chart [26] (Figure 1).

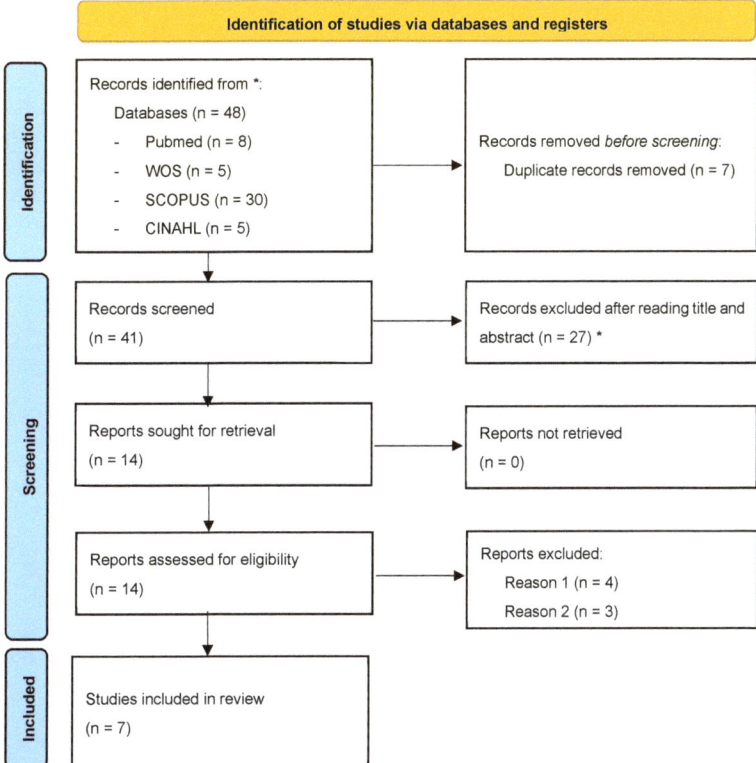

Figure 1. Flow diagram. * Did not meet the inclusion criteria. Reason 1: RCT protocols; Reason 2: systematic reviews of RCTs.

These seven studies included a total of 840 pregnant women. The intervention groups included 417 pregnant women at term, while the control groups included 423 pregnant women.

Five articles assessed pain during the first stage of labor using the visual analog scale (VAS) as a method, and two articles assessed pain during the first stage of labor using the percentage of analgesic medication use.

Table 1 summarizes the articles selected for the systematic review and meta-analysis.

Overall, the use of hydrotherapy reduced pain in the first stage of labor compared with the control group, showing considerable heterogeneity between studies (Pain, −0.97; 95% CI, −1.91 to −0.03; I^2 = 97.32%, p < 0.001 and n = 840) (Figure 2).

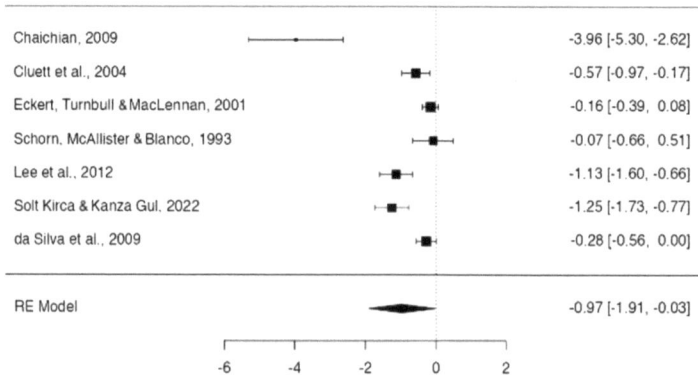

Figure 2. Forest plot use of hydrotherapy for pain [16–22].

The study with the largest effect size concerning pain assessment was that of Chaichian et al. [16], (d = −3.964). The studies by Lee et al. [20] and Solt Kirca and Kanza Gul [21] also presented large effects, with values of −1.127 and −1.2467, respectively. Cluett et al. [11] found a moderate effect (d = −0.5693), while da Silva et al. [22] found a small effect (d = −0.2789). Eckert, Turnbull, and MCallister [18] along with Schorn, McAllister, and Blanco [19] showed no effect on the intervention, with a Cohen's d of less than 0.20 (−0.1552 and −0.0736, respectively) (Figure 3).

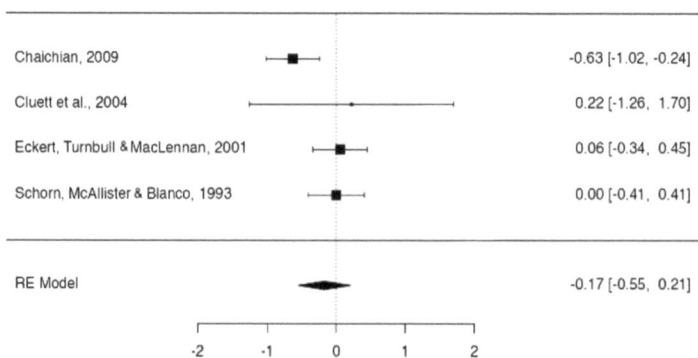

Figure 3. Forest plot use of hydrotherapy versus times in the first stage of labor [16–19].

However, the use of hydrotherapy did not significantly affect the duration of the first stage of labor, with moderate heterogeneity between studies (duration of the first stage of labor −0.17; 95% CI, −0.55 to 0.21; I^2 = 56.75%, p = 0.059 and n = 572) (Figure 3).

Regarding the physical condition of the newborn, it was observed that the use of hydrotherapy does not affect the physical condition of the newborn, with homogeneity in the studies (Apgar 5 min, 0.18; 95% CI, −0.48 to 0.85; I^2 = 2.15%, p = 0.939 and n = 654) (Figure 4).

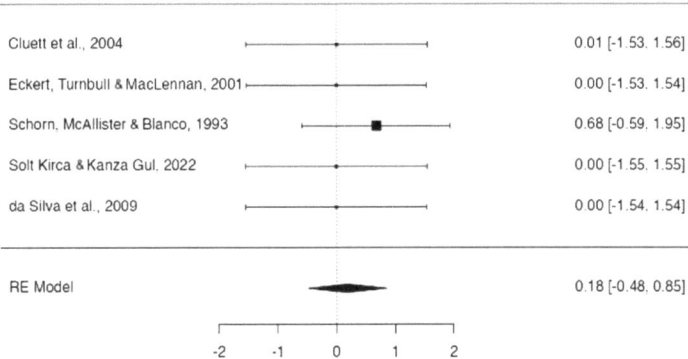

Figure 4. Forest plot use of hydrotherapy against the physical condition of newborns [17–19,21,22].

The assessment of methodological quality revealed that most of the information was obtained from trials with good methodological quality (Supplementary Table S2). However, all articles noted that blinding of participants, researchers, and groups was impossible due to the nature of the intervention performed during the first stage of labor.

Figure 5 shows the funnel plot used to assess publication bias in the studies included in the meta-analysis. The results of the conducted tests are as follows: the fail-safe N, which indicates the number of additional studies needed to nullify the meta-analysis results, is 48 ($p < 0.001$), suggesting a high robustness of the findings. Kendall's tau test yielded a value of -1.000 with a p-value of 0.003, indicating significant publication bias. Additionally, Egger's regression produced a coefficient of -4.553 with a p-value of less than 0.001, confirming the presence of publication bias. These combined results suggest that although the meta-analysis shows a significant effect, the potential impact of publication bias must be considered when interpreting the findings.

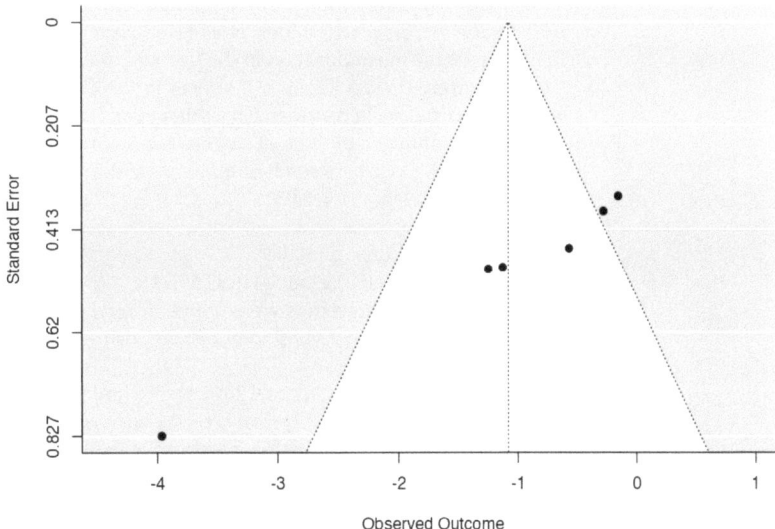

Figure 5. Funnel plot.

4. Discussion

This meta-analysis has enabled us to synthesize the current relevant findings on the use of hydrotherapy during the first stage of labor. The findings of this study contribute to the evidence demonstrating significant differences in pain control during this stage between the groups using hydrotherapy and those following standard hospital procedures.

In this work, we found that the most studied outcome was pain during the first stage of labor among groups that used hydrotherapy compared with those that did not. These results indicated that hydrotherapy during labor was associated with lower pain scores in the hydrotherapy group. It should be noted that the measurement tools used in these studies varied, with most employing the visual analog pain scale [17,18,20–22], while some assessed pain through analgesic use [16,19]. Da Silva et al. [22] reported decreased pain in the water immersion groups compared with those that did not use hydrotherapy, combining this assessment with a behavioral pain scale between the two groups. Other studies also reported decreased pain in hydrotherapy groups at various times during the dilation phase compared with non-hydrotherapy groups that received conventional procedures such as amniotomy and oxytocin infusion [20,21]. However, no significant differences in mean scores for clinical or laboratory pain indicators were found in two articles [17,18]. A meta-analysis of the data shows that the effect size of hydrotherapy during the first stage of labor is significant compared with conventional procedures.

Although pain was perceived to be less in some studies, Eckert, Turnbull, and MCallister [18] noted that women's use of analgesia was greater in the hydrotherapy group. When contractions intensified, they needed to exit the water and discontinue hydrotherapy. However, in general, neither group demonstrated significant differences in the amount of pharmacological analgesia administered [17,19]. Conversely, Cluett et al. [17] showed that women using water immersion had a lower rate of epidural analgesia compared with those undergoing amniotomy and oxytocin without hydrotherapy.

In non-hydrotherapy groups, conventional management of labor, including amniotomy and oxytocin administration, was performed more frequently than in hydrotherapy groups [17,19,21].

This review found no differences in delivery types between hydrotherapy and non-hydrotherapy groups [16–19]. In a randomized controlled study by Chaichian et al. [16] involving 106 women, all women using hydrotherapy had natural birth, whereas 79.2% of those receiving conventional treatment had natural birth, although the differences were not significant. Similarly, Cluett et al. [17] found no significant differences in operative deliveries or the mean duration of the first stage of labor. Schorn et al. [19] also concluded that there were no significant differences in the duration of the first stage of labor with respect to minutes. In contrast, Chaichian et al. [16] found a significant difference in the active phase duration of the first stage of labor. The meta-analysis showed no statistically significant difference between hydrotherapy and conventional treatment in the duration of the first stage of labor ($p = 0.059$).

Neonatal outcome measures, including maternal infection rates related to neonatal infection, Apgar scores, fetal distress, or abnormal fetal cardiotocographic recordings, were similar between the two groups [16,17,19,21].

Although no differences were noted, Eckert, Turnbull, and MCallister [18] reported more use of oxygen masks and intermittent positive pressure ventilation in infants whose mothers used hydrotherapy.

Admissions to the neonatal unit were similar in both groups, with no significant differences. Cluett et al. [17] analyzed six admissions of infants born to women using water immersion and terminated in operative delivery, concluding that they experienced no subsequent problems.

Regarding maternal outcomes, Chaichian et al. [16] recorded 23% episiotomies in the non-hydrotherapy group, although tears were 12% higher in the water immersion group; however, the differences were minimal and not significant [16,17]. No differences were observed for hospital readmissions, postpartum endometritis, or postpartum pain at 24–48 h and at 8 months [17,19].

Eckert, Turnbull, and MCallister [18] assessed the birth experience, finding it more positive in the conventionally managed group in terms of relationship with staff, social support, information, choices and decisions, and satisfaction.

Birth using hydrotherapy has been shown to be more satisfying for women, which is attributed to the freedom of movement, intimacy, and reduced labor pain intensity, all positively influencing women's wellbeing and comfort [19]. However, studies such as Cluett et al. [17] mention this satisfaction but find no significant differences.

The main limitations of this study are closely related to the existing scientific literature on this topic. Given that hydrotherapy is an innovative technique, the current knowledge on it is limited.

Additionally, the impact of publication bias was evaluated using several statistical and visual tests. The analysis included the calculation of the fail-safe N, Kendall's tau test, and Egger's regression. The fail-safe N was 48 ($p < 0.001$), indicating that 48 additional studies with null effects would be needed to render the meta-analysis results non-significant. Kendall's tau test and Egger's regression showed values suggesting a significant presence of publication bias. These results, along with the funnel plot, indicate that although the meta-analysis results are statistically significant, the magnitude of the observed effect may be influenced by publication bias. Therefore, it is crucial to interpret the results with caution and consider this potential bias when drawing conclusions.

Future research lines have emerged from this study. A project involving four hospitals in the province of Granada will study births and pain control in pregnant women, with subsequent follow-up during the postpartum period. A control group will be established to compare results.

Additionally, the possible benefits of hydrotherapy in deliveries of pregnant women diagnosed with hypermobile Ehlers–Danlos syndrome, a rare disease, will be investigated.

5. Conclusions

Based on the provided information from the systematic review, several conclusions can be drawn:

Hydrotherapy as a non-pharmacological method for pain relief: The systematic review suggests that hydrotherapy during labor can serve as an effective non-pharmacological method for pain relief. This implies that it could offer an alternative or complementary approach to traditional pharmacological methods, potentially reducing the need for epidurals.

Improved coping mechanisms and satisfaction: Women who utilize hydrotherapy during labor may experience an enhanced ability to cope with pain, leading to a greater sense of control, satisfaction, and comfort. These psychological benefits can contribute positively to the overall childbirth experience.

No significant impact on labor duration or newborn health: The use of hydrotherapy does not seem to affect the duration of labor or the physical condition of the newborn. This suggests that while it provides pain relief and psychological benefits, it does not interfere with the natural progression of labor or compromise the health of the newborn.

Potential reduction in instrumental deliveries and cesarean sections: Some authors suggest that hydrotherapy may even facilitate the natural completion of labor, resulting in fewer instrumental deliveries and cesarean sections. This has significant implications for addressing concerns about the increasing rates of cesarean sections and reducing interventionism in clinical practice.

Need for further research: Despite the positive findings, there is a need for further research, particularly research focusing on the use of hydrotherapy in the second stage of labor. Additionally, the lack of reported adverse neonatal outcomes in many articles contrasts with the caution expressed by some pediatric associations, highlighting the necessity for more comprehensive studies to assess safety concerns.

Importance of correct management and training: Proper management of hydrotherapy during labor involves training and updating midwives, as well as developing clinical practice protocols and guidelines that are supported by scientific evidence. This ensures that women receive optimal care during childbirth and mitigates potential risks associated with hydrotherapy.

Overall, this systematic review suggests that hydrotherapy during labor offers promising benefits for pain relief and childbirth outcomes, but further research and proper management are necessary to fully understand its implications and ensure safe implementation.

Supplementary Materials: The following supporting information can be downloaded at: https://www.mdpi.com/article/10.3390/jcm13113260/s1, Supplementary Material Table S1 provides the search strategies used in each of the databases and the filters applied. Supplementary Material Table S2 provides the results of the application of the PEDro scale to each of the articles included in this meta-analysis.

Author Contributions: Conceptualization, E.M.-G., J.C.-M., J.C.S.-G. and R.R.-B.; data curation, M.M.P.F. and J.C.S.-G.; methodology, J.C.-M., E.M.-G., B.P.-S. and L.D.-R.; investigation, R.R.-B. and B.P.-S.; resources, J.C.-M. and J.C.S.-G.; writing—original draft preparation, E.M.-G., R.R.-B. and B.P.-S.; writing—review and editing, J.C.-M., J.C.S.-G., E.M.-G., L.D.-R., M.M.P.F. and R.R.-B.; visualization, B.P.-S. and R.R.-B.; supervision, J.C.S.-G. and R.R.-B.; project administration, L.D.-R. All authors have read and agreed to the published version of the manuscript.

Funding: This research received no external funding.

Institutional Review Board Statement: The review protocol is registered on the PROSPERO website (http://www.crd.york.ac.uk/PROSPERO/ (accessed on 25 February 2023)), and its registration number is CRD42023399625.

Informed Consent Statement: Not applicable.

Data Availability Statement: Data are available upon request from the corresponding author.

Acknowledgments: This study was carried out within the framework of the research project "Effects of hydrotherapy during labour in terms of maternal and neonatal health", which is part of the Doctoral Programme in Clinical Medicine and Public Health at the University of Granada. We are grateful to the Official College of Nursing of Granada (CODEGRA) for their help in the research support program and to the Chair of Research in Nursing Care of the University of Granada and the Official College of Nursing of Granada.

Conflicts of Interest: The authors declare no conflicts of interest.

References

1. Cluett, E.R.; Burns, E.; Cuthbert, A. Immersion in Water during Labour and Birth. *Cochrane Database Syst. Rev.* **2018**, *2018*, CD000111. [CrossRef] [PubMed]
2. Hinkson, L.; Henrich, W. Intrapartum Care. *J. Perinat. Med.* **2018**, *46*, 571–572. [CrossRef] [PubMed]
3. Grupo de trabajo de la Guía de Práctica Clínica sobre atención al parto normal. *Guía de Práctica Clínica Sobre la Atención al Parto Normal*. Plan de Calidad Para el Sistema Nacional de Salud del Ministerio de Sanidad y Política Social, 1st ed.; Servicio Central de Publicaciones del Gobierno Vasco, Ed.; Ministerio de Sanidad y Política Social: Madrid, Spain, 2010; ISBN 9788445730904.
4. Labour and Birth—Warm Water Immersion and Water Birth—Patient Information Brochures—Mater Group. Available online: https://brochures.mater.org.au/brochures/mater-mothers-hospital/labour-and-birth-warm-water-immersion-and-water-bi (accessed on 28 May 2024).
5. Mellado-García, E.; Díaz-Rodríguez, L.; Cortés-Martín, J.; Sánchez-García, J.C.; Piqueras-Sola, B.; Higuero Macías, J.C.; Rodríguez-Blanque, R. Systematic Reviews and Synthesis without Meta-Analysis on Hydrotherapy for Pain Control in Labor. *Healthcare* **2024**, *12*, 373. [CrossRef] [PubMed]
6. Fair, C.D.; Crawford, A.; Houpt, B.; Latham, V. "After Having a Waterbirth, I Feel like It's the Only Way People Should Deliver Babies": The Decision Making Process of Women Who Plan a Waterbirth. *Midwifery* **2020**, *82*, 102622. [CrossRef] [PubMed]
7. Bailey, J.M.; Zielinski, R.E.; Emeis, C.L.; Kane Low, L. A Retrospective Comparison of Waterbirth Outcomes in Two United States Hospital Settings. *Birth* **2020**, *47*, 98–104. [CrossRef] [PubMed]
8. Chaillet, N.; Belaid, L.; Crochetière, C.; Roy, L.; Gagné, G.P.; Moutquin, J.M.; Rossignol, M.; Dugas, M.; Wassef, M.; Bonapace, J. Nonpharmacologic Approaches for Pain Management during Labor Compared with Usual Care: A Meta-Analysis. *Birth* **2014**, *41*, 122–137. [CrossRef] [PubMed]
9. Kavosi, Z.; Keshtkaran, A.; Setoodehzadeh, F.; Kasraeian, M.; Khammarnia, M.; Eslahi, M. A Comparison of Mothers' Quality of Life after Normal Vaginal, Cesarean, and Water Birth Deliveries. *Int. J. Community Based Nurs. Midwifery* **2015**, *3*, 198.

10. Burns, E.; Feeley, C.; Hall, P.J.; Vanderlaan, J. Systematic Review and Meta-Analysis to Examine Intrapartum Interventions, and Maternal and Neonatal Outcomes Following Immersion in Water during Labour and Waterbirth. *BMJ Open* **2022**, *12*, e056517. [CrossRef] [PubMed]
11. Cluett, E.R.; Burns, E. Immersion in Water in Labour and Birth. *Sao Paulo Med. J.* **2013**, *131*, 364. [CrossRef]
12. Camargo, J.C.S.; Varela, V.; Ferreira, F.M.; Pougy, L.; Ochiai, A.M.; Santos, M.E.; Grande, M.C.L.R. The Waterbirth Project: São Bernardo Hospital Experience. *Women Birth* **2018**, *31*, e325–e333. [CrossRef]
13. AMERICAN ACADEMY OF PEDIATRICS Committee on Fetus and Newborn; Papile, L.-A.; Baley, J.E.; Benitz, W.; Carlo, W.A.; Cummings, J.; Kumar, P.; Polin, R.A.; Tan, R.C.; Watterberg, K.L.; et al. Immersion in Water during Labor and Delivery. *Pediatrics* **2014**, *133*, 758–761. [CrossRef] [PubMed]
14. Davies, R.; Davis, D.; Pearce, M.; Wong, N. The Effect of Waterbirth on Neonatal Mortality and Morbidity: A Systematic Review and Meta-Analysis. *JBI Database Syst. Rev. Implement. Rep.* **2015**, *13*, 180–231. [CrossRef]
15. Jacoby, S.; Becker, G.; Crawford, S.; Wilson, R.D. Water Birth Maternal and Neonatal Outcomes Among Midwifery Clients in Alberta, Canada, from 2014 to 2017: A Retrospective Study. *J. Obstet. Gynaecol. Can.* **2019**, *41*, 805–812. [CrossRef]
16. Chaichian, S.; Akhlaghi, A.; Rousta, F.; Safavi, M. Experience of Water Birth Delivery in Iran. *Arch. Iran. Med.* **2009**, *12*, 468–471. [PubMed]
17. Cluett, E.R.; Pickering, R.M.; Getliffe, K.; Saunders, N.J.S.G. Randomised Controlled Trial of Labouring in Water Compared with Standard of Augmentation for Management of Dystocia in First Stage of Labour. *Br. Med. J.* **2004**, *328*, 314–318. [CrossRef] [PubMed]
18. Eckert, K.; Turnbull, D.; Clin, M.; Maclennan, A. Immersion in Water in the First Stage of Labor: A Randomized Controlled Trial. *Birth* **2001**, *28*, 84–93. [CrossRef]
19. Schorn, M.; McAllister, J.; Blanco, J. Water Immersion and the Effect on Labor. *J. Nurse-Midwifery* **1993**, *38*, 336–342. [CrossRef]
20. Lee, S.L.; Liu, C.Y.; Lu, Y.Y.; Gau, M.L. Efficacy of Warm Showers on Labor Pain and Birth Experiences During the First Labor Stage. *J. Obstet. Gynecol. Neonatal Nurs.* **2013**, *42*, 19–28. [CrossRef]
21. Solt, A.; Kanza, D. European Journal of Obstetrics & Gynecology and Reproductive Biology Effects of Acupressure and Shower Applied in the Delivery on the Intensity of Labor Pain and Postpartum Comfort. *Eur. J. Obstet. Gynecol. Reprod. Biol.* **2022**, *273*, 98–104. [CrossRef]
22. da Silva, F.M.B.; de Oliveira, S.M.J.V.; Nobre, M.R.C. A Randomised Controlled Trial Evaluating the Effect of Immersion Bath on Labour Pain. *Midwifery* **2009**, *25*, 286–294. [CrossRef]
23. Jacob, C. *Statistical Power Analysis for the Behavioral Sciences*; Academic Press: Cambridge, MA, USA, 2013.
24. Higgins, J.P.T.; Thompson, S.G. Quantifying Heterogeneity in a Meta-Analysis. *Stat. Med.* **2002**, *21*, 1539–1558. [CrossRef] [PubMed]
25. Sterne, J.A.C.; Egger, M.; Smith, G.D. Systematic Reviews in Health Care: Investigating and Dealing with Publication and Other Biases in Meta-Analysis. *Br. Med. J.* **2001**, *323*, 101–105. [CrossRef] [PubMed]
26. Page, M.J.; McKenzie, J.E.; Bossuyt, P.M.; Boutron, I.; Hoffmann, T.C.; Mulrow, C.D.; Shamseer, L.; Tetzlaff, J.M.; Akl, E.A.; Brennan, S.E.; et al. The PRISMA 2020 Statement: An Updated Guideline for Reporting Systematic Reviews. *Int. J. Surg.* **2021**, *88*, 105906. [CrossRef] [PubMed]

Disclaimer/Publisher's Note: The statements, opinions and data contained in all publications are solely those of the individual author(s) and contributor(s) and not of MDPI and/or the editor(s). MDPI and/or the editor(s) disclaim responsibility for any injury to people or property resulting from any ideas, methods, instructions or products referred to in the content.

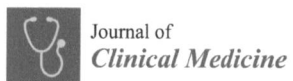

Article

Performance of the First-Trimester Cervical Consistency Index to Predict Preterm Birth

Carlos H. Becerra-Mojica [1,2,3,*], Miguel A. Parra-Saavedra [4], Ruth A. Martínez-Vega [5], Luis A. Díaz-Martínez [1], Raigam J. Martínez-Portilla [6], Johnatan Torres-Torres [6] and Bladimiro Rincon-Orozco [1,*]

1. School of Medicine, Universidad Industrial de Santander, Bucaramanga 680002, Colombia; ladimar@uis.edu.co
2. Maternal-Fetal Medicine Unit, Hospital Universitario de Santander, Bucaramanga 680002, Colombia
3. Centro de Atención Materno-Fetal INUTERO, Floridablanca 681004, Colombia
4. Departamento Ginecologia y Obstetricia, Universidad Libre, Barranquilla 080003, Colombia; miguelparra51@hotmail.com
5. Escuela de Medicina, Universidad de Santander, Bucaramanga 680003, Colombia; rutharam@yahoo.com
6. Clinical Research Division, National Institute of Perinatology, Mexico City 11000, Mexico; raifet@hotmail.com (R.J.M.-P.); torresmmf@gmail.com (J.T.-T.)
* Correspondence: cbecerra@uis.edu.co (C.H.B.-M.); blrincon@uis.edu.co (B.R.-O.)

Citation: Becerra-Mojica, C.H.; Parra-Saavedra, M.A.; Martínez-Vega, R.A.; Díaz-Martínez, L.A.; Martínez-Portilla, R.J.; Torres-Torres, J.; Rincon-Orozco, B. Performance of the First-Trimester Cervical Consistency Index to Predict Preterm Birth. *J. Clin. Med.* **2024**, *13*, 3906. https://doi.org/10.3390/jcm13133906

Academic Editors: Ioannis Tsakiridis and Apostolos Mamopoulos

Received: 6 May 2024
Revised: 16 June 2024
Accepted: 16 June 2024
Published: 3 July 2024

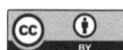

Copyright: © 2024 by the authors. Licensee MDPI, Basel, Switzerland. This article is an open access article distributed under the terms and conditions of the Creative Commons Attribution (CC BY) license (https://creativecommons.org/licenses/by/4.0/).

Abstract: Background/Objectives: Preterm birth (PTB) remains a significant global health challenge. Previous attempts to predict preterm birth in the first trimester using cervical length have been contradictory. The cervical consistency index (CCI) was introduced to quantify early cervical changes and has shown promise across various clinical scenarios in the mid-trimester, though testing in the first trimester is lacking. This study aims to assess the cervical consistency index performance in predicting preterm birth during the first trimester of pregnancy. **Methods**: In this prospective cohort study, focused exclusively on research, women with singleton pregnancies, both with and without a history of spontaneous preterm birth (sPTB), were included. The primary outcome was sPTB before 37 weeks, with a secondary outcome of sPTB before 34 weeks. CCI measurements were taken between 11^{+0} to 13^{+6} weeks of gestation. Receiver operating characteristic (ROC) curves were generated, and sensitivity and specificity were calculated for the optimal cut-off and for the 5th, 10th, and 15th percentile. Intraobserver and interobserver agreements were assessed using the intraclass correlation coefficient (ICC). **Results**: Among the 667 patients analyzed, the rates of sPTB before 37 and 34 weeks were 9.2% (61/667) and 1.8% (12/667), respectively. The detection rates (DRs) for CCI predicting PTB before 37 and 34 weeks were 19.7% (12/61) and 33.3% (4/12). Negative predictive values were 91.8% (546/595) and 98.7% (588/596), while the areas under the curve (AUC) for sPTB before 37 and 34 weeks were 0.62 (95% CI: 0.54–0.69) and 0.80 (95% CI: 0.71–0.89), respectively. Of the 61 patients with preterm birth, 13 (21.3%) had a preterm birth history; in this group, the CCI percentile 10th identified 39% (5/13). Intraobserver ICC was 0.862 (95% CI: 0.769–0.920), and interobserver ICC was 0.833 (95% CI: 0.722–0.902). **Conclusions**: This study suggests that utilizing CCI in the first trimester of pregnancy could serve as a valuable tool for predicting preterm birth before 34 weeks of gestation, demonstrating robust intraobserver and interobserver reliability.

Keywords: preterm birth; cervical consistency index; cervical length; preterm birth prediction

1. Introduction

Preterm birth (PTB), defined as childbirth occurring before 37 weeks of gestation, remains a significant global health challenge [1]. According to WHO estimates, approximately 15 million PTB cases occur annually [2]. Colombia has the highest PTB rates (10%) in Latin America, as reported by UNICEF [3,4]. This alarming statistic underscores PTB's status as a leading cause of neonatal and under-five mortality, contributing to the death of approximately one million neonates annually due to PTB-related complications [5]. Numerous investigations have been conducted to predict and prevent PTB, resulting in substantial evidence supporting the use of cervical length measurement between 18 and 22 weeks of gestation. This currently stands as the standard method to identify pregnant women at risk of PTB, identifying 28% of pregnant women who will deliver between 34 to 37 weeks using a cut-off of 25 mm and a false positive rate of 10% [6]. Through a tailored approach, the detection rate of spontaneous preterm birth (sPTB) before 37 weeks using cervical length can be substantially enhanced, reaching as high as 50% [7].

To address the need to search for better predictive tools for sPTB, Parra et al. introduced the Cervical Consistency Index (CCI) as an ultrasound measurement for identifying accelerated cervical softening in 2011 [8]. The CCI quantifies the change of the anteroposterior diameter of the uterine cervix after deformation induced with the transvaginal probe by the operator. Notably, CCI has displayed good performance in various clinical scenarios, including low-risk pregnant women [9], high-risk pregnant women [10], and twin pregnancies [11], outperforming the cervical length measurements typically conducted during mid-trimester evaluations. However, CCI requires specific training to perform adequate measurements. Despite its promise, a recent review showed that more evidence is needed about CCI performance in order to achieve robust results in different clinical scenarios, especially in a prospective cohort developed for research purposes [12].

In an effort to tackle the PTB rates and to look for better prediction in the first trimester of pregnancy, we sought to assess the predictive capability of CCI measured during the first trimester for the prediction of sPTB before 37 weeks of gestation.

2. Materials and Methods

2.1. Study Design and Participants

This is a prospective cohort of singleton pregnant women between 11^{+0} to 13^{+6} weeks of gestation recruited from November 2019 to September 2022. Participants were recruited from the maternal–fetal units of two health institutions in Bucaramanga, Colombia, namely Hospital Universitario de Santander and Centro de Atencion Maternal-Fetal INUTERO. The Committee on Ethics and Research from the Universidad Industrial de Santander and participating centers approved the study (CEINCI: Act No. 17, 17 October 2019. Project code 254). All pregnant women signed informed consent for participation in this study. Criteria for inclusion were pregnant women between 11^{+0} to 13^{+6} weeks with a singleton pregnancy, including previous sPTB and nulliparous women. Criteria for exclusion were women with history of cervical surgery or Mullerian anomalies, PTB due to fetal or maternal indications (non-spontaneous), or pregnancies that ended before 22 weeks of gestation.

2.2. Recruitment

All eligible women who attended the 11^{+0} to 13^{+6} screening were invited to participate. Data were obtained from pregnant women using a standard survey at enrollment, including age, obstetric history, history of preterm birth, and cervical procedures. Anthropometric data were obtained before the ultrasound evaluation to determine typical risk calculations for chromosomal abnormalities and risk of preeclampsia.

2.3. Ultrasound Evaluation

Highly skilled maternal–fetal specialists, each with over five years of experience in 11^{+0} to 13^{+6} ultrasound screening scans, conducted the examinations. The medical team underwent rigorous training to master the CCI measurement technique, led by Dr. Parra-Saavedra, the creator of the method. Following the acquisition of ten practice images, feedback was provided, and a predetermined format was applied to assess competence. The assessment process involved registering a transabdominal image in the longitudinal middle plane of the uterus and cervix to evaluate cervical canal orientation. Subsequently, a transvaginal ultrasound, utilizing a 4–9 MHz endocavitary probe (Voluson E6, S8 General Electric, Milwaukee, MI, USA), was conducted.

As described elsewhere [13,14], cervical length measurement was executed by tracing a line between the internal and external os as reference points, avoiding the isthmus while ensuring proper orientation. For the CCI measurement, the double-screen image was activated, maintaining the same plane, and after freezing the left image, pressure with the probe was applied in an anteroposterior direction until the minimum diameter was obtained. AP diameters at the mid-third of the cervix were recorded for both images, and a second measurement of AP diameters was obtained to estimate intraobserver agreement (Figure 1). The CCI was calculated by dividing the AP diameter after probe pressure by the pre-pressure diameter, generating a value between 0 and 1, which was duly registered. Another team member, ensuring operator blinding, obtained the CCI value posteriorly.

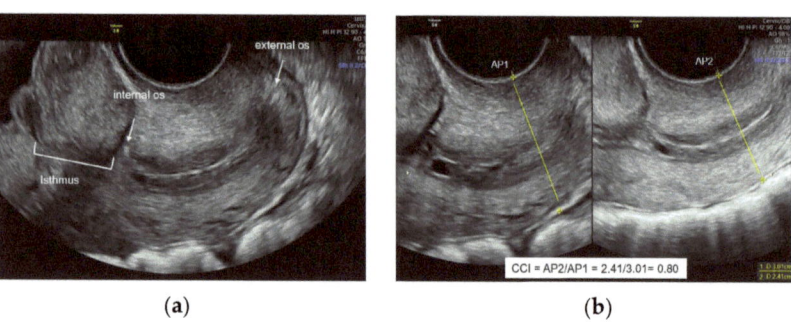

Figure 1. Cervical measurements. (**a**) Ultrasound image characteristics for first-trimester cervical length measurement. (**b**) Anteroposterior diameter before pressure (AP1) and anteroposterior diameter after probe pressure (AP2) to obtain the cervical consistency index (CCI).

Interobserver agreement was assessed by two independent operators in a subset of patients, with image evaluations and measurements conducted by experts MPS and CB. Importantly, the results of CCI measurements did not influence clinical decisions, and operators remained blinded to both CCI values and patient outcomes, maintaining scientific integrity throughout the study and avoiding bias. None of the patients received progesterone prescriptions, ensuring unbiased assessment and objective evaluation.

2.4. Follow Up

After the baseline evaluation, we performed a monthly telephone call to monitor the pregnancy's evolution until delivery. A record was kept with the date of delivery, the delivery route, the delivery characteristics; and if it was spontaneous or was indicated by fetal or maternal conditions, the reason was also recorded. These data were obtained from the medical records of each patient.

2.5. Data Collection

Clinical data were stored in a password-protected, web-based electronic database, REDCap, with the de-identification capability to protect patient information. After extraction from the ultrasound machine, the deidentified ultrasound images were stored in a repository and linked through the unique assigned code.

2.6. Outcomes

The primary outcome was the occurrence of preterm birth, defined as childbirth before 37 weeks of gestation. The secondary outcome was preterm birth before 34 weeks of gestation.

2.7. Statistical Analysis

Mean and standard deviation were used for normally distributed data while the median and interquartile range (IQR) was used for non-parametric data. Categoric data were expressed as proportions and percentages. ROC curves were generated for the CCI, for PTB before 37 weeks and for PTB before 34 weeks. The sensitivity, specificity, positive (PPV) and negative (NPV) predictive values, and positive (LR+) and negative (LR−) likelihood ratios were calculated for the best cut-off obtained from the ROC curves and for intended additional cut-offs as the percentile 5, 10, and 15. The association between PTB, CCI, CL, and history of PTB was performed by multiple logistic regression analysis, while the performance was assessed using sensitivity, specificity, PPV and NPV, LR+ and LR−, and area under the curve (AUC). In addition, the intraobserver and the interobserver reliability were evaluated with the intraclass correlation coefficient (ICC) (two-way random effect model). Intraobserver agreement was calculated as the difference between two CCI measurements by the same observer, and the interobserver agreement as the difference between the CCI measurements obtained by different observers. The magnitude of the differences was estimated as described by Bland–Altman [15]. (StataCorp. 2020, Stata Statistical Software: Release 16. StataCorp LLC: College Station, TX, USA).

3. Results

3.1. Description of the Cohort and Characteristics of the Study Population

Among the 786 pregnant women initially recruited, 45 were excluded due to miscarriages (16), iatrogenic preterm birth (40), and cases with incomplete perinatal outcomes (63) (Figure 2).

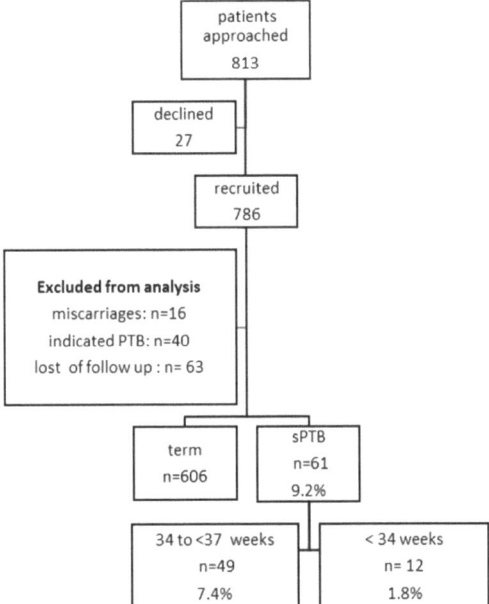

Figure 2. Patient flowchart.

For the 667 women left for analysis, the median maternal age was 28 years. History of PTB was present in 8.1% (54/667) of the population, 55% (371/667) had a previous term birth, and the rest were nulliparous. The rate of sPTB < 37 and <34 weeks was 9.2% (61/667) and 1.8% (12/667), respectively. Women delivering < 37 weeks had a higher prevalence of history of PTB compared to patients delivering at term (21.3% vs. 6.8%: $p < 0.001$) and a lower CCI (0.80 vs. 0.83; $p = 0.003$) at first trimester, with no significant difference in CL (35 mm vs. 35 mm; $p = 0.845$) (Table 1).

Supplementary Table S1 contains the clinical and demographic characteristics of the entire cohort.

Table 1. Characteristics of the included population by groups of PTB < 37 weeks.

Characteristic	Term Birth n = 606	sPTB < 37 Weeks n = 61	p-Value
Maternal age (years) *	28 (24–32)	27(25–32)	0.118
Preterm birth history	41 (6.8%)	13 (21.3%)	<0.001
Smoking history	70 (11.5%)	4 (6.6%)	0.244
Body mass index *	25.3 (22.6–28.1)	26.5 (23.4–29.7)	0.224
GA at scan (weeks) *	13.1(12.5–13.5)	13.2 (12.5–13.5)	0.671
Cervical length (mm) *	35 (35–38)	35 (33–37)	0.845
CCI *	0.83 (0.78–0.87)	0.80 (0.76–0.85)	0.003
GA at delivery(weeks) *	38.6 (38–39.4)	36.2(34.5–36.4)	<0.001
Without previous pregnancies	223 (37%)	16 (26.2%)	0.097
Health care system			
Subsidized	78 (28.2%)	10 (29.4%)	
Contributive	172 (62.1%)	17 (50.0%)	0.537
Special	16 (5.8%)	5 (14.7%)	0.146
Not in the system	11 (3.1%)	2 (5.9%)	0.677
Marital status			
Married	189 (31.2%)	13(21.3%)	
Live with partner	334 (55.1%)	44 (72.1%)	0.480
Single	83 (13.7%)	4 (6.5%)	0.544
Residence place			
Metropolitan area	460 (76.0%)	42(68.8%)	
Outside	145(24.0%)	19 (31.2%)	0.217
Nationality			
Colombian	576 (95.1%)	58 (95.1%)	
Venezuelan	30 (4.9%)	3 (4.9%)	0.991

The control group consisted of pregnant women who delivery at term. * Median (IQR); sPTB: spontaneous preterm birth; CCI: cervical consistency index; GA: gestational age.

3.2. Cervical Consistency Index as Predictor of sPTB

A first-trimester CCI < 10th percentile (CCI < 0.74) has 20% sensitivity and 90% specificity for the prediction of sPTB < 37 weeks. Meanwhile, the same percentile has a 33% sensitivity and 90% specificity for sPTB < 34 weeks. The positive and negative LRs for the 10th percentile were 2.05 and 0.89 for sPTB < 37 weeks, and 3.35 and 0.74 for sPTB < 34 weeks. The cut-off point with the best LR+ for sPTB < 37 weeks was 0.70 CCI with a 9.8% detection rate (DR) at a 4% FPR and positive and negative LRs of 3.4 and 0.87, respectively. The best cut-off point for sPTB < 34 weeks was 0.69 CCI with a DR of 17% at a 3.7% FPR and 4.53 and 0.87 positive and negative LRs (Table 2).

Table 2. Predictive performance of the CCI for the prediction of sPTB.

Cut-Off	Sensitivity % (n/N)	Specificity % (n/N)	PPV % (n/N)	NPV % (n/N)	LR+ 95% CI	LR− 95% CI
sPTB < 37 weeks						
CCI (centile)						
0.71 (5th)	9.8 (6/61)	95.4 (576/604)	17.6 (6/34)	76.2 (576/631)	2.12 (0.91–4.92)	0.95 (0.85–1.06)
0.74 (10th)	19.7 (12/61)	90.4 (546/604)	17.1 (12/70)	91.8(546/595)	2.05 (1.17–3.60)	0.89 (0.77–1.03)
0.76 (15th)	24.6 (15/61)	85.9 (519/604)	15.0(15/100)	91.9 (519/565)	1.75 (1.08–2.83)	0.88 (0.75–1.03)
CCI < 0.70 *	9.8 (6/34)	96.2 (581/604)	20.7 (23/29)	91.4 (581/636)	3.40 (1.09–6.10)	0.87 (0.84–1.05)
sPTB < 34 weeks						
CCI (centile)						
0.71 (5th)	16.7 (2/12)	95.1 (621/653)	5.9 (2/34)	98.4 (621/631)	3.40 (0.92–12.60)	0.88 (0.67–1.14)
0.74 (10th)	33.3 (4/12)	90.0 (588/653)	5.8 (4/69)	98.7 (588/596)	3.35 (1.46–7.70)	0.74 (0.49–1.11)
0.76 (15th)	50.0 (6/12)	85.6 (559/653)	6.0 (6/100)	98.9 (559/565)	3.47 (1.91–6.30)	0.58 (0.33–1.03)
CCI < 0.69 *	16.7 (2/12)	96.3 (629/653)	7.7 (2/26)	98.4 (629/639)	4.53 (1.21–17.06)	0.87 (0.66–1.13)

* the best cut-off point.

3.3. Cervical Consistency Index as Predictor of sPTB According to History of sPTB

Using the same 10th percentile of CCI (CCI < 0.74) as a cut-off point, we divided the women in the study into two groups, namely those with preterm birth histories and those without. CCI sensitivity was better in women with previous sPTB compared to those without history of sPTB. However, specificity was lower in women with history of sPTB. The best sensitivity was found among women with history of sPTB that delivered before 34 weeks (67%), while the highest specificity was the same for women without history of sPTB overall (Table 3).

Table 3. Performance of CCI for the prediction of sPTB according to history of preterm birth.

No History of sPTB	Sensitivity % (n/N)	Specificity % (n/N)	PPV % (n/N)	NPV % (n/N)	LR+	LR−
sPTB < 37 weeks CCI at 10th percentile	15 (7/48)	91 (516/565)	13 (7/49)	93 (516/557)	1.68	0.94
sPTB < 34 weeks CCI at 10th percentile	22 (2/9)	91 (550/604)	4 (2/56)	99 (550/557)	2.49	0.85
History of sPTB						
sPTB < 37 weeks CCI at 10th percentile	39 (5/13)	90 (37/41)	56 (5/9)	82 (37/45)	3.94	0.68
sPTB < 34 weeks CCI at 10th percentile	67 (2/3)	82 (44/51)	22 (2/9)	98 (44/45)	4.86	0.40

3.4. Association between sPTB, CCI, Cervical Length, and History of PTB

In a multiple regression analysis, the two independent variables associated with sPTB < 37 weeks were CCI (OR: 2.55; 95% CI: 1.28–5.10; $p = 0.008$) and history of sPTB (OR: 3.73; 95% CI: 1.87–7.44; $p < 0.001$). For sPTB < 34 weeks, the two independent variables were CCI below the 10th percentile (OR: 4.87; 95% CI: 1.42–16.63; $p = 0.012$), and history of sPTB (OR: 3.94; 95% CI: 1.03–15.09; $p = 0.044$). When measuring the performance of the different covariates for the prediction of sPTB, the best AUC was obtained by CCI (0.62; 95% CI: 0.48–0.76). There was no significant association between sPTB and CL (Table 4).

Table 4. Association between sPTB, CCI, cervical length, and history of PTB.

PTB < 37 Weeks	OR	5% CI	95% CI	p-Value	AUC
CCI <10th percentile	2.55	1.28	5.10	0.008	0.55 (0.50–0.60)
Cervical Length	1.00	0.95	1.06	0.843	0.50 (0.43–0.58)
History of PTB	3.73	1.87	7.44	<0.001	0.57 (0.52–0.62)
PTB < 34 weeks					
CCI < 10th percentile	4.87	1.42	16.63	0.012	0.62 (0.48–0.76)
Cervical Length	0.95	0.83	1.08	0.475	0.41 (0.22–0.60)
History of PTB	3.94	1.03	15.09	0.044	0.58 (0.45–0.71)

3.5. Intraobserver and Interobserver Agreement of the Cervical Consistency Index

Two measurements were evaluated in 109 cases by the same operator to establish the intraobserver variability, and two operators evaluated 49 patients to establish the interobserver variability. The relationship between the differences and means of the intraobserver and interobserver measurements are represented in the Bland–Altman plots (Figures 3 and 4). The intraobserver ICC was 0.862 (95% CI, 0.769–0.920), and the interobserver ICC was 0.833 (95% CI, 0.722–0.902).

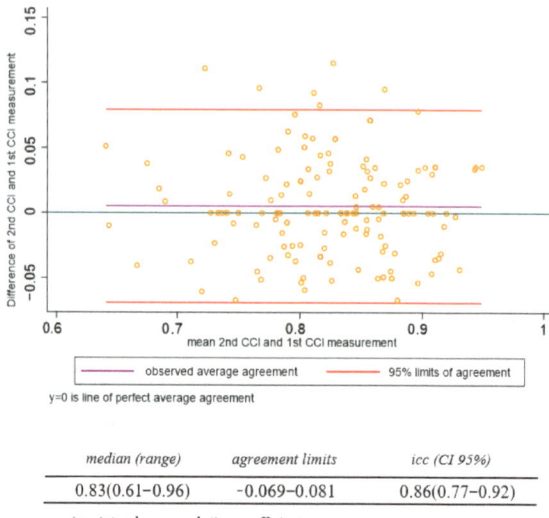

Figure 3. Intraobserver agreement of the cervical consistency index.

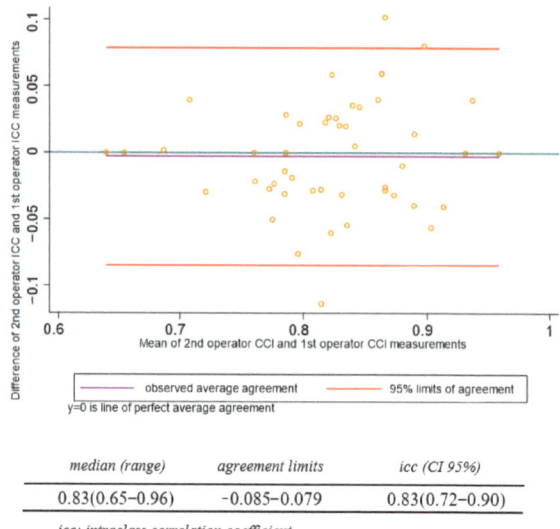

Figure 4. Interobserver agreement of the cervical consistency index.

The Bland–Altman plot shows the magnitude of differences for the intraobserver CCI measurements.

The Bland–Altman plot shows the magnitude of differences for the interobserver CCI measurements.

4. Discussion

There are two main findings from the study. This first is that first-trimester CCI below the 10th percentile (CCI < 0.74) demonstrated a significant association with sPTB before 37 weeks, exhibiting 20% sensitivity and 90% specificity. The same percentile had a 33% sensitivity and 90% specificity for predicting sPTB before 34 weeks. The second finding is that women with a history of PTB who delivered before 34 weeks showed the highest sensitivity (67%) for CCI < 0.74, while the overall best predictor for sPTB was CCI, with an area under the curve (AUC) of 0.62. Also, we found a robust intraobserver and interobserver agreement, affirming the reliability of CCI measurements in predicting preterm birth. These results are in line with our previous observations, which other researchers have confirmed: the cervix softens before it shortens [16,17].

Many studies have evaluated CL performance early in pregnancy to select the population at risk of sPTB [18–26]. In the Conoscenti study [18], the authors evaluated the role of CL in the early second trimester (13–15 weeks) to predict sPTB; they did not find differences between groups. Carvalho et al. [19] evaluated CL at two points in the pregnancy; no differences were found between groups at 11–14 weeks. However, when comparing the outcome with CL at 22–24 weeks, the association was significant (39.3 mm vs. 26.7 mm, $p = 0.0001$), concluding that the cervix shortens more rapidly between the first and the second trimester in those patients who deliver prematurely. In the Berghella study [20], in pregnant women with a high risk of preterm birth, a short cervix (CL < 25 mm) at 10–14 weeks identified 14% of women who delivered preterm. Antsaklis et al. [21] used 27 mm and 30 mm as cut-offs at 11–14 weeks to predict PTB; the authors did not find predictive values for sPTB < 35 weeks and the predictive value for sPTB before 37 weeks (AUC 0.60; 95% CI 0.54–0.66, $p = 0.001$). Other studies arguing that the CL measurement technique may influence the results have reported an association between the first-trimester short cervix and sPTB. Souka et al. [22] evaluated the predictive value of a model including maternal characteristics and CL at 11–13 weeks; they did not include the uterine isthmus in the measurement. A cut-off of 27 mm identified 25% (3/12) of the patients who presented a cervix < 15 mm at 20–24 weeks. Greco et al. [23], measuring the CL at 11–13 weeks, found significant differences between patients who delivered preterm compared to patients who delivered at term (27,5 mm vs. 32.5 mm $p < 0.0001$); the prediction was not evaluated. Souka et al. [24] reported that median CL at 11–13 weeks was significantly shorter in the women who subsequently delivered preterm; CL predicted PTB before 37 weeks (OR 0.90; 95% CI, 0.522–0.671; AUC 0.596) and before 34 weeks (OR, 0.74; 95% CI, 0.649–0.869; AUC 0.759). The sensitivity for predicting 37 weeks was 27% for a fixed 25% screen positive rate. Recently, Feng et al. [25] found that CL was significantly shorter in women who delivered < 34 weeks compared to women who delivered at term ($p < 0.001$) with the two-line method, following the curvature of the cervical canal (AUC 0.658; 95% CI 0.637–0.677). In our study, the uterine isthmus was excluded in the CL measurement, and we did not find differences between cervical length in women who delivered at term 35 mm (33–38) and women who delivered preterm 35 mm (33–37) $p = 0.845$.

Regarding the other cervical characteristic considered, such as softness for the prediction of PTB, many techniques have been tested at different gestational ages; the characteristics of each are reviewed in detail by Feltovich et al. [26]. The author discusses the techniques' limitations, and finally emphasizes the necessity of integrating quantitative techniques. Shear wave elastography (SWE) is one of the most evaluated. Hernandez-Andrade et al. [27] found that a soft cervix evaluated by SWE between 18 to 24 weeks of gestation increased the risk of sPTB < 37 weeks and <34 weeks. A soft cervix defined as an SWE at the internal OS < 25th percentile for the gestational age is a risk factor for sPTB < 34 weeks (OR 7.7; 95% CI 1.8–29.6) and for sPTD < 37 weeks (OR 4.4; 95% CI 1.4–12.0), independent of cervical length.

For the first trimester, Feng et al. [25] explored the potential value for the SWE to predict sPTB; the mean cervical SWE scores were significantly lower in women who delivered < 37 weeks (28.0 kPa vs. 30.6 kPa, $p < 0.05$). Women with a mean cervical SWE MoM <10th percentile had a RR of 2.42 (95% CI 1.29–4.55) and 7.81 (95% CI 2.13–28.60) for spontaneous delivery at <37 weeks and <34 weeks of gestation, respectively. The detection rate was 20.4% and 44.4% for sPTB at 37 and 34 weeks, respectively. In our study, the CCI showed a detection rate of 20% for sPTB < 37 weeks and 33% for sPTB < 34 weeks.

Taking all these results together, we consider, for the case of first-trimester sPTB prediction, that cervical softening is the characteristic that identifies early changes in the course of the disease, and the CCI is an efficient technique for detecting premature softening. Early intervention strategies, such as pharmacologic interventions (progesterone), targeted monitoring, and personalized care plans, can be implemented for women identified with a low CCI, potentially reducing the incidence of PTB and improving maternal and neonatal outcomes. Studies in larger populations are required to validate these findings.

We acknowledge that the first trimester CCI has limited ability to identify patients at risk of preterm birth, and considering the multiple pathways that cause preterm birth, it is unlikely that a single test will achieve better figures. Therefore, it will be necessary to add other measurements and biomarkers to build a model that improves its predictive capacity.

The study's strengths lie in its prospective nature, the operator blindness for the cervical consistency index result, and the fact that the research team did not make clinical or therapeutic decisions based on the cervical measurements; additionally, the gestational age based on the CRL adds robustness to our findings. Reproducibility challenges were minimized by our approach, considering the cervical tissue's biomechanical characteristics.

We recognize that the study has limitations, including a low prevalence of sPTB before 34 weeks, which impacted precision. We must be cautious with the sensitivity to identify patients with a history of preterm birth (67%) based on three cases. Additionally, a slight loss of participants to follow-up was observed, which affected accuracy; however, the study's prospective design, the operator blinding, and the diverse participant pool from multiple institutions ensured a rigorous methodology and enhanced its credibility.

5. Conclusions

This study establishes the CCI as a promising and early predictive marker for sPTB risk, particularly before 34 weeks of gestation. This manuscript shows that a CCI below the 10th percentile in the first trimester significantly correlates with an increased likelihood of preterm birth. This research re-opens the question of first-trimester research for the prediction of sPTB.

Supplementary Materials: The following supporting information can be downloaded at: https://www.mdpi.com/article/10.3390/jcm13133906/s1, Table S1: Demographic and clinical characteristics of the entire cohort ($n = 667$).

Author Contributions: Conceptualization: C.H.B.-M., B.R.-O., M.A.P.-S., R.A.M.-V., L.A.D.-M. and R.J.M.-P.; methodology: C.H.B.-M., B.R.-O., R.A.M.-V., L.A.D.-M., R.J.M.-P. and J.T.-T.; software: R.A.M.-V., L.A.D.-M., R.J.M.-P., J.T.-T. and C.H.B.-M., validation: C.H.B.-M., B.R.-O., M.A.P.-S., R.A.M.-V., L.A.D.-M., R.J.M.-P. and J.T.-T.; formal analysis: C.H.B.-M., B.R.-O., M.A.P.-S., R.A.M.-V., L.A.D.-M., R.J.M.-P. and J.T.-T.; data curation: C.H.B.-M., R.A.M.-V. and B.R.-O.; writing—original draft preparation: C.H.B.-M., B.R.-O., M.A.P.-S., R.A.M.-V., L.A.D.-M., R.J.M.-P. and J.T.-T.; writing—review and editing C.H.B.-M., B.R.-O., M.A.P.-S., R.A.M.-V., L.A.D.-M., R.J.M.-P. and J.T.-T.; Project administration: B.R.-O. and C.H.B.-M.; funding acquisition: B.R.-O., L.A.D.-M. and C.H.B.-M.; teaching the CCI technique and evaluating the competence: M.A.P.-S. and C.H.B.-M. All authors have read and agreed to the published version of the manuscript.

Funding: This project was partially funded by grants from: Universidad Industrial de Santander projects code 2542 and 2841. Ministry of Science, Technology, and Innovation of Colombia (MINCIENCIAS, project code 110291891745).

Institutional Review Board Statement: The study was conducted in accordance with the Declaration of Helsinki and approved by the Research Ethics Committee of Universidad Industrial de Santander (CEINCI: Act No. 17, 17 October 2019). Project code 254.

Informed Consent Statement: Informed consent was obtained from all subjects involved in the study.

Data Availability Statement: The data that support the findings of this study are available on request from the corresponding author.

Acknowledgments: The authors would like to acknowledge the contributions of Carolina Parra and Mónica Beltran. The authors also would like to thank the health institutions that have facilitated the recruitment. They also would like to thank the mothers who participated in the cohort study.

Conflicts of Interest: The authors declare no conflicts of interest. The funders had no role in the design of the study; in the collection, analyses, or interpretation of data; in the writing of the manuscript; or in the decision to publish the results.

References

1. Walani, S.R. Global burden of preterm birth. *Int. J. Gynaecol. Obstet.* **2020**, *150*, 31–33. [CrossRef] [PubMed]
2. March of Dimes, pmNch, Save the Children, WHO. Born Too Soon: The Global Action Report on Preterm Birth. eds cp howson, mV Kinney, Je lawn. World Health Organization. Geneva. 2012. Available online: https://apps.who.int/iris/bitstream/handle/10665/44864/9789241503433_eng.pdf;jsessionid=C221360BA148E228A7A079C1EE4261E8?sequence=1 (accessed on 15 June 2024).
3. De Costa, A.; Moller, A.B.; Blencowe, H.; Johansson, E.W.; Hussain-Alkhateeb, L.; Ohuma, E.O.; Okwaraji, Y.B.; Cresswell, J.; Requejo, J.H.; Bahl, R.; et al. Study protocol for WHO and UNICEF estimates of global, regional, and national preterm birth rates for 2010 to 2019. *PLoS ONE* **2021**, *16*, e0258751. [CrossRef] [PubMed]
4. Blencowe, H.; Cousens, S.; Oestergaard, M.Z.; Chou, D.; Moller, A.B.; Narwal, R.; Adler, A.; Vera Garcia, C.; Rohde, S.; Say, L.; et al. National, regional, and worldwide estimates of preterm birth rates in the year 2010 with time trends since 1990 for selected countries: A systematic analysis and implications. *Lancet* **2012**, *379*, 2162–2172. [CrossRef] [PubMed]
5. Liu, L.; Oza, S.; Hogan, D.; Chu, Y.; Perin, J.; Zhu, J.; Lawn, J.E.; Cousens, S.; Mathers, C.; Black, R.E. Global, regional, and national causes of under-5 mortality in 2000–15: An updated systematic analysis with implications for the Sustainable Development Goals. *Lancet* **2016**, *388*, 3027–3035, published correction appears in *Lancet* **2017**, *389*, 1884. [CrossRef] [PubMed]
6. Celik, E.; To, M.; Gajewska, K.; Smith, G.C.; Nicolaides, K.H.; Fetal Medicine Foundation Second Trimester Screening Group. Cervical length and obstetric history predict spontaneous preterm birth: Development and validation of a model to provide individualized risk assessment. *Ultrasound Obstet. Gynecol.* **2008**, *31*, 549–554. [CrossRef] [PubMed]
7. Gudicha, D.W.; Romero, R.; Kabiri, D.; Hernandez-Andrade, E.; Pacora, P.; Erez, O.; Kusanovic, J.P.; Jung, E.; Paredes, C.; Berry, S.M.; et al. Personalized assessment of cervical length improves prediction of spontaneous preterm birth: A standard and a percentile calculator. *Am. J. Obstet. Gynecol.* **2021**, *224*, 288.e1–288.e17. [CrossRef] [PubMed]
8. Parra-Saavedra, M.; Gómez, L.; Barrero, A.; Parra, G.; Vergara, F.; Navarro, E. Prediction of preterm birth using the cervical consistency index. *Ultrasound Obstet. Gynecol.* **2011**, *38*, 44–51. [CrossRef] [PubMed]
9. Baños, N.; Murillo-Bravo, C.; Julià, C.; Migliorelli, F.; Perez-Moreno, A.; Ríos, J.; Gratacós, E.; Valentin, L.; Palacio, M. Mid-trimester sonographic cervical consistency index to predict spontaneous preterm birth in a low-risk population. *Ultrasound Obstet. Gynecol.* **2018**, *51*, 629–636. [CrossRef] [PubMed]
10. Baños, N.; Julià, C.; Lorente, N.; Ferrero, S.; Cobo, T.; Gratacos, E.; Palacio, M. Mid-Trimester Cervical Consistency Index and Cervical Length to Predict Spontaneous Preterm Birth in a High-Risk Population. *AJP Rep.* **2018**, *8*, e43–e50. [CrossRef] [PubMed]
11. van der Merwe, J.; Couck, I.; Russo, F.; Burgos-Artizzu, X.P.; Deprest, J.; Palacio, M.; Lewi, L. The Predictive Value of the Cervical Consistency Index to Predict Spontaneous Preterm Birth in Asymptomatic Twin Pregnancies at the Second-Trimester Ultrasound Scan: A Prospective Cohort Study. *J. Clin. Med.* **2020**, *9*, 1784. [CrossRef] [PubMed]
12. Wharton, L.K.; Anumba, D.O.C. Techniques for detecting cervical remodeling as a predictor for spontaneous preterm birth: Current evidence and future research avenues in patients with multiple pregnancies. *J. Matern. Fetal Neonatal Med.* **2023**, *36*, 2262081. [CrossRef] [PubMed]
13. Sonek, J.; Shellhaas, C. Cervical sonography: A review. *Ultrasound Obstet. Gynecol.* **1998**, *11*, 71–78. [CrossRef] [PubMed]
14. Becerra-Mojica, C.H.; Parra-Saavedra, M.A.; Diaz-Martinez, L.A.; Martinez-Portilla, R.J.; Rincon Orozco, B. Cohort profile: Colombian Cohort for the Early Prediction of Preterm Birth (COLPRET): Early prediction of preterm birth based on personal medical history, clinical characteristics, vaginal microbiome, biophysical characteristics of the cervix and maternal serum biochemical markers. *BMJ Open* **2022**, *12*, e060556. [PubMed]
15. Bland, J.M.; Altman, D.G. Statistical methods for assessing agreement between two methods of clinical measurement. *Lancet* **1986**, *1*, 307–310. [CrossRef] [PubMed]
16. Torres, J.; Faris, I.; Callejas, A. Histobiomechanical Remodeling of the Cervix during Pregnancy: Proposed Framework. *Math. Probl. Eng.* **2019**, *2019*, 5957432. [CrossRef]
17. McFarlin, B.L.; Bigelow, T.A.; Laybed, Y.; O'Brien, W.D.; Oelze, M.L.; Abramowicz, J.S. Ultrasonic attenuation estimation of the pregnant cervix: A preliminary report. *Ultrasound Obstet. Gynecol.* **2010**, *36*, 218–225. [CrossRef]
18. Conoscenti, G.; Meir, Y.J.; D'Ottavio, G.; Rustico, M.A.; Pinzano, R.; Fischer-Tamaro, L.; Stampalija, T.; Natale, R.; Maso, G.; Mandruzzato, G. Does cervical length at 13–15 weeks' gestation predict preterm delivery in an unselected population? *Ultrasound Obstet. Gynecol.* **2003**, *21*, 128–134. [CrossRef]
19. Carvalho, M.H.; Bittar, R.E.; Brizot, M.L.; Maganha, P.P.; Borges da Fonseca, E.S.; Zugaib, M. Cervical length at 11–14 weeks' and 22-24 weeks' gestation evaluated by transvaginal sonography, and gestational age at delivery. *Ultrasound Obstet. Gynecol.* **2003**, *21*, 135–139. [CrossRef] [PubMed]

20. Berghella, V.; Talucci, M.; Desai, A. Does transvaginal sonographic measurement of cervical length before 14 weeks predict preterm delivery in high-risk pregnancies? *Ultrasound Obstet. Gynecol.* **2003**, *21*, 140–144. [CrossRef] [PubMed]
21. Antsaklis, P.; Daskalakis, G.; Pilalis, A.; Papantoniou, N.; Mesogitis, S.; Antsaklis, A. The role of cervical length measurement at 11–14 weeks for the prediction of preterm delivery. *J. Matern. Fetal Neonatal Med.* **2011**, *24*, 465–470. [CrossRef] [PubMed]
22. Souka, A.P.; Papastefanou, I.; Michalitsi, V.; Papadopoulos, G.K.; Kassanos, D. A predictive model of short cervix at 20–24 weeks using first-trimester cervical length measurement and maternal history. *Prenat. Diagn.* **2011**, *31*, 202–206. [CrossRef] [PubMed]
23. Greco, E.; Lange, A.; Ushakov, F.; Calvo, J.R.; Nicolaides, K.H. Prediction of spontaneous preterm delivery from endocervical length at 11 to 13 weeks. *Prenat. Diagn.* **2011**, *31*, 84–89. [CrossRef] [PubMed]
24. Souka, A.P.; Papastefanou, I.; Michalitsi, V.; Salambasis, K.; Chrelias, C.; Salamalekis, G.; Kassanos, D. Cervical length changes from the first to second trimester of pregnancy, and prediction of preterm birth by first-trimester sonographic cervical measurement. *J. Ultrasound Med.* **2011**, *30*, 997–1002, published correction appears in *J. Ultrasound Med.* **2011**, *30*, 1753. [CrossRef] [PubMed]
25. Feng, Q.; Chaemsaithong, P.; Duan, H.; Ju, X.; Appiah, K.; Shen, L.; Wang, X.; Tai, Y.; Leung, T.Y.; Poon, L.C. Screening for spontaneous preterm birth by cervical length and shear-wave elastography in the first trimester of pregnancy. *Am. J. Obstet. Gynecol.* **2022**, *227*, 500.e1–500.e14. [CrossRef] [PubMed]
26. Feltovich, H.; Carlson, L. New techniques in evaluation of the cervix. *Semin. Perinatol.* **2017**, *41*, 477–484. [CrossRef] [PubMed]
27. Hernandez-Andrade, E.; Maymon, E.; Luewan, S.; Bhatti, G.; Mehrmohammadi, M.; Erez, O.; Pacora, P.; Done, B.; Hassan, S.S.; Romero, R. A soft cervix, categorized by shear-wave elastography, in women with short or with normal cervical length at 18–24 weeks is associated with a higher prevalence of spontaneous preterm delivery. *J. Perinat. Med.* **2018**, *46*, 489–501. [CrossRef] [PubMed]

Disclaimer/Publisher's Note: The statements, opinions and data contained in all publications are solely those of the individual author(s) and contributor(s) and not of MDPI and/or the editor(s). MDPI and/or the editor(s) disclaim responsibility for any injury to people or property resulting from any ideas, methods, instructions or products referred to in the content.

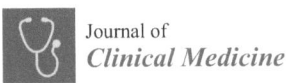 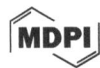

Article

Comparison of Fetal Crown-Rump Length Measurements between Thawed and Fresh Embryo Transfer

Kyriaki Mitta, Ioannis Tsakiridis *, Evaggelia Giougi, Apostolos Mamopoulos, Ioannis Kalogiannidis, Themistoklis Dagklis and Apostolos Athanasiadis

Third Department of Obstetrics and Gynaecology, School of Medicine, Faculty of Health Sciences, Aristotle University of Thessaloniki, 54642 Thessaloniki, Greece; kmittb@auth.gr (K.M.); egiougi@gmail.com (E.G.); amamop@auth.gr (A.M.); ikalogia@auth.gr (I.K.); dagklis@auth.gr (T.D.); apathana@auth.gr (A.A.)
* Correspondence: iotsakir@gmail.com

Citation: Mitta, K.; Tsakiridis, I.; Giougi, E.; Mamopoulos, A.; Kalogiannidis, I.; Dagklis, T.; Athanasiadis, A. Comparison of Fetal Crown-Rump Length Measurements between Thawed and Fresh Embryo Transfer. *J. Clin. Med.* 2024, *13*, 2575. https://doi.org/10.3390/jcm13092575

Academic Editors: Alberto Revelli and Tailang Yin

Received: 12 March 2024
Revised: 8 April 2024
Accepted: 23 April 2024
Published: 27 April 2024

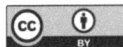

Copyright: © 2024 by the authors. Licensee MDPI, Basel, Switzerland. This article is an open access article distributed under the terms and conditions of the Creative Commons Attribution (CC BY) license (https://creativecommons.org/licenses/by/4.0/).

Abstract: Background and Objectives: Neonates born from thawed embryo transfers tend to have a significantly higher birthweight compared to those from fresh embryo transfers. The aim of this study was to compare the crown-rump length (CRL) between thawed and fresh embryos to investigate the potential causes of different growth patterns between them. **Materials and Methods:** This was a retrospective study (July 2010–December 2023) conducted at the Third Department of Obstetrics and Gynecology, School of Medicine, Faculty of Health Sciences, Aristotle University of Thessaloniki, Greece. In total, 3082 assisted reproductive technology (ART) pregnancies (4044 embryos) underwent a routine scan at 11^{+0}–13^{+6} gestational weeks and were included in the study. Maternal age, the type of embryo transfer (thawed vs. fresh, donor vs. their own oocytes), CRL, twin and singleton gestations were analyzed. **Results:** The mean maternal age in thawed was significantly higher than in fresh embryos (39.8 vs. 35.8 years, *p*-value < 0.001). The mean CRL z-score was significantly higher in thawed compared to fresh embryo transfers (0.309 vs. 0.199, *p*-value < 0.001). A subgroup analysis on singleton gestations showed that the mean CRL z-score was higher in thawed blastocysts compared to fresh (0.327 vs. 0.215, *p*-value < 0.001). Accordingly, an analysis on twins revealed that the mean CRL z-score was higher in thawed blastocysts (0.285 vs. 0.184, *p*-value: 0.015) and in oocytes' recipients compared to own oocytes' cases (0.431 vs. 0.191, *p*-value: 0.002). **Conclusions:** The difference in CRL measurements between thawed and fresh embryos may be a first indication of the subsequent difference in sonographically estimated fetal weight and birthweight. This finding highlights the need for additional research into the underlying causes, including maternal factors and the culture media used.

Keywords: ART; thawed; fresh; embryo; CRL; measurement

1. Introduction

The use of assisted reproductive technology (ART) is constantly rising, and thus associated fetal, maternal and neonatal complications have been investigated over the past few years. Recent findings have indicated an increased risk of low birthweight in infants born after fresh cycle in vitro fertilization (IVF)/intracytoplasmic sperm injection (ICSI) treatments [1]. Studies comparing the outcomes of pregnancies resulting from thawed and fresh blastocysts following IVF/ICSI have shown that infants born from thawed blastocysts have significantly higher birthweight than those born from fresh embryo transfers [2].

Regarding the health outcomes of infants conceived via ART, the current literature suggests that IVF/ICSI is associated with an increased likelihood of small-for-gestational age (SGA) neonates, as well as higher incidences of low-birthweight and preterm births [1,3]. Notably, thawed embryos are associated with large-for-gestational age (LGA) neonates and a higher risk of gestational hypertension and preeclampsia [4]. Moreover, the risks of antepartum hemorrhage, SGA, preterm birth, low birthweight and perinatal mortality are all significantly lower in pregnancies from thawed embryo transfers [3]. Thawed embryo transfer at the blastocyst stage is suggested to be the most suitable method in terms of optimal fetal growth [5].

In most settings, a first-trimester scan is offered at 11^{+0}–13^{+6} gestational weeks for dating, screening for preeclampsia and chromosomal abnormalities and the early detection of severe fetal defects [6,7]. The aim of this study was to compare the crown-rump length (CRL) between thawed and fresh embryos at a routine first-trimester scan. Taking into consideration the different fetal growth patterns and birthweights between the two types of embryos, an investigation of the potential differences in CRL measurements could clarify the reasons for these discrepancies and signify when these changes occur.

2. Materials and Methods

This was a retrospective study (July 2010–December 2023) conducted at the Third Department of Obstetrics and Gynecology, School of Medicine, Faculty of Health Sciences, Aristotle University of Thessaloniki, Greece. Maternal age, type of embryo transfer (thawed vs. fresh, donor vs. own oocytes), CRL and type of pregnancy (twin vs. singleton gestations) were recorded, as well. Inclusion criteria were women who underwent IVF using either fresh or frozen embryo blastocysts, regardless of the ovarian stimulation protocol, the number of embryos transferred or hormone levels involved. The pregnancies were confirmed to be between 11^{+0} and 13^{+6} weeks of gestation and all the participants had undergone a first-trimester scan performed by an expert sonographer. Any cases with anatomical or chromosomal abnormalities during the first-trimester scan, as well as all monochorionic twin gestations, were excluded from the study, as these may affect fetal growth. Those with missing data (i.e., type of embryo transfer) were also excluded.

All women had given their informed consent that their anonymized data could be used for future research. As per standard policy for audit or observational database studies not involving any intervention or modification of the management of the participants, no institutional review was required or obtained [8]. Of note, no incentives were provided to the participants. All first-trimester scans were performed by experienced maternal–fetal medicine specialists, according to the International Society of Ultrasound in Obstetrics and Gynecology guideline for first-trimester scans [9].

Qualitative variables were described as n (%), and quantitative data as mean (SD). An independent Student's t-test was employed to compare the means of quantitative variables (maternal age, CRL z-score). CRL was expressed as z-scores of a reference population of 11–13^{+6} weeks (45–84 mm) in fresh and thawed/thawed blastocysts after ART conceptions [10]. CRL z-scores were calculated using the formula Z-score = (XGA − MGA)/SDGA, where XGA was the actual fetal CRL measurement at a given gestation and MGA and SDGA were the expected mean and SD according to the international standards for early fetal size and pregnancy dating based on an ultrasound measurement of crown-rump length in the first trimester of pregnancy, obtained from the general population [11]. Further, subgroup analyses were conducted according to the type of oocyte used (own vs. donor) and the type of pregnancy (singletons vs. twins). A chi-squared test (x^2) was also employed to investigate any association between the types of gestations (twin vs. singleton) and the types of embryos transferred (thawed vs. fresh embryo transfer). It was also employed to examine any association between the type of gestation and the type of embryo (embryos from donor oocytes vs. their own ones). The level of statistical significance was set at $p = 0.05$. The statistical package IBM SPSS Statistics 29.0 was used.

3. Results

In total, 3082 ART pregnancies, including 4044 embryos, underwent a first-trimester scan during the study period. Of these embryos, 1255 (40.7%) originated from thawed transfers, whereas 1827 (59.3%) originated from fresh ones. The thawed embryos included 892 (71%) singleton pregnancies and 363 pairs of twins (726 embryos) (29%). The fresh embryos included 1228 (67.2%) singleton pregnancies and 599 pairs of twins (1198 embryos)

(32.8%) (Table 1a,b). Of note, 1725 (56%) pregnancies were from donor and 1357 (44%) from own oocytes. The donor embryo transfers included 600 (35%) twin and 1125 (65%) singleton gestations. The own oocyte embryo transfers included 362 (27%) twin and 995 (73%) singleton gestations.

Table 1. (**a**) Baseline characteristics according to type of embryo transfer (thawed vs. fresh) for the whole sample. (**b**) Baseline characteristics according to type of embryo transfer (thawed vs. fresh) for the whole sample (chi-squared test).

(a)					
Characteristics	**Thawed Cycles**	**Fresh Cycles**	***p*-Value**		
Number of embryos	1618 (40%)	2426 (60%)	N/A		
Maternal age (mean/SD)	39.8 (5.7)	35.8 (4.3)	**<0.001**		
CRL z-score (mean/SD)	0.309 (0.806)	0.199 (0.805)	**<0.001**		
(b)					
Characteristics	**Thawed Cycles**	**Fresh Cycles**	***p*-Value**	**OR**	**95% CI**
Number of singleton gestations	892 (71%)	1228 (67.2%)			
Number of twin gestations	363 (29%)	599 (32.8%)	**0.005**	1.20	1.06–1.36

CRL: crown-rump length; N/A: not applicable. OR: odds ratio; 95% CI: 95% confidence interval.

The mean age of women who underwent thawed embryo transfer was higher compared to those following fresh embryo transfer (39.8 years vs. 35.8 years, $p < 0.001$). The incidence of twin gestations was significantly higher in fresh compared to thawed embryo transfer (OR:1.20, 95% CI: 1.06–1.36, p-value= 0.005). The CRL z-score was higher in thawed compared to fresh embryos in the total sample population (0.309 vs. 0.199, $p < 0.001$) (Table 1a,b, Figure 1).

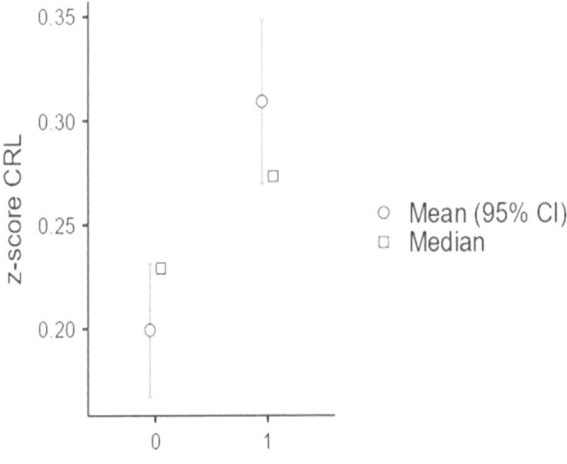

Figure 1. CRL z-score according to type of embryo transfer (ET) in the whole sample (0: fresh embryo transfer; 1: thawed embryo transfer).

A subgroup analysis on twin gestations found that the mean CRL z-score was significantly higher in both thawed cycles (0.285 vs. 0.184, p-value: 0.015) and in donor oocytes (0.431 vs. 0.191, p-value: 0.002) (Table 2, Figure 2). An analysis on singletons also showed that the mean CRL z-score was significantly higher in thawed compared to fresh cycles (0.327 vs. 0.215, p-value < 0.001) (Table 3, Figure 3).

Table 2. Subgroup analysis on twin gestations.

Characteristics	Thawed Cycles	Fresh Cycles	p-Value
Maternal age (mean/SD)	40.1 (6.1)	35.1 (4.3)	<0.001
CRL z-score (mean/SD)	0.285 (0.869)	0.184 (0.893)	0.015
Characteristics	**Own Oocytes**	**Donor Oocytes**	**p-Value**
Maternal age (mean/SD)	37.5 (5.1)	43.5 (4.7)	<0.001
CRL z-score (mean/SD)	0.191 (1.05)	0.431 (0.813)	0.002

CRL: crown-rump length.

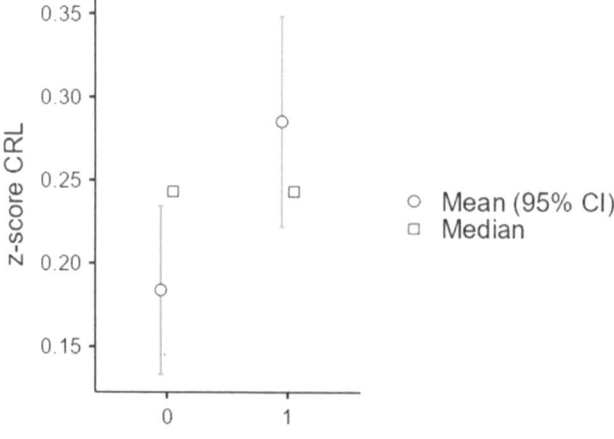

Figure 2. CRL z-score, according to type of embryo transfer (ET) in twin gestations (0: own oocytes; 1: donor oocytes).

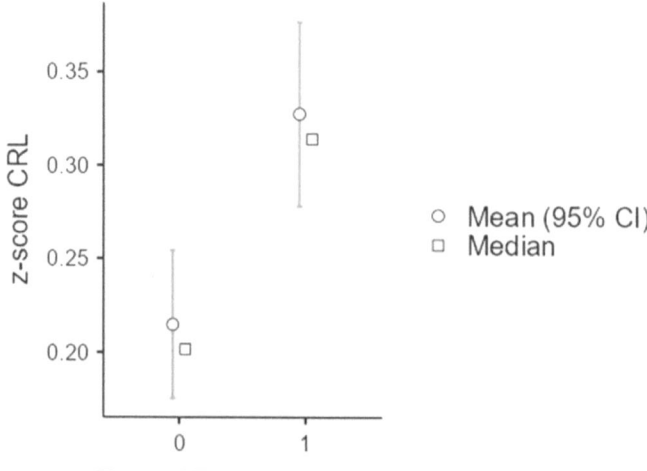

Figure 3. CRL z-scores according to type of embryo transfer in singleton gestations (0: fresh embryo transfer; 1: thawed embryo transfer).

Table 3. Subgroup analysis on singleton gestations.

Characteristics	Thawed Cycles	Fresh Cycles	p-Value
Maternal age (mean/SD)	39.6 (5.3)	36.4 (4.3)	<0.001
CRL z-score (mean/SD)	0.327 (0.751)	0.215 (0.709)	<0.001
Characteristics	Own Oocytes	Donor Oocytes	p-Value
Maternal age (mean/SD)	37.6 (4.5)	43.7 (4.1)	<0.001
CRL z-score (mean/SD)	0.455 (1.17)	0.314 (0.919)	0.412

CRL: crown-rump length.

4. Discussion

The main findings of this study were that (i) the mean maternal age in thawed embryo transfers was significantly higher than in fresh embryo transfers in the total sample, in singleton and twin gestations; (ii) the mean CRL z-score at 11^{+0}–13^{+6} weeks was significantly higher in thawed embryos compared to fresh embryos in both singleton and twin gestations; (iii) the mean maternal age of donor oocytes cases was significantly higher than those who used their own oocytes in both singleton and twin gestations; (iv) twin gestations were significantly higher in fresh blastocysts; and (v) the mean CRL z-score was significantly higher in twin gestations, arising from donor oocytes.

The conventional IVF/ICSI procedure consists of a fresh embryo transfer, followed by thawed embryo transfers in subsequent cycles in the case of failure at the first attempt. However, an alternative approach consists of the "freeze-all" strategy, in which case all embryos are thawed and transferred in subsequent cycles. A meta-analysis, comparing the two approaches, showed that the cumulative live birth rate and ongoing pregnancy rate are the same in the two methods [12]. However, a decreased risk of ovarian hyperstimulation syndrome (OHSS) seems to be associated with the "freeze-all" strategy. The same meta-analysis showed that in large-for-gestational age neonates, birthweight and incidence of hypertensive disorders may be increased in the "freeze-all" strategy [12]. New evidence suggests that hypertensive disorders are increased only in frozen cycles after hormone-replacement therapy, due to the absence of the corpus luteum and the absence of relaxin; the latter is associated with systematic vasodilation and increased arterial compliance [13]. However, the available data in the literature suggest that the maternal and perinatal outcomes are, in general, improved in thawed compared to fresh embryo transfer [14]. Therefore, there is an increased tendency towards thawed embryo transfer, nowadays.

Higher maternal age is related to more obstetric and maternal complications; therefore, it is reasonable to proceed with thawed embryo transfer [14]. The maternal age is higher in thawed compared to fresh embryo transfers, according to a retrospective cohort study [15]. The same finding was supported by other published data [16], which were in agreement with the results of our study. Pregnancies resulting from thawed embryos have become increasingly prevalent in Europe, resulting in about half of the ART cycles in numerous countries [17], especially in cases involving oocyte donation [18]. The use of thawed embryo transfer offers several clinical advantages, including the avoidance of endometrial asynchrony [19,20].

A retrospective analysis of 5406 embryos, revealed that the birthweight of neonates from thawed embryos was higher than in those arising from fresh embryos, but the potential mechanisms of this difference were not elucidated [21]. Therefore, investigating any difference in CRL measurement between thawed and fresh embryos could partially clarify these mechanisms. According to a secondary analysis of a prospective cohort study, the average CRL z-score between 6 and 14 weeks was notably higher in thawed compared to fresh transfers; the likelihood of having a CRL below the fifth percentile was 68% for fresh versus 40% for thawed embryos at 6 weeks, and 2% versus 1% at 14 weeks, respectively [22]. Similarly, in our study, CRL measurement during the first trimester anomaly scan was significantly increased in thawed compared to fresh embryos. This difference remained significant in subgroup analyses in singletons and twins. Several factors could contribute to the observed differences in CRL growth, such as changes in the condition of the endometrium [23,24], epigenetic modifications in the trophoblast [25], variations in ovarian hormone levels during the peri-implantation phase [26], the quality of the embryo, differences in blood flow to the uterus and disparities in cardiovascular health among the groups studied [27]. Another factor that could explain this difference in CRL measurements between thawed vs. fresh embryos could be the freezing and thawing process itself; embryos that survive this process are often considered to be more robust, potentially contributing to the observed differences in early growth as measured by CRL. Notably, the high levels of hormones after ovarian stimulation in fresh cycles compared to frozen cycles may contribute to these discrepancies in CRL measurement, as well. The association between fetal growth and the type of embryo transfer in the first trimester of pregnancy indicates that there might be a link between endometrial environment, hormonal milieu and fetal growth, as suggested by published data [28]. Nonetheless, a definitive causal relationship explaining the growth patterns and abnormalities in fetuses from thawed or fresh embryos has not been established, suggesting the causes are likely varied and complex. Of note, the CRL measurement has been suggested in the literature as a potential prognostic factor for pregnancy outcome; pregnancies following spontaneous conception with higher CRL measurements had a significantly lower risk of stillbirth [29].

According to the results of our study, the maternal age of oocyte recipients was significantly increased compared to those who used their own, which is reasonably explained; in 2014, up to 12% of all IVF cycles in the U.S. were performed using donor oocytes and a high pregnancy rate from women in their 50s was observed (>35%) [30]. Oocyte donation currently represents the main option for aging-related infertility [30].

Twin gestations are still a relatively common occurrence in ART [31]. The results of our study indicated a higher prevalence of twin gestations in fresh compared to thawed embryo transfer; this could be explained by the number of embryos transferred in each case. Furthermore, a comparative study on the cost-effectiveness of single embryo transfer followed by an additional thawed embryo transfer, compared to double embryo transfer, showed that in women above 32 years of age, double embryo transfer was more effective in fresh cycles [32], explaining the higher prevalence of twins in fresh embryo transfer. Increasing the success rate in the area of ART is crucial, taking into consideration the high cost of the procedure [33]. A meta-analysis of individual patient data analysis from randomized trials showed that elective single embryo transfer is related to a higher chance of delivering a full-term, healthy neonate compared to double embryo transfer, yet it is also associated with a lower pregnancy rate in fresh cycles [13]. Even though this difference is completely overcome by an additional thawed embryo transfer, there is still a tendency towards maximizing the chances of live birth at the first attempt and not cumulatively [13]. Elective single embryo transfer is the only effective way of minimizing the risk of multiple gestations and can also be applied in women 36–39 years old [34]. Preimplantation genetic testing for aneuploidies (PGT) could also enhance the strategy of elective single embryo transfer, without compromising the results of ART. Although evidence suggests that PGT improves live birth rates in women above 35, the Greek legislation does not allow its implementation in women before 40 years of age, without any other indication, thus discouraging elective single embryo transfer [35].

Notably, the mean CRL z-score was significantly higher in cases of twin gestations arising from donor oocytes, which was not observed in singletons. The current literature suggests that CRL is higher in heterologous embryos, derived from donor oocytes, compared to homologous embryos, derived from the parent's own gametes [36]. This could be attributed to the fact that donor gametes might be selected based on certain desirable traits, and overall vitality, which could have an impact on early embryonic growth, as indicated by CRL measurement. Furthermore, the age of the oocytes might have an impact, as well, since donor oocytes arise typically from young women. Therefore, oocytes from young donors may have a higher quality and better growth pattern due to the lack of genetic abnormalities. Sperm quality might affect the embryo's early growth and development, as well. Sperm donors are selected through thorough screening processes. Regarding embryological techniques, differences in culture conditions between homologous and heterologous embryos could also play a role. Techniques might vary in donor programs within IVF clinics. Selection and embryo transfer practices might influence early growth, as well. The best-quality embryos are chosen more rigorously in donor cycles, compared to homologous cycles, due to the associated costs and implications. The hormonal environment, endometrial receptivity and hormonal preparation for IVF in donor–recipient cycles may be different, contributing to a more favorable environment for optimal early embryo growth. Further research is needed to determine the reasons why these differences in early growth exist. Moreover, in twin gestations, there might be interactions between embryos that influence their developmental capacity; these interactions might enhance growth patterns, such as CRL, especially in a highly optimized environment of donor embryo transfer. Maternal hormonal and immune system adaptations in response to embryo implantation could differ significantly between one and two embryos and might be influenced further by the genetic unfamiliarity of donor embryos. In twin pregnancies resulting from IVF, particularly with heterologous embryos, there may be a selection bias towards implanting the best-quality embryos, given the increased complexity of managing twin pregnancies. This selection could be even more pronounced with donor embryos, where there might be a higher availability of high-quality embryos due to factors like donor age and health. Differences in the genetics between heterologous and homologous embryos could be more pronounced in twins. Each embryo expresses different traits strongly influenced by the donor's genetics, which might not be as evident in singleton pregnancies where intrauterine competition and resources are not factors.

The major strength of our study is its sample, which provides significant statistical power regarding the results. To date, this is the only study providing data on the differences between CRL in thawed and fresh embryos during the nuchal translucency scan. The main limitation of this study is its retrospective nature and other maternal co-factors (confounders) that could be a potential explanation for the findings, such as comorbidities, i.e., cardiovascular disease, including hypertension, body mass index and smoking. Of note, the risk of bias was eliminated because of the electronic recording of the data. Furthermore, with regard to the process, the patients underwent varying ovarian stimulation protocols and embryo transfer policies at different IVF units. Most of these patients did not provide comprehensive written medical information about the procedures, leading to a lack of accurate data on hormone levels, the number of oocytes retrieved and the type of ovarian stimulation used. As a result, this information was not included in our study.

5. Conclusions

A higher CRL measurement was found in cases of thawed compared to fresh embryos in both singleton and twin gestations. Knowing the precise day of conception in pregnancies achieved via ART, due to the specific timing of oocyte retrieval and subsequent embryo transfer, provides a strong reason to avoid dating these pregnancies using first-trimester sonographic measurements of CRL. A significant difference in the measurement of CRL between thawed and fresh embryos renders it necessary to further investigate the potential reasons for this, in terms of maternal factors and culture material. More longitudinal studies are encouraged to evaluate the impact of thawed embryos on the incidence of LGA fetuses.

Author Contributions: Conceptualization, K.M. and I.T.; Methodology, K.M. and I.T.; Validation, T.D. and A.A.; Investigation, A.M.; Resources, E.G.; Data Curation, E.G.; Writing—Original Draft Preparation, K.M.; Writing—Review and Editing, I.T. and T.D.; Visualization, I.K. and A.M.; Supervision, T.D. and A.A.; Project Administration, K.M. and E.G. All authors have read and agreed to the published version of the manuscript.

Funding: This research received no external funding.

Institutional Review Board Statement: As per standard policy for audit or observational database studies not involving any intervention or modification of the management of the participants, no institutional review was required or obtained.

Informed Consent Statement: Informed consent was obtained for future research using the data and no incentives were provided for the participation in the study.

Data Availability Statement: Data are available upon request.

Conflicts of Interest: The authors declare that they have no conflicts of interest.

References

1. McDonald, S.D.; Han, Z.; Mulla, S.; Murphy, K.E.; Beyene, J.; Ohlsson, A.; Knowledge Synthesis, G. Preterm birth and low birth weight among in vitro fertilization singletons: A systematic review and meta-analyses. *Eur. J. Obstet. Gynecol. Reprod. Biol.* **2009**, *146*, 138–148. [CrossRef] [PubMed]
2. Shih, W.; Rushford, D.D.; Bourne, H.; Garrett, C.; McBain, J.C.; Healy, D.L.; Baker, H.W. Factors affecting low birthweight after assisted reproduction technology: Difference between transfer of fresh and cryopreserved embryos suggests an adverse effect of oocyte collection. *Hum. Reprod.* **2008**, *23*, 1644–1653. [CrossRef] [PubMed]
3. Maheshwari, A.; Pandey, S.; Shetty, A.; Hamilton, M.; Bhattacharya, S. Obstetric and perinatal outcomes in singleton pregnancies resulting from the transfer of frozen thawed versus fresh embryos generated through in vitro fertilization treatment: A systematic review and meta-analysis. *Fertil. Steril.* **2012**, *98*, 368–377.e9. [CrossRef] [PubMed]
4. Ishihara, O.; Araki, R.; Kuwahara, A.; Itakura, A.; Saito, H.; Adamson, G.D. Impact of frozen-thawed single-blastocyst transfer on maternal and neonatal outcome: An analysis of 277,042 single-embryo transfer cycles from 2008 to 2010 in Japan. *Fertil. Steril.* **2014**, *101*, 128–133. [CrossRef] [PubMed]
5. Nakashima, A.; Araki, R.; Tani, H.; Ishihara, O.; Kuwahara, A.; Irahara, M.; Yoshimura, Y.; Kuramoto, T.; Saito, H.; Nakaza, A.; et al. Implications of assisted reproductive technologies on term singleton birth weight: An analysis of 25,777 children in the national assisted reproduction registry of Japan. *Fertil. Steril.* **2013**, *99*, 450–455. [CrossRef]
6. Syngelaki, A.; Chelemen, T.; Dagklis, T.; Allan, L.; Nicolaides, K.H. Challenges in the diagnosis of fetal non-chromosomal abnormalities at 11–13 weeks. *Prenat. Diagn.* **2011**, *31*, 90–102. [CrossRef]
7. Santorum, M.; Wright, D.; Syngelaki, A.; Karagioti, N.; Nicolaides, K.H. Accuracy of first-trimester combined test in screening for trisomies 21, 18 and 13. *Ultrasound Obstet. Gynecol.* **2017**, *49*, 714–720. [CrossRef] [PubMed]
8. Wade, D.T. Ethics, audit, and research: All shades of grey. *BMJ* **2005**, *330*, 468–471. [CrossRef] [PubMed]
9. Salomon, L.J.; Alfirevic, Z.; Bilardo, C.M.; Chalouhi, G.E.; Ghi, T.; Kagan, K.O.; Lau, T.K.; Papageorghiou, A.T.; Raine-Fenning, N.J.; Stirnemann, J.; et al. ISUOG practice guidelines: Performance of first-trimester fetal ultrasound scan. *Ultrasound Obstet. Gynecol.* **2013**, *41*, 102–113. [CrossRef] [PubMed]
10. Robinson, H.P.; Fleming, J.E. A critical evaluation of sonar "crown-rump length" measurements. *Br. J. Obstet. Gynaecol.* **1975**, *82*, 702–710. [CrossRef] [PubMed]
11. Papageorghiou, A.T.; Kennedy, S.H.; Salomon, L.J.; Ohuma, E.O.; Cheikh Ismail, L.; Barros, F.C.; Lambert, A.; Carvalho, M.; Jaffer, Y.A.; Bertino, E.; et al. International standards for early fetal size and pregnancy dating based on ultrasound measurement of crown-rump length in the first trimester of pregnancy. *Ultrasound Obstet. Gynecol.* **2014**, *44*, 641–648. [CrossRef] [PubMed]
12. Zaat, T.; Zagers, M.; Mol, F.; Goddijn, M.; van Wely, M.; Mastenbroek, S. Fresh versus frozen embryo transfers in assisted reproduction. *Cochrane Database Syst. Rev.* **2021**, *2*, CD011184. [CrossRef] [PubMed]
13. Singh, B.; Reschke, L.; Segars, J.; Baker, V.L. Frozen-thawed embryo transfer: The potential importance of the corpus luteum in preventing obstetrical complications. *Fertil. Steril.* **2020**, *113*, 252–257. [CrossRef] [PubMed]
14. Bhattacharya, S. Maternal and perinatal outcomes after fresh versus frozen embryo transfer-what is the risk-benefit ratio? *Fertil. Steril.* **2016**, *106*, 241–243. [CrossRef] [PubMed]
15. Zhang, J.; Du, M.; Li, Z.; Wang, L.; Hu, J.; Zhao, B.; Feng, Y.; Chen, X.; Sun, L. Fresh versus frozen embryo transfer for full-term singleton birth: A retrospective cohort study. *J. Ovarian Res.* **2018**, *11*, 59. [CrossRef] [PubMed]
16. Spijkers, S.; Lens, J.W.; Schats, R.; Lambalk, C.B. Fresh and Frozen-Thawed Embryo Transfer Compared to Natural Conception: Differences in Perinatal Outcome. *Gynecol. Obstet. Investig.* **2017**, *82*, 538–546. [CrossRef] [PubMed]
17. De Geyter, C.; Calhaz-Jorge, C.; Kupka, M.S.; Wyns, C.; Mocanu, E.; Motrenko, T.; Scaravelli, G.; Smeenk, J.; Vidakovic, S.; Goossens, V.; et al. ART in Europe, 2014: Results generated from European registries by ESHRE: The European IVF-monitoring Consortium (EIM) for the European Society of Human Reproduction and Embryology (ESHRE). *Hum. Reprod.* **2018**, *33*, 1586–1601. [CrossRef] [PubMed]
18. Kawwass, J.F.; Monsour, M.; Crawford, S.; Kissin, D.M.; Session, D.R.; Kulkarni, A.D.; Jamieson, D.J.; National ART Surveillance System (NASS) Group. Trends and outcomes for donor oocyte cycles in the United States, 2000–2010. *JAMA* **2013**, *310*, 2426–2434. [CrossRef] [PubMed]
19. Wong, K.M.; van Wely, M.; Mol, F.; Repping, S.; Mastenbroek, S. Fresh versus frozen embryo transfers in assisted reproduction. *Cochrane Database Syst. Rev.* **2017**, *3*, CD011184. [CrossRef] [PubMed]

20. Shapiro, B.S.; Daneshmand, S.T.; Restrepo, H.; Garner, F.C.; Aguirre, M.; Hudson, C. Matched-cohort comparison of single-embryo transfers in fresh and frozen-thawed embryo transfer cycles. *Fertil. Steril.* **2013**, *99*, 389–392. [CrossRef]
21. Laval, M.; Garlantezec, R.; Guivarc'h-Leveque, A. Birthweight difference of singletons conceived through in vitro fertilization with frozen versus fresh embryo transfer: An analysis of 5406 embryo transfers in a retrospective study 2013–2018. *J. Gynecol. Obstet. Hum. Reprod.* **2020**, *49*, 101644. [CrossRef] [PubMed]
22. Cavoretto, P.I.; Farina, A.; Girardelli, S.; Gaeta, G.; Spinillo, S.; Morano, D.; Amodeo, S.; Galdini, A.; Vigano, P.; Candiani, M. Greater fetal crown-rump length growth with the use of in vitro fertilization or intracytoplasmic sperm injection conceptions after thawed versus fresh blastocyst transfers: Secondary analysis of a prospective cohort study. *Fertil. Steril.* **2021**, *116*, 147–156. [CrossRef] [PubMed]
23. Pinborg, A.; Henningsen, A.A.; Loft, A.; Malchau, S.S.; Forman, J.; Andersen, A.N. Large baby syndrome in singletons born after frozen embryo transfer (FET): Is it due to maternal factors or the cryotechnique? *Hum. Reprod.* **2014**, *29*, 618–627. [CrossRef] [PubMed]
24. Ishii, R.; Shoda, A.; Kubo, M.; Okazaki, S.; Suzuki, M.; Okawa, R.; Enomoto, M.; Shitanaka, M.; Fujita, Y.; Nakao, K.; et al. Identifying a possible factor for the increased newborn size in singleton pregnancies after assisted reproductive technology using cryopreserved embryos, in comparison with fresh embryos. *Reprod. Med. Biol.* **2018**, *17*, 307–314. [CrossRef]
25. Senapati, S.; Wang, F.; Ord, T.; Coutifaris, C.; Feng, R.; Mainigi, M. Superovulation alters the expression of endometrial genes critical to tissue remodeling and placentation. *J. Assist. Reprod. Genet.* **2018**, *35*, 1799–1808. [CrossRef] [PubMed]
26. Conrad, K.P.; Baker, V.L. Corpus luteal contribution to maternal pregnancy physiology and outcomes in assisted reproductive technologies. *Am. J. Physiol. Regul. Integr. Comp. Physiol.* **2013**, *304*, R69–R72. [CrossRef] [PubMed]
27. Conrad, K.P.; Petersen, J.W.; Chi, Y.Y.; Zhai, X.; Li, M.; Chiu, K.H.; Liu, J.; Lingis, M.D.; Williams, R.S.; Rhoton-Vlasak, A.; et al. Maternal Cardiovascular Dysregulation During Early Pregnancy After In Vitro Fertilization Cycles in the Absence of a Corpus Luteum. *Hypertension* **2019**, *74*, 705–715. [CrossRef]
28. Weinerman, R. Growth differences after fresh and frozen embryo transfers: When do they begin? *Fertil. Steril.* **2021**, *116*, 75–76. [CrossRef]
29. Bilagi, A.; Burke, D.L.; Riley, R.D.; Mills, I.; Kilby, M.D.; Katie Morris, R. Association of maternal serum PAPP-A levels, nuchal translucency and crown-rump length in first trimester with adverse pregnancy outcomes: Retrospective cohort study. *Prenat. Diagn.* **2017**, *37*, 705–711. [CrossRef] [PubMed]
30. Ubaldi, F.M.; Cimadomo, D.; Vaiarelli, A.; Fabozzi, G.; Venturella, R.; Maggiulli, R.; Mazzilli, R.; Ferrero, S.; Palagiano, A.; Rienzi, L. Advanced Maternal Age in IVF: Still a Challenge? The Present and the Future of Its Treatment. *Front. Endocrinol.* **2019**, *10*, 94. [CrossRef]
31. Leon, G.; Papetta, A.; Spiliopoulou, C. Overview of the Greek legislation regarding assisted reproduction and comparison with the EU legal framework. *Reprod. Biomed. Online* **2011**, *23*, 820–823. [CrossRef]
32. van Loendersloot, L.L.; Moolenaar, L.M.; van Wely, M.; Repping, S.; Bossuyt, P.M.; Hompes, P.G.A.; van der Veen, F.; Mol, B.W.J. Cost-effectiveness of single versus double embryo transfer in IVF in relation to female age. *Eur. J. Obstet. Gynecol. Reprod. Biol.* **2017**, *214*, 25–30. [CrossRef] [PubMed]
33. Medical Advisory, S. In vitro fertilization and multiple pregnancies: An evidence-based analysis. *Ont. Health Technol. Assess. Ser.* **2006**, *6*, 1–63.
34. Veleva, Z.; Vilska, S.; Hyden-Granskog, C.; Tiitinen, A.; Tapanainen, J.S.; Martikainen, H. Elective single embryo transfer in women aged 36-39 years. *Hum. Reprod.* **2006**, *21*, 2098–2102. [CrossRef] [PubMed]
35. Simopoulou, M.; Sfakianoudis, K.; Maziotis, E.; Tsioulou, P.; Grigoriadis, S.; Rapani, A.; Giannelou, P.; Asimakopoulou, M.; Kokkali, G.; Pantou, A.; et al. PGT-A: Who and when? Alpha systematic review and network meta-analysis of RCTs. *J. Assist. Reprod. Genet.* **2021**, *38*, 1939–1957. [CrossRef] [PubMed]
36. Iuculano, A.; Stagnati, V.; Serrenti, M.; Peddes, C.; Monni, G.; Sole, G.; Cucca, F. Crown-rump length: Are they different or similar after homologous vs heterologous oocyte/embryo donation? *Am. J. Obstet. Gynecol.* **2017**, *217*, 224–225. [CrossRef]

Disclaimer/Publisher's Note: The statements, opinions and data contained in all publications are solely those of the individual author(s) and contributor(s) and not of MDPI and/or the editor(s). MDPI and/or the editor(s) disclaim responsibility for any injury to people or property resulting from any ideas, methods, instructions or products referred to in the content.

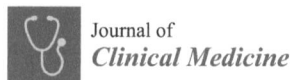 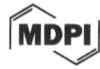

Perspective

Incidence and Risk Factors of Perianal Pathology during Pregnancy and Postpartum Period: A Prospective Cohort Study

Zivile Sabonyte-Balsaitiene [1,*], Tomas Poskus [2], Eugenijus Jasiunas [3], Diana Ramasauskaite [1] and Grazina Drasutiene [1]

1. Clinic of Obstetrics and Gynaecology, Institute of Clinical Medicine, Vilnius University Faculty of Medicine, 03101 Vilnius, Lithuania; diana.ramasauskaite@santa.lt (D.R.); grazina.drasutiene@mf.vu.lt (G.D.)
2. Clinic of Gastroenterology, Nephrourology and Surgery, Institute of Clinical Medicine, Vilnius University Faculty of Medicine, 03101 Vilnius, Lithuania; tomas.poskus@santa.lt
3. Centre for Informatics and Development, Vilnius University Hospital Santaros Klinikos, 08661 Vilnius, Lithuania; eugenijus.jasiunas@santa.lt
* Correspondence: zivile.sabonyte@gmail.com; Tel.: +370-68785607

Abstract: Objective: We aimed to identify the incidence and risk factors of perianal pathology during pregnancy and the postpartum period. Methods: A prospective cohort study was conducted in three institutions in Lithuania. A total of 190 patients were examined and interviewed three times (<12, 18–20 weeks of gestation, and during the first 2 months after delivery). They completed a questionnaire including demographic, obstetric, coloproctological, and birth data. Results: A total of 73 (34.59%) women developed hemorrhoidal disease after delivery, and 120 (56.87%) developed perianal pathology. Multivariate analysis identified a neonatal birth weight $\geq$3380 g (OR 4.22; 95% CI 1.83–9.71, $p < 0.001$) and consumption of eggs (OR 3.10; 95% CI 1.13–8.53, $p = 0.028$) or cereals (OR 2.87; 95% CI 1.32–6.25, $p = 0.008$) several times per week as significant risk factors for hemorrhoidal disease. Neonatal birth weight $\geq$3380 g (OR 3.95; 95% CI 1.47–10.59, $p = 0.006$), maternal BMI $\geq$ 21.48 (OR 3.58; 95% CI 1.51–8.47, $p = 0.004$), the duration of the second labor period $\geq$38 min (OR 2.81; 95% CI 1.09–7.23, $p = 0.032$), and consumption of flour products several times per week (OR 2.77; 95% CI 1.10–6.98, $p = 0.030$) were associated with a higher risk of perianal pathology. Daily consumption of fruits and vegetables (OR 0.35; 95% CI 0.15–0.81, $p = 0.014$) and less frequent consumption of eggs were protective factors (OR 0.18; 95% CI 0.06–0.56, $p = 0.003$). Conclusions: Perianal diseases, especially hemorrhoidal disease, are common during pregnancy and the postpartum period. A neonatal birth weight $\geq$ 3380 g, a maternal BMI of $\geq$21.48, duration of the second labor period of $\geq$38 min, and consumption of flour products and cereals several times a week are risk factors for developing these diseases.

Keywords: pregnancy; hemorrhoidal disease; perianal diseases; risk factors

Citation: Sabonyte-Balsaitiene, Z.; Poskus, T.; Jasiunas, E.; Ramasauskaite, D.; Drasutiene, G. Incidence and Risk Factors of Perianal Pathology during Pregnancy and Postpartum Period: A Prospective Cohort Study. *J. Clin. Med.* **2024**, *13*, 2371. https://doi.org/10.3390/jcm13082371

Academic Editor: Christian Selinger

Received: 16 February 2024
Revised: 14 April 2024
Accepted: 15 April 2024
Published: 18 April 2024

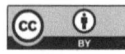

Copyright: © 2024 by the authors. Licensee MDPI, Basel, Switzerland. This article is an open access article distributed under the terms and conditions of the Creative Commons Attribution (CC BY) license (https://creativecommons.org/licenses/by/4.0/).

1. Introduction

Perianal diseases are common and can require referral to gastroenterologists and proctologists. The incidence of these conditions in the general Western population ranges from 4% to 10% [1]. The most common benign anal conditions include hemorrhoidal disease (HD), anal fissures, perianal abscesses, fecal incontinence, functional rectal pain, anal itching, and perineal prolapse [2,3].

HD is a common complaint in the general population which is more prevalent in the 45–65-year-old population and women of childbearing age [4]. This condition often develops during pregnancy and the postpartum period [5,6]. The incidence varies from 15% to 41% [7]. Clinical reports have shown that HD is most widespread in the last trimester of pregnancy and the first month after delivery, and approximately 25–35% of pregnant women suffer from it [8].

Pregnancy and childbirth are known to be some of the most critical risk factors for HD and perianal pathologies. The actual cause of HD remains unknown, but there are several theories that physiological factors may trigger it in pregnancy. At the end of pregnancy, the mechanical effect of the enlarging uterus on the digestive system is most pronounced [9]. The growing uterus affects intestinal movements, especially of hard stool, making bowel movements difficult and causing constipation [9,10]. In addition, the increase in intra-abdominal pressure due to the enlargement of the uterus leads to venous stasis in the perianal region and decreased blood circulation to the internal anal sphincter [7,11]. Furthermore, the 25–40% increase in circulating blood volume leads to vasodilatation and venous stasis in the pelvis [11]. During pregnancy, certain hormonal factors also favor the development of disease. A myorelaxant effect characterizes the increasing amount of progesterone in the blood serum. It inhibits the movement of calcium ions in smooth muscle cells and slows down the motility of the entire digestive system [12]. Furthermore, a higher concentration of progesterone in blood serum is associated with 30–50% slower peristalsis in the stomach and intestines [13]. The longest duration of intestinal peristalsis is observed in the second and third trimesters of pregnancy [14].

Some risk factors for perianal pathology and HD have already been demonstrated and recognized in several prospective studies. These include constipation, diarrhea, pregnancy, and delivery [11]. Poskus et al. reported that a personal history of perianal disease, straining during delivery for more than 20 min, newborn birth weight >3800 g, and constipation are independent risk factors for HD and anal fissures [5]. Ferdinande et al. found that constipation and a history of anal problems are significant risk factors for developing perianal disease during pregnancy [15]. Other reported risk factors in pregnant women include obesity and overweight before pregnancy, dyschezia, smoking, unhealthy diet, and a family history of oncologic diseases of the digestive system [6,15–18]. This study aimed to identify the most important risk factors for the development of HD and perianal pathology in pregnant women to assist in the possible prevention of those conditions during pregnancy and after delivery.

2. Materials and Methods

2.1. Study Design

A prospective cohort study was carried out in 3 hospitals (Vilnius University Hospital Santaros Klinikos, Vilnius City Clinical Hospital, and Vilnius Maternity Hospital) in Lithuania. Participants were enrolled in the study between June 2016 and June 2019. The study was approved by the institutional ethics committee (158200-16-843-357).

2.2. Inclusion and Exclusion Criteria

Women with an early viable pregnancy (less than 12 weeks' gestation) between the ages of 18 and 45 years who gave written informed consent were included in this study. All other women who did not meet all inclusion criteria were excluded.

2.3. Study Visits and Data Collection

Each participant experienced a total of three visits during the study: during the first trimester of pregnancy (<12 weeks of gestation), the second trimester of pregnancy (18–20 weeks of gestation), and two months after childbirth.

The first visit coincided with enrolment in this study, during which a detailed questionnaire was completed based on a comprehensive review of previous reports. It included demographic factors, physical activity and dietary data, anthropometric maternal measurements, and obstetrical and coloproctological anamnesis.

During each visit, a proctology questionnaire was completed. It included the most common symptoms of anal disorders (pain, bleeding from the anus, lumps in the anus, constipation and its type, and fecal and gas incontinence) and the most common anal disorders—HD, anal fissures, and constipation. Additionally, a physical examination was performed. A gynecologist was prepared by a colorectal surgeon to recognize and diagnose the perianal pathology using a standardized methodology before the study began. Constipation was defined by the Rome III criteria. Birth and neonatal data were obtained from medical records at the third visit. The frequency of these risk factors in patients with HD (HD group) was compared with that in patients who did not have HD (control group). In addition, to exclude falsely undiagnosed perianal disease, we examined whether subjects had symptoms characteristic of these conditions even though they had not been diagnosed with HD or constipation. We combined the indicators "postpartum HD", "symptoms characteristic of perianal disease", and "constipation during pregnancy" and named the resulting indicator "perianal pathology".

2.4. Sample Size Calculation

This was a non-probabilistic sample. A total of 405 pregnant women were screened for eligibility for this study. Of them, 194 were excluded: 182 declined to participate, 5 did not meet inclusion criteria (were <18 years of age), and 7 had spontaneous miscarriages. We presumed the baseline risk of HD during pregnancy to be 35% from our previous experience. Based on a statistical power of 80% and a level of significance set at 6%, we calculated the total sample size to be 210 mothers. The ratio of women who had HD and who did not was 73:137 = 0.53, so the groups of the study consisted of 73 and 137 participants, respectively. We also presumed the baseline risk of perianal pathology after childbirth to be 35%. Based on a statistical power of 80% and a level of significance set at 5%, we calculated the total sample size to be 208 mothers. The ratio of women who had perianal pathology and who did not was 120:91 = 1.32; the groups of this study consisted of 118 and 90 participants, respectively.

2.5. Statistical Analysis

We performed statistical data analysis with the software package R statistical V 4.2.2 (31 October 2022) (© The R Foundation for Statistical Computing), RStudio 2022.07.2 Build 576 © 2024–2022 RStudio, PBC, IBM SPSS Statistics V.23, G*Power V. 3.1.9.4 University of Duesseldorf, Germany).

In describing the subjects' characteristics, quantitative variables were reported as the mean with standard deviation (SD), median, first quartile (Q1), and third quartile (Q3). Qualitative variables were reported in absolute numbers and percentages.

We used the Shapiro–Wilk test to test the normality assumption of the quantitative variables.

We used the nonparametric Mann–Whitney U test for quantitative data that did not meet the normality conditions for comparisons between two independent groups.

We used the Welch parametric F test and the Bayes factor as an additional measure of hypothesis validity for comparisons of three or more independent groups when the variables met the conditions of normality.

When comparing two groups of variables, we used the rank biserial correlation coefficient (rpb) to estimate the effect size between interval (discrete) quantitative variables that did not meet the conditions of normality. We considered the effect size to be small if $rpb < 0.05$, very small if $0.05 \leq rpb < 0.20$, small if $0.20 \leq rpb < 0.30$, medium if $0.30 \leq rpb < 0.40$, and large if $rpb > 0.41$.

When comparing two or more groups of nominal variables, we used Cramer's V to estimate the effect size.

3. Results

A total of 405 pregnant women were screened for eligibility for this study. The analysis of risk factors related to HD and perianal pathology included 70 (33.2%) and 120 (56.9%) women, respectively, after excluding women with missing information regarding relevant variables. In total, 70 patients were diagnosed with postpartum HD, and only 2 (0.95%) of them had thrombosed HD.

The study groups' baseline demographic, obstetric, and coloproctological parameters are shown in Tables 1 and 2. There were a few minor differences between the groups. We did not find statistically significant differences between groups comparing postpartum HD in demographic and obstetric data. However, we discovered a statistically significant strong association between this condition and a history of HD (ES = 0.36 (CI 95% 24–100, $p < 0.001$). Women diagnosed with this disease more frequently felt perianal discomfort (ES = 0.20 (CI 95% 8–100, $p = 0.002$), pain (ES = 0.15 (CI 95% 0–100, $p = 0.021$), and lumps (ES = 0.30 (CI 95% 18–100, $p < 0.001$) during the study period.

Table 1. Baseline characteristics by groups with and without postpartum hemorrhoidal disease.

	No PHD * (N = 138)	PHD * (N = 73)	p-Value **	ES *** (95% CI)
	Demographic variables			
Age [mean ± SD]	30.3 ±4.4	30.9 ±4.4	0.2	−0.12 (−0.27, 0.05)
Median [Q1, Q3]	30.0 [27.0, 32.0]	31.0 [27.0, 34.0]		
BMI (before pregnancy) [mean ± SD]	21.5 [20.1, 24.2]	22.0 [20.9, 24.6]	0.12	−0.13 (−0.29, 0.03)
Median [Q1, Q3]	21.5 [20.1, 24.2]	22.0 [20.9, 24.6]		
BMI evaluation (before pregnancy) [n (%)]			0.5	0.00 (0.00, 1.0)
Too low	13 (9.4%)	3 (4.1%)		
Normal	97 (70.0%)	54 (74.0%)		
Overweight	20 (14.0%)	10 (14.0%)		
Obese	8 (5.8%)	6 (8.2%)		
Marital status [n (%)]			0.7	0.00 (0.00, 1.0)
Married	106 (77.0%)	61 (84.0%)		
Partnership	23 (17.0%)	9 (12.0%)		
Single	8 (5.8%)	3 (4.1%)		
Education [n (%)]			0.8	0.00 (0.00, 1.0)
Secondary	16 (12.0%)	6 (8.2%)		
Special secondary	19 (14.0%)	8 (11.0%)		
Unfinished higher	16 (12.0%)	8 (11.0%)		
Higher	87 (63.0%)	51 (70.0%)		
Living conditions [n (%)]			0.7	0.00 (0.00, 1.0)
Satisfactory	23 (17.0%)	14 (19.0%)		
Good	115 (83.0%)	59 (81.0%)		
Living area [n (%)]			0.6	0.00 (0.00, 1.0)
Rural	31 (22.0%)	14 (19.0%)		
Urban	107 (78.0%)	59 (81.0%)		
Monthly income [n (%)]			0.7	0.00 (0.00, 1.0)
<EUR 300	12 (8.7%)	4 (5.5%)		
EUR 300–500	31 (22.0%)	18 (25.0%)		
>EUR 500	95 (69.0%)	51 (70.0%)		
Physical activity [n (%)]			0.6	0.00 (0.00, 1.0)

Table 1. Cont.

	No PHD * (N = 138)	PHD * (N = 73)	p-Value **	ES *** (95% CI)
Too low	77 (56.0%)	35 (48.0%)		
Enough	61 (44.4%)	36 (49.4%)		
Sports [n (%)]			0.076	0.10 (0.00, 1.0)
No	40 (29.0%)	30 (41.0%)		
Yes	98 (71.0%)	43 (59.0%)		
Obstetric variables				
Menarche [mean ± SD]	11.6 ± 4.5	12.2 ± 4.0	0.4	−0.07 (−0.23, 0.10)
Median [Q1, Q3]	13.0 [12.0, 14.0]	13.0 [12.0, 14.0]		
Number of previous pregnancies [n (%)]			0.4	0.00 (0.00, 1.0)
0	66 (48.0%)	29 (40.0%)		
1	41 (30.0%)	24 (33.0%)		
2	26 (19.0%)	14 (19.0%)		
3 and more	5 (3.6%)	6 (8.2%)		
Outcomes of previous delivery [n (%)]			0.4	0.00 (0.00, 1.0)
Did not give birth	75 (54.0%)	37 (51.0%)		
Vaginal delivery	47 (33.7%)	32 (42.8%)		
Cesarean delivery	16 (12.0%)	5 (6.8%)		
Previous vaginal tear [n (%)]			0.7	0.00 (0.00, 1.0)
No	132 (96.0%)	69 (95.0%)		
Yes	6 (4.3%)	4 (5.5%)		
Previous perineal tear [n (%)]			0.2	0.07 (0.00, 1.0)
No	115 (83.0%)	55 (75.0%)		
Yes	23 (17.0%)	18 (25.0%)		
Previous episiotomy [n (%)]			0.4	0.00 (0.00, 1.0)
No	94 (69.0%)	54 (74.0%)		
Yes	43 (31.0%)	19 (26.0%)		
Coloproctological variables				
History of HD [n (%)]			<0.001	0.36 (0.24, 1.0)
No	136 (99.0%)	56 (77.0%)		
Yes	2 (1.4%)	17 (23.0%)		
Current perianal discomfort [n (%)]			0.002	0.20 (0.08, 1.0)
No	118 (86.0%)	49 (67.0%)		
Yes	20 (14.0%)	24 (33.0%)		
Current perianal pain [n (%)]			0.021	0.15 (0.00, 1.0)
No	133 (96.0%)	64 (88.0%)		
Yes	5 (3.6%)	9 (12.0%)		
Current perianal bleeding [n (%)]			0.051	0.13 (0.00, 1.0)

Table 1. Cont.

	No PHD * (N = 138)	PHD * (N = 73)	p-Value **	ES *** (95% CI)
No	134 (97.0%)	66 (90.0%)		
Yes	4 (2.9%)	7 (9.6%)		
Current perianal lumps [n (%)]			<0.001	0.30 (0.18, 1.0)
No	134 (97.0%)	57 (78.0%)		
Yes	4 (2.9%)	16 (22.0%)		
Constipation [n (%)]			0.11	0.08 (0.00, 1.0)
No	121 (88.0%)	58 (79.0%)		
Yes	17 (12.0%)	15 (21.0%)		
History of perianal operations [n (%)]			0.11	0.12 (0.00, 1.0)
No	138 (100%)	69 (97.0%)		
Yes	0 (0.0%)	2 (2.8%)		
Family history of perianal disease [n (%)]			0.4	0.00 (0.00, 1.0)
No	114 (83.0%)	57 (78.0%)		
Yes	24 (17.0%)	16 (22.0%)		

* PHD—postpartum hemorrhoidal disease. ** Wilcoxon rank sum test; Fisher's exact test; Pearson's Chi-squared test. *** Cramer's V effect size; rank biserial correlation coefficient (ES—effect size).

Table 2. Baseline characteristics by groups with and without perianal pathology after childbirth.

	No PP * (N = 91)	PP * (N = 120)	p-Value **	ES *** (95% CI)
	Demographic variables			
Age [mean ± SD]	30.3 ± 4.4	30.3 ± 4.5	>0.9	0.00 (−0.16, 0.15)
Median [Q1, Q3]	31.0 [27.5, 32.5]	30.0 [27.0, 34.0]		
BMI (before pregnancy) [mean ± SD]	22.6 ± 4.1	23.1 ± 3.4	0.001	−0.26 (−0.40, −0.11)
median [Q1, Q3]	21.4 [19.8, 24.4]	22.1 [20.9, 24.5]		
BMI evaluation (before pregnancy) [n (%)]			0.5	0.00 (0.00, 1.0)
Too low	14 (9.9%)	2 (2.9%)		
Normal	97 (69%)	52 (76%)		
Overweight	19 (13%)	11 (16%)		
Obese	11 (7.8%)	3 (4.4%)		
Marital status [n (%)]			0.2	0.08 (0.00, 1.0)
Married	69 (76.0%)	98 (82.0%)		
Partnership	18 (20.0%)	14 (12.0%)		
Single	4 (4.4%)	8 (6.6%)		
Education [n (%)]			>0.9	0.00 (0.00, 1.0)
Secondary	10 (11.0%)	12 (10.0%)	0.3	0.05 (0.00, 1.0)
Special secondary	10 (11.0%)	13 (11.0%)		

Table 2. *Cont.*

	No PP * (N = 91)	PP * (N = 120)	*p*-Value **	ES *** (95% CI)
Unfinished higher	11 (12.0%)	13 (11.0%)		
Higher	60 (66.0%)	78 (65.0%)		
Living conditions [n (%)]			0.6	0.00 (0.00, 1.0)
Satisfactory	14 (15.0%)	23 (19.0%)		
Good	77 (85.0%)	97 (81.0%)		
Living area [n (%)]			0.6	0.00 (0.00, 1.0)
Rural	18 (20.0%)	27 (22.0%)		
Urban	73 (80.0%)	93 (78.0%)		
Monthly income [n (%)]			0.13	0.10 (0.00, 1.0)
<EUR 300	8 (8.8%)	8 (6.7%)		
EUR 300–500	15 (16.0%)	34 (28.0%)		
>EUR 500	68 (75.0%)	78 (65.0%)		
Physical activity [n (%)]			0.7	0.00 (0.00, 1.0)
Too low	48 (53.0%)	64 (53.0%)		
Enough	43 (47.2%)	56 (46.8%)		
Sports [n (%)]			0.13	0.00 (0.00, 1.0)
No	25 (27.0%)	45 (38.0%)		
Yes	66 (73.0%)	75 (62.0%)		
Obstetric variables				
Menarche [mean ± SD]	11.2 ± 4.8	12.2 ± 3.8	0.3	−0.09 (−0.24, 0.07)
median [Q1, Q3]	13.0 [11.5, 14.0]	13.0 [12.0, 14.0]		
Number of previous pregnancies [n (%)]			0.075	0.14 (0.00, 1.0)
0	50 (55.0%)	45 (38.0%)		
1	25 (27.0%)	40 (33.0%)		
2	13 (14.0%)	27 (22.0%)		
3 and more	11 (5.2%)	8 (6.7%)		
Outcomes of previous delivery [n (%)]			0.038	0.15 (0.00, 1.0)
Did not give birth	56 (62.0%)	56 (47.0%)		
Vaginal delivery	24 (26.0%)	54 (44.5%)		
Cesarean delivery	11 (12.0%)	10 (8.3%)		
Previous vaginal tear [n (%)]			0.7	0.00 (0.00, 1.0)
No	86 (95.0%)	115 (96.0%)		
Yes	5 (5.5%)	5 (4.2%)		
Previous perineal tear [n (%)]			0.019	0.15 (0.00, 1.0)
No	80 (88.0%)	90 (75.0%)		
Yes	11 (12.0%)	30 (25.0%)		
Previous episiotomy [n (%)]			0.7	0.00 (0.00, 1.0)
No	62 (69.0%)	86 (72.0%)		
Yes	28 (31.0%)	34 (28.0%)		

Table 2. Cont.

	No PP * (N = 91)	PP * (N = 120)	p-Value **	ES *** (95% CI)
	Coloproctological variables			
History of HD [n (%)]			<0.001	0.23 (0.11, 1.0)
No	90 (99.0%)	102 (85.0%)		
Yes	1 (1.1%)	18 (15.0%)		
Current perianal discomfort [n (%)]			<0.001	0.27 (0.15, 1.0)
No	84 (92.0%)	83 (69.0%)		
Yes	7 (7.7%)	37 (31.0%)		
Current perianal pain [n (%)]			0.09	0.09 (0.00, 1.0)
No	88 (97.0%)	109 (91.0%)		
Yes	3 (3.3%)	11 (9.2%)		
Current perianal bleeding [n (%)]			0.12	0.10 (0.00, 1.0)
No	89 (98.0%)	111 (92.0%)		
Yes	2 (2.2%)	9 (7.5%)		
Current perianal lumps [n (%)]			<0.001	0.27 (0.15, 1.0)
No	91 (100%)	100 (83.0%)		
Yes	0 (0.0%)	20 (17.0%)		
Constipation [n (%)]			0.003	0.20 (0.07, 1.0)
No	85 (93.0%)	94 (78.0%)		
Yes	6 (6.6%)	26 (22.0%)		
History of perianal operations [n (%)]			0.5	0.05 (0.00, 1.0)
No	91 (100%)	116 (98.0%)		
Yes	0 (0.0%)	2 (1.7%)		
Family history of perianal disease [n (%)]			0.7	0.00 (0.00, 1.0)
No	75 (82.0%)	96 (80.0%)		
Yes	16 (18.0%)	24 (20.0%)		

* PP—perianal pathology. ** Wilcoxon rank sum test; Fisher's exact test; Pearson's Chi-squared test. *** Cramer's V effect size; rank biserial correlation coefficient (ES—effect size).

The women in the group with perianal pathology had a higher BMI before pregnancy than the healthy women (ES = −0.26 (CI 95% −0.40, −0.11), $p = 0.001$). Additionally, most of them had a history of vaginal delivery (ES = 0.15 (CI 95% 0–100, $p = 0.038$) and perineal tears (ES = 0.15 (CI 95% 0–100, $p = 0.019$). They were more likely to have a history of HD (ES = 0.23 (CI 95% 11–100, $p < 0.001$), perianal discomfort (ES = 0.27 (CI 95% 15–100, $p < 0.001$), lumps (ES = 0.27 (CI 95% 15–100, $p < 0.001$), and constipation (ES = 0.20 (CI 95% 7–100, $p = 0.003$) during pregnancy and the period after childbirth. Otherwise, there were no other statistically significant differences between the groups.

The pregnancy outcomes of women who fully completed the study are shown in Table 3.

Table 3. Pregnancy characteristics by groups according to the presence of postpartum hemorrhoidal disease and perianal pathology.

	HDP *			
	No HDP * (N = 138)	HDP * (N = 73)	*p*-Value **	ES *** (95% CI)
Birth week [mean ± SD]	38.78 ± 2.17	38.97 ± 1.78	0.8	−0.02 (−0.18, 0.14)
Median [Q1, Q3]	39.0 [39.0, 40.0]	39.0 [38.0, 40.0]		
Preterm birth [n (%)]			0.3	0.02 (0.00, 1.0)
Yes	18 (13.0%)	6 (8.2%)		
No	120 (87.0%)	67 (92.0%)		
Birth assistance [n (%)]			0.017	0.19 (0.00, 1.0)
Vaginal birth without assistance	92 (66.3%)	62 (85.4%)		
Vaginal birth with assistance	8 (5.8%)	2 (2.7%)		
Cesarean delivery	38 (28.0%)	9 (12.0%)		
Newborn weight [mean ± SD]	3375 ± 722	3586 ± 509	0.05	−0.16 (−0.32, 0.00)
Median [Q1, Q3]	3500.0 [3100.0, 3855.0]	3610.0 [3380.0, 3870.0]		
Newborn height [mean ± SD]	51.7 ± 4.5	53.2 ± 2.9	0.018	−0.20 (−0.35, −0.04)
Median [Q1, Q3]	53.0 [51.0, 55.0]	54.0 [52.0, 55.0]		
Head circumference [mean ± SD]	34.72 ± 2.13	35.27 ± 1.78	0.055	−0.16 (−0.31, 0.01)
Median [Q1, Q3]	35.0 [34.0, 36.0]	36.0 [34.0, 36.0]		
Duration of second labor period [mean ± SD]	31 ± 34	39 ± 30	0.019	−0.22 (−0.38, −0.04)
Median [Q1, Q3]	25.0 [2, 44]	36.0 [16, 52]		
	PP ****			
	No PP **** (N = 91)	PP **** (N = 120)	*p*-value **	ES *** (95% CI)
Birth week [mean ± SD]	39.0 [38.0, 40.0]	39.5 [39.0, 40.0]	0.12	−0.13 (−0.29, 0.04)
Median [Q1, Q3]				
Preterm birth [n (%)]			0.2	0.06 (0.00, 1.0)
Yes	19 (13.0%)	5 (7.4%)		
No	122 (87.0%)	64 (93.0%)		
Birth assistance [n (%)]			0.1	0.12 (0.00, 1.0)
Vaginal birth without assistance	96 (68.1%)	57 (83.9%)		
Vaginal birth with assistance	8 (5.6%)	2 (3.0%)		
Cesarean delivery	37 (26.0%)	9 (13.0%)		
Newborn weight [mean ± SD]	3383 ± 694	3586 ± 579	0.028	−0.19 (−0.34, 0.02)
Median [Q1, Q3]	3476 [3130.0, 3840.0]	3655.0 [3322.0, 3975.0]		
Newborn height [mean ± SD]	51.8 ± 4.3	53.0 ± 3.4	0.021	−0.20 (−0.35, 0.03)
Median [Q1, Q3]	53.0 [51.0, 54.0]	54.0 [52.0, 55.0]		
Head circumference [mean ± SD]	34.86 ± 2.08	35.03 ± 1.95	0.6	−0.04 (−0.20, 0.13)
Median [Q1, Q3]	35.0 [34.0, 36.0]	35.0 [34.0, 36.0]		

Table 3. *Cont.*

	HDP *			
	No HDP * (N = 138)	HDP * (N = 73)	*p*-Value **	ES *** (95% CI)
Duration of second labor period [mean ± SD]	31 ± 32	40 ± 34	0.04	−0.20 (−0.37, −0.01)
Median [Q1, Q3]	25.0 [3, 44]	32.0 [19, 52]		

* PHD—postpartum hemorrhoidal disease. ** Wilcoxon rank sum test; Fisher's exact test; Pearson's Chi-squared test. *** Cramer's V effect size; rank biserial correlation coefficient (ES—effect size). **** PP—perianal pathology.

We found that vaginal delivery without support was more common among women in the group diagnosed with postpartum HD (62 (85.4%) vs. 92 (66.3%), $p = 0.017$). In addition, women in this group delivered larger newborns (54 cm vs. 53 cm, $p = 0.018$), and the median duration of their second labor, in minutes, was longer (25 min. vs. 36 min., $p = 0.019$). All dependencies were statistically significant and moderately strong.

Women diagnosed with perianal pathology delivered heavier (3655 g vs. 3476 g, $p = 0.028$) and larger (53 cm vs. 54 cm, $p = 0.021$) neonates, and their second stage of labor was longer (32 min. vs. 25 min., $p = 0.04$) than that of healthy women.

Women who had postpartum HD were statistically more likely to suffer from symptoms characteristic of perianal disease during their pregnancy (22 (16%) vs. 46 (63%), $p < 0.001$) and constipation (32 (27%) vs. 34 (50%), $p < 0.001$).

Statistically significant differences in dietary data were found between women diagnosed with postpartum HD and healthy pregnant women. They consumed eggs daily or more frequently (97 (75%) vs. 62 (87%)) compared to less frequently than several times per week (30 (23%) vs. 7 (9.9%), $p = 0.046$), respectively. They were more likely to consume fruits and vegetables several times per week (87 (65%) vs. 61 (85%)) than daily (46 (35%) vs. 11 (15%)), $p = 0.003$, respectively, and salted products several times per week (49 (38%) vs. 41 (56%)) compared to daily, respectively. A total of 41 (56%)) were more likely to consume products cooked in oil daily (54 (42%) vs. 20 (27%)) compared to never (27 (21%) vs. 12 (16%), $p = 0.037$) (88 (70%) vs. 53 (73%)) or several times per week (26 (21%) vs. 6 (8.2%), $p = 0.02$).

While constipation during pregnancy and postpartum HD are the most important factors influencing perianal pathology, we constructed a logistic regression prognostic model to predict this condition. Before that, we used Youden's method to determine the critical values for the most important indicators that make up the optimized logistic equations (Table 4).

Table 4. Critical points for the development of perianal pathology and postpartum hemorrhoidal disease.

Variable	Critical Value of the PHD *	Critical Value of the PP **
Newborn weight (g)	3380	3380
Newborn height (cm)	52	58
Duration of the second labor period (min)	38	38
Maternal BMI before pregnancy	20.57	21.48
Duration of pregnancy (wks)	41	38

* PHD—postpartum hemorrhoidal disease. ** PP—perianal pathology.

After constructing and optimizing the logistic equation for postpartum HD (Table 5), we obtained that a newborn weight greater than 3380 g increases the probability of this disease by 4.22 times compared to a newborn weight lower than 3380 g (OR 4.22, CI 95% 1.83–9.71, $p < 0.001$). Moreover, smoking increases the probability of this disease by 6,59 times compared to non-smoking (OR 6.59, CI 95% 0.95–46.01, $p = 0.057$). Some dietary habits were associated with a higher risk of postpartum HD: consumption of eggs several times per week increased the probability of disease by 3.1 times compared to daily consumption of those products (OR 3.10, CI 95% 1.31–8.53, $p = 0.028$) and consumption of grain several times per week increased this probability by 2,87 times compared to daily consumption (OR 2.87, CI 95% 1.32–6.25, $p = 0.008$). Consumption of fruits and vegetables several times per week had the opposite effect: it reduced the probability of development of this disease by 2,86 times compared to daily consumption (OR 0.35, CI 95% 0.15–0.81, $p = 0.014$).

Table 5. Coefficients of the regression analysis of postpartum hemorrhoidal disease.

Variable	Value	HDP *		OR ** (Univariate Analysis)	OR ** (Multivariate Analysis)
		No, N = 129	Yes, N = 70		
Average newborn weight	<3380	54 (41.9%)	16 (22.9%)		
	≥3380	75 (58.1%)	54 (77.1%)	2.43 (1.26–4.69, $p = 0.008$)	4.22 (1.83–9.71, $p < 0.001$)
Consumption of eggs	daily or more frequently	30 (23.3%)	7 (10%)		
	several times a week	97 (75.2%)	61 (87.1%)	2.70 (1.11–6.52, $p = 0.028$)	3.10 (1.13–8.53, $p = 0.028$)
	never	2 (1.6%)	2 (2.9%)	4.29 (0.51–35.91, $p = 0.180$)	5.45 (0.46–64.31, $p = 0.178$)
Consumption of fruits and vegetables	daily or more frequently	84 (65.1%)	59 (84.3%)		
	several times a week	45 (34.9%)	11 (15.7%)	0.35 (0.17–0.73, $p = 0.005$)	0.35 (0.15–0.81, $p = 0.014$)
Consumption of grain	daily or more frequently	86 (66.7%)	40 (57.1%)		
	several times a week	42 (32.6%)	30 (42.9%)	1.54 (0.84–2.80, $p = 0.161$)	2.87 (1.32–6.25, $p = 0.008$)
	never	1 (0.8%)	0 (0%)	0.00 (0.00, $p = 0.988$)	0.00 (0.00, $p = 0.990$)
Smoking	no	95 (73.6%)	44 (62.9%)		
	smoked before	32 (24.8%)	21 (30%)	1.42 (0.74–2.73, $p = 0.298$)	1.85 (0.84–4.08, $p = 0.126$)
	yes	2 (1.6%)	5 (7.1%)	5.40 (1.01–28.91, $p = 0.049$)	6.59 (0.95–46.01, $p = 0.057$)

* PHD—postpartum hemorrhoidal disease. ** OR—odds ratio.

After constructing and optimizing the logistic equation for perianal pathology (Table 6), we found that newborn weight greater than 3380 g increases the probability of this disease by 3.95 times compared to newborn weight lower than 3380 g (OR 3.95, CI 95% 1.47–10.59, $p = 0.006$). Moreover, a BMI of more than 21.48 increases the probability (OR 3.56, CI 95% 1.51–8.47, $p = 0.004$) of this disease. Some dietary habits were associated with a higher risk of postpartum HD: consumption of eggs several times per week decreased the probability of disease by 5.56 times compared to daily consumption of those products (OR 0.18, CI 95% 0.06–0.56, $p = 0.003$) and consumption of flour several times per week increased this probability by 2.77 times compared to daily consumption (OR 2.77, CI 95% 1.10–6.98, $p = 0.030$).

Table 6. Coefficients of the regression analysis of perianal pathology.

Variable	Value	PP *		OR ** (Univariate Analysis)	OR ** (Multivariate Analysis)
		No, N = 54	Yes, N = 86		
Average newborn weight	<3380	23 (42.6%)	22 (25.6%)		
	≥3380	31 (57.4%)	64 (74.4%)	2.16 (1.05–4.46, $p = 0.037$)	3.95 (1.47–10.59, $p = 0.006$)
Average newborn height	<58	51 (94.4%)	85 (98.8%)		
	≥58	3 (5.6%)	1 (1.2%)	0.20 (0.02–1.97, $p = 0.168$)	0.03 (0.00–0.47, $p = 0.013$)
BMI ***	<21.48	32 (59.3%)	29 (33.7%)		
	≥21.48	22 (40.7%)	57 (66.3%)	2.86 (1.42–5.78, $p = 0.003$)	3.58 (1.51–8.47, $p = 0.004$)

Table 6. Cont.

Variable	Value	PP * No, N = 54	PP * Yes, N = 86	OR ** (Univariate Analysis)	OR ** (Multivariate Analysis)
Duration of second labor period	<38	38 (70.4%)	49 (57%)		
	≥38	16 (29.6%)	37 (43%)	1.79 (0.87–3.70, $p = 0.114$)	2.81 (1.09–7.23, $p = 0.032$)
Gestation	<38	5 (9.3%)	14 (16.3%)		
	≥38	49 (90.7%)	72 (83.7%)	0.52 (0.18–1.55, $p = 0.244$)	0.09 (0.02–0.39, $p = 0.001$)
Sports	no	16 (29.6%)	31 (36%)		
	yes	38 (70.4%)	55 (64%)	0.75 (0.36–1.55, $p = 0.434$)	0.41 (0.15–1.13, $p = 0.085$)
Consumption of eggs	daily or more frequently	40 (74.1%)	76 (88.4%)		
	several times a week	14 (25.9%)	10 (11.6%)	0.38 (0.15–0.92, $p = 0.033$)	0.18 (0.06–0.56, $p = 0.003$)
Consumption of flour products	daily or more frequently	40 (74.1%)	50 (58.1%)		
	several times a week	14 (25.9%)	36 (41.9%)	2.06 (0.98–4.33, $p = 0.058$)	2.77 (1.10–6.98, $p = 0.030$)
Consumption of water	more, than 2 l/d	43 (79.6%)	76 (88.4%)		
	less, than 2 l/d	11 (20.4%)	10 (11.6%)	0.51 (0.20–1.31, $p = 0.163$)	0.33 (0.10–1.15, $p = 0.083$)

* PHD—postpartum hemorrhoidal disease. ** OR—odds ratio. *** BMI—body mass index.

The logistic regression equation model for postpartum HD fitted the included indicators well (AU ROC 0.801, CI 95% 73–86%, $p < 0.001$, pseudo-R^2 (Cragg–Uhler) = 0.33, pseudo-R^2 (McFadden) = 0.21, sensitivity = 60%, CI 95% (48–72%), specificity = 84%, CI 95% (76–90%), positive prognostic value = 67%, CI 95% (54–78%), negative prognostic value = 79%, CI 95% (72–86%), and prevalence = 35%, CI 95% (29–42%).

The prognostic equation allows fairly accurate prediction of the development of anal pathology during pregnancy (AU ROC 0.821, $\chi^2(10) = 48.05$, $p = 0.00$, Pseudo-R^2 (Cragg-Uhler) = 0.39, Pseudo-R^2 (McFadden) = 0.26, sensitivity = 90%, CI 95% (81–95%), specificity = 59%, CI 95% (45–72%), positive prognostic value = 78%, CI 95% (68–86%), negative prognostic value = 78%, CI% (62–89%), prevalence = 61%, CI% (53–70%).

Figure 1 shows the decision curve analysis for postpartum HD and Figure 2 shows the decision curve analysis for perianal pathology.

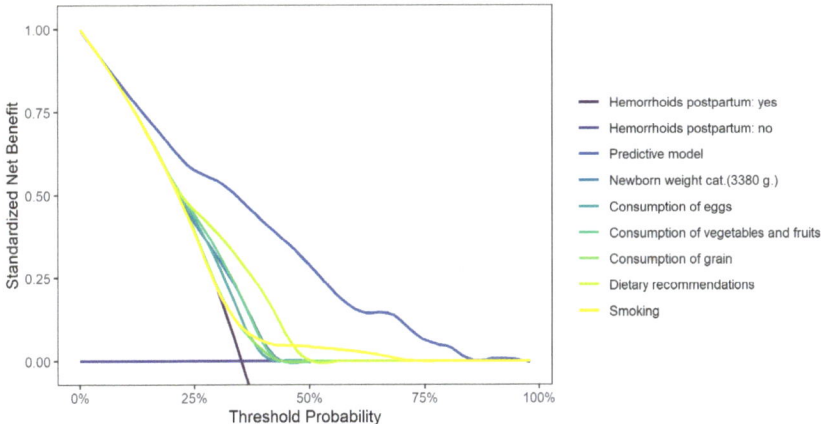

Figure 1. A decision curve analysis for postpartum hemorrhoidal disease.

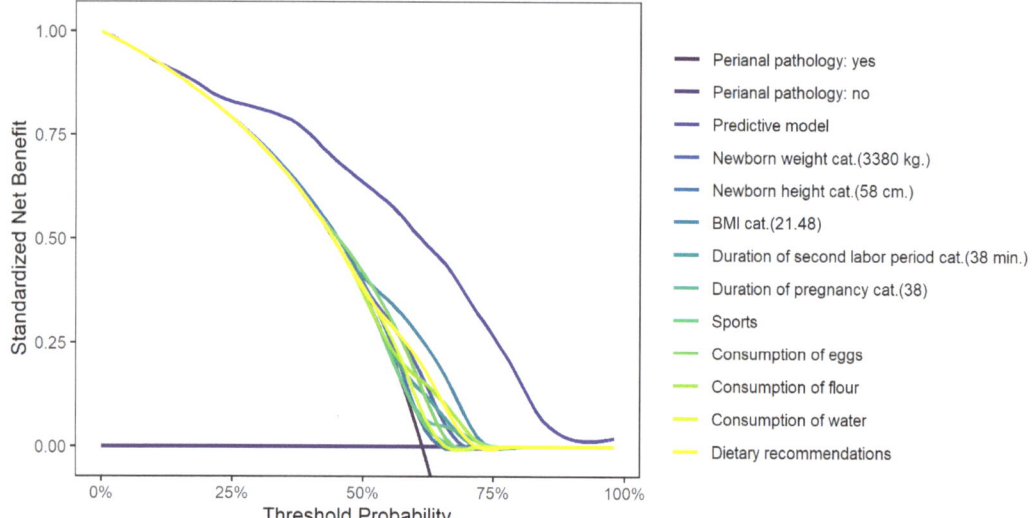

Figure 2. A decision curve analysis for the development of perianal pathology.

4. Discussion

4.1. Main Findings

This study identified an incidence of perianal pathology of 61.4% and postpartum HD of 35.1%. Multivariate analysis identified a neonatal birth weight ≥3380 g (OR 4.22; CI 95% 1.83–9.71, $p < 0.001$) and consumption of eggs (OR 3.10; CI 95% 1.13–8.53, $p = 0.028$) or cereals (OR 2.87; CI 95% 1.32–6.25, $p = 0.008$) several times a week as significant risk factors for hemorrhoidal disease. Neonatal birth weight ≥3380 g (OR 3.95; CI 95% 1.47–10.59, $p = 0.006$), maternal BMI ≥ 21.48 (OR 3.58; CI 95% 1.51–8.47, $p = 0.004$), duration of the second labor period ≥ 38 min (OR 2.81; CI 95% 1.09–7.23, $p = 0.032$), and consumption of flour products several times per week (OR 2.77; CI 95% 1.10–6.98, $p = 0.030$) were associated with a higher risk of perianal pathology. Daily consumption of fruits and vegetables (OR 0.35; CI 95% 0.15–0.81, $p = 0.014$) and less frequent consumption of eggs were protective factors (OR 0.18; CI 95% 0.06–0-0.56, $p = 0.003$).

4.2. Strengths and Limitations

This study has significant strengths. For instance, this was a prospective cohort study that was conducted in three institutions. The main weak point of the study was that we used only questionnaire assessment and physical examination and no other perianal pathology diagnostic procedures like colonoscopy. However, our aim was to avoid any unnecessary interventions as our study population was pregnant and postpartum women. Moreover, all participants who developed perianal symptoms were consulted by a colorectal surgeon and anoscopy was performed. Another potential limitation may be the relatively small sample size.

4.3. Interpretation

Maternal perianal pathologies, especially HD, are common during pregnancy and after delivery. They affect maternal health and quality of life. Although there are several studies on HD and perianal disease in the general population, these data are sparse for women during pregnancy and the postpartum period.

The incidence of postpartum HD in this study was 35.1%. This is consistent with the 43.9% rate observed by Buzinskiene and Poskus and the 38.1% rate observed in a similar population by Hong et al. [2,5,19]. The incidence of thrombosed external HD in our study was lower than that estimated by Ferdinande et al. (0.95% vs. 14.6%) [15].

The incidence of perianal pathology was 61.4%. Unadkat conducted a prospective study involving 217 pregnant women. They found that 27% of the participants had at least one symptom of perianal disease [20].

In the general population, constipation, a low-fiber diet, a high body mass index, pregnancy, and a sedentary lifestyle are defined as major risk factors for HD development [21]. Previous studies reported that Caucasians are affected 1.5 times more often [4]. We could not compare this risk factor because, in our study, all participants were Caucasian. Moreover, increased prevalence rates of HD were associated with higher socioeconomic status [4,19]. We did not find statistically significant differences in demographic data between groups with and without postpartum HD. A variety of diagnoses are associated with HD: depression, allergy, type I or II diabetes, Crohn's disease, hematological diseases or blood cancer, psoriasis, asthma, varicose veins of the legs, restless leg syndrome, personal HD anamnesis, hypertension, spinal cord injury, and various diseases of the rectum and anus [22,23]. Although we did not confirm HD's association with other diseases, we found a statistically significant strong association between this condition and a personal history of HD. Previous studies report overweight and obesity as HD risk factors [15,24–26]. Overweight persons are 2.6 times more likely to be ill [26]. In our study, women diagnosed with HD and perianal pathology had a higher BMI before pregnancy than the healthy ones. However, only a small number of participants developed these outcomes, and critical values for developing those pathologies were in normal BMI ranges (20.57 in the perianal pathology group and 21.48 in the postpartum HD group). This makes BMI a very questionable risk factor.

This study is the first study in which dietary impact on perianal pathology and HD is evaluated. We found that consumption of eggs (OR 3.10; CI 95% 1.13–8.53, $p = 0.028$) or cereals (OR 2.87; CI 95% 1.32–6.25, $p = 0.008$) several times a week were significant risk factors for developing HD. Moreover, consumption of flour products several times per week (OR 2.77; CI 95% 1.10–6.98, $p = 0.030$) was associated with a higher risk of perianal pathology. Daily consumption of fruits and vegetables (OR 0.35; CI 95% 0.15–0.81, $p = 0.014$) and less frequent consumption of eggs were protective factors (OR 0.18; CI 95% 0.06–0–0.56, $p = 0.003$). Those dietary changes can be easily recommended to pregnant and postpartum women to reduce the risk of those pathologies without causing any complications or negative outcomes.

Previous studies have compared women diagnosed with HD and perianal pathology with healthy pregnant women. Poskus (2014) conducted a prospective observational cohort study that surveyed 280 women who had given birth in Lithuania. In a multivariate analysis, he identified a personal history of perianal disease (OR 11.93; CI 95% 2.18–65.30), constipation (OR 18.98; CI 95% 7.13–50.54), straining during labor for more than 20 min (OR 29.75; CI 95% 4.00–221.23), and newborn birth weight >3800 g (OR 17.99; CI 95% 3.29–98.49) as significant predictors of HD and anal fissures during pregnancy and the perinatal period [5]. We found that lower neonatal weight (3380 g) may also be a risk factor for developing HD after birth. However, only a small number of participants developed the outcome, which makes it a very questionable risk factor.

However, we did not observe that constipation before the first trimester and a history of perianal disease were associated with HD after delivery. Moreover, the duration of the second birth period in our study was longer and was not estimated for the development of HD but rather for perianal pathology.

Abramowitz (2002) compared 165 women during the last 3 months of pregnancy and after delivery (within 2 months). The independent risk factors for anal lesions were dyschezia, with an odds ratio of 5.7 (CI 95% 2.7–12), and late delivery, with an odds ratio of 1.4 (CI 95% 1.05–1.9). Furthermore, thrombosed external HD was often observed after superficial perineal tears and in heavier babies ($p < 0.05$). Only 1 of the 33 patients with thrombosed external HD underwent Cesarean section [6]. The results of our study show that vaginal delivery without assistance was more prevalent among women in the group diagnosed with postpartum HD. However, we found no association between this condition and perineal tears.

Ferdinande (2018) found that 68% of 94 patients developed anal symptoms. The most common diagnoses were hemorrhoidal thrombosis (immediately after birth), hemorrhoidal prolapse (in the third trimester and immediately after birth), and anal fissure (not episode-related). The two independent risk factors for anal symptoms were constipation, with an odds ratio of 6.3 (CI 95% 2.08–19.37), and a history of anal problems, with an odds ratio of 3.9 (CI 95% 1.2–13) [15]. The results of our study were similar: women who had postpartum HD were more likely to suffer symptoms characteristic of perianal disease and constipation during their pregnancy.

Our results confirm that bigger neonatal weight is a risk factor for the development of HD and perianal pathology. Our data also show that length of labor and maternal BMI before pregnancy are risk factors for the development of perianal pathology. Our final independent risk factor for postpartum HD, more frequent consumption of eggs and cereals, has not yet been demonstrated and requires additional investigation. Based on our findings, we recommend paying more attention to normal maternal body mass index and eating habits while planning and during pregnancy. Counseling about healthy eating and keeping physically active during pregnancy is essential for preventing various health disorders. The results of our study show that perianal pathology and especially HD are also associated with healthy living habits. However, future research should consider the potential effects of maternal BMI and neonatal weight more carefully since, in our study, only a small number of participants developed the outcome, which makes them very questionable risk factors. Moreover, future research could examine the association between eating habits and perianal pathology since those diseases affect almost half of all pregnant women and some dietary interventions could reverse this trend. This research indicates the necessity of monitoring and evaluating dietary behaviors, which will enable the early diagnosis and prevention of perianal diseases.

5. Conclusions

Perianal pathology and especially HD are common during pregnancy and the postpartum period. In conclusion, neonatal birth weight $\geq$ 3380 g and daily consumption of eggs and cereals were identified as independent risk factors for postpartum HD. A newborn birth weight of $\geq$3380 g, a maternal BMI of $\geq$21.48, duration of the second labor period of $\geq$38 min, and consumption of cereals several times per week increased the likelihood of developing perianal pathology. Daily consumption of fruits and vegetables and less frequent consumption of eggs could be protective factors for perianal pathology development. Future studies should aim to replicate these results in a larger sample.

Author Contributions: Conceptualization, Z.S.-B., T.P. and G.D.; methodology, T.P., Z.S.-B. and G.D.; software, Z.S.-B.; validation, T.P., Z.S.-B. and G.D.; formal analysis, E.J.; investigation, Z.S.-B., T.P., Z.S.-B., E.J. and D.R.; resources, Z.S.-B., T.P. and G.D.; data curation, Z.S.-B.; writing—original draft preparation, Z.S.-B.; writing—review and editing, T.P., Z.S.-B. and D.R.; visualization, E.J. and Z.S.-B.; supervision T.P., Z.S.-B., D.R. and G.D.; project administration, T.P., Z.S.-B., D.R. and G.D.; funding acquisition, N/A. All authors have read and agreed to the published version of the manuscript.

Funding: The authors have not declared a specific grant for this research from any funding agency in the public, commercial, or not-for-profit sectors. This study was initiated and conducted by the Faculty of Medicine, Vilnius University, Vilnius, Lithuania, and is part of a Ph.D. research project by Zivile Sabonyte-Balsaitiene.

Institutional Review Board Statement: This study was approved by the Vilnius Regional Bioethics Committee, Vilnius, Lithuania, on 10 May 2016, registration number 158200-16-843-357. Registration site URL: https://www.mf.vu.lt/mokslas/vilniaus-regioninis-biomedicininiu-tyrimu-etikos-komitetas#isduoti-vrbtek-leidimai, accessed on 9 May 2016.

Informed Consent Statement: Not applicable.

Data Availability Statement: The datasets used and analyzed during this study are available from the corresponding author upon reasonable request. All data relevant to the study are included in the article or uploaded as supplemental online information. Unidentified data underlying the findings reported in this article will be released to third parties upon written request to the corresponding author describing the intent of the data use and the full affiliation of the requesting organization. A data access agreement must be signed to gain access to the data.

Conflicts of Interest: The authors declare that they have no competing interests.

References

1. Barleben, A.; Mills, S. Anorectal anatomy and physiology. *Surg. Clin. N. Am.* **2010**, *90*, 1–15. [CrossRef] [PubMed]
2. Bužinskienė, D. Nėščiųjų ir Gimdyvių Išangės Ligų Dažnis, Rizikos Veiksniai ir Įtaka Moters Gyvenimo Kokybei. Doctoral Dissertation, Vilniaus Universitetas, Vilnius, Lithuania, 2015.
3. Foxx-Orenstein, A.E.; Umar, S.B.; Crowell, M.D. Common anorectal disorders. *Gastroenterol. Hepatol.* **2014**, *10*, 294–301.
4. Johanson, J.F.; Sonnenberg, A. The prevalence of hemorrhoids and chronic constipation. An epidemiologic study. *Gastroenterology* **1990**, *98*, 380–386. [CrossRef]
5. Poskus, T.; Buzinskienė, D.; Drasutiene, G.; Samalavicius, N.; Barkus, A.; Barisauskiene, A.; Tutkuviene, J.; Sakalauskaite, I.; Drasutis, J.; Jasulaitis, A.; et al. Haemorrhoids and anal fissures during pregnancy and after childbirth: A prospective cohort study. *BJOG Int. J. Obstet. Gynaecol.* **2014**, *121*, 1666–1671. [CrossRef] [PubMed]
6. Abramowitz, L.; Sobhani, I.; Benifla, J.L.; Vuagnat, A.; Daraï, E.; Mignon, M.; Madelenat, P. Anal Fissure and Thrombosed External Hemorrhoids Before and After Delivery. *Dis. Colon Rectum* **2002**, *45*, 650–655. [CrossRef] [PubMed]
7. Poskus, T.; Sabonyte-Balsaitiene, Z.; Jakubauskiene, L.; Jakubauskas, M.; Stundiene, I.; Barkauskaite, G.; Smigelskaite, M.; Jasiunas, E.; Ramasauskaite, D.; Strupas, K.; et al. Preventing hemorrhoids during pregnancy: A multicenter, randomized clinical trial. *BMC Pregnancy Childbirth* **2022**, *22*, 374. [CrossRef]
8. Shirah, B.H.; Shirah, H.A.; Fallata, A.H.; Alobidy, S.N.; Hawsawi, M.M.A. Hemorrhoids during pregnancy: Sitz bath vs. ano-rectal cream: A comparative prospective study of two conservative treatment protocols. *Women Birth* **2018**, *31*, e272–e277. [CrossRef]
9. Gomes, C.F.; Sousa, M.; Lourenço, I.; Martins, D.; Torres, J. Gastrointestinal diseases during pregnancy: What does the gastroenterologist need to know? *Ann. Gastroenterol.* **2018**, *31*, 385–394. [PubMed]
10. Cullen, G.; O'Donoghue, D. Constipation and pregnancy. *Best Pract. Res. Clin. Gastroenterol.* **2007**, *21*, 807–818. [CrossRef]
11. Bužinskienė, D.; Sabonytė-Balšaitienė, Ž.; Poškus, T. Perianal Diseases in Pregnancy and After Childbirth: Frequency, Risk Factors, Impact on Women's Quality of Life and Treatment Methods. *Front. Surg.* **2022**, *9*, 788823. [CrossRef]
12. Everson, G.T. Gastrointestinal motility in pregnancy. *Gastroenterol. Clin. N. Am.* **1992**, *21*, 751–776. [CrossRef]
13. Costantine, M.M. Physiologic and pharmacokinetic changes in pregnancy. *Front. Pharmacol.* **2014**, *5*, 65. [CrossRef] [PubMed]
14. Chiloiro, M.; Darconza, G.; Piccioli, E.; De Carne, M.; Clemente, C.; Riezzo, G. Gastric emptying and orocecal transit time in pregnancy. *J. Gastroenterol.* **2001**, *36*, 538–543. [CrossRef] [PubMed]
15. Ferdinande, K.; Dorreman, Y.; Roelens, K.; Ceelen, W.; De Looze, D. Anorectal symptoms during pregnancy and postpartum: A prospective cohort study. *Colorectal. Dis.* **2018**, *20*, 1109–1116. [CrossRef] [PubMed]
16. Abramowitz, L.; Batallan, A. Epidemiology of anal lesions (fissure and thrombosed external hemorroid) during pregnancy and postpartum. *Gynecol. Obstet. Fertil.* **2003**, *31*, 546–549. [CrossRef] [PubMed]
17. Vazquez, J.C. Constipation, haemorrhoids, and heartburn in pregnancy. *BMJ Clin. Evid.* **2010**, *2010*, 1411. [PubMed]
18. Gaj, F.; Trecca, A.; Crispino, P. La malattia emorroidaria durante la gestazione: Focus sulle sale parto [Haemorrhoid disease during pregnancy: Focus on delivery unit]. *Clin. Ter.* **2007**, *158*, 285–289. [PubMed]
19. Hong, Y.S.; Jung, K.U.; Rampal, S.; Zhao, D.; Guallar, E.; Ryu, S.; Chang, Y.; Kim, H.O.; Kim, H.; Chun, H.-K.; et al. Risk factors for hemorrhoidal disease among healthy young and middle-aged Korean adults. *Sci. Rep.* **2022**, *12*, 129. [CrossRef]
20. Unadkat, S.N.; Leff, D.R.; Teoh, T.G.; Rai, R.; Darzi, A.W.; Ziprin, P. Anorectal symptoms during pregnancy: How important is trimester? *Int. J. Colorectal. Dis.* **2010**, *25*, 375–379. [CrossRef]
21. De Marco, S.; Tiso, D. Lifestyle and Risk Factors in Hemorrhoidal Disease. *Front. Surg.* **2021**, *8*, 729166. [CrossRef]
22. Sheikh, P.; Régnier, C.; Goron, F.; Salmat, G. The prevalence, characteristics and treatment of hemorrhoidal disease: Results of an international web-based survey. *J. Comp. Eff. Res.* **2020**, *9*, 1219–1232. [CrossRef] [PubMed]
23. Delco, F.; Sonnenberg, A. Associations between hemorrhoids and other diagnoses. *Dis. Colon Rectum* **1998**, *41*, 1534–1541, discussion 1541–1542. [CrossRef] [PubMed]
24. Sandler, R.S.; Peery, A.F. Rethinking What We Know About Hemorrhoids. *Clin. Gastroenterol. Hepatol.* **2019**, *17*, 8–15. [CrossRef] [PubMed]
25. Lohsiriwat, V. Hemorrhoids: From basic pathophysiology to clinical management. *World J. Gastroenterol.* **2012**, *18*, 2009–2017. [CrossRef]
26. Kibret, A.A.; Oumer, M.; Moges, A.M. Prevalence and associated factors of hemorrhoids among adult patients visiting the surgical outpatient department in the University of Gondar Comprehensive Specialized Hospital, Northwest Ethiopia. *PLoS ONE* **2021**, *16*, e0249736. [CrossRef]

Disclaimer/Publisher's Note: The statements, opinions and data contained in all publications are solely those of the individual author(s) and contributor(s) and not of MDPI and/or the editor(s). MDPI and/or the editor(s) disclaim responsibility for any injury to people or property resulting from any ideas, methods, instructions or products referred to in the content.

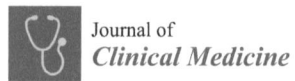

Article

Gastrointestinal Disorders and Atopic Dermatitis in Infants in the First Year of Life According to ROME IV Criteria—A Possible Association with the Mode of Delivery and Early Life Nutrition

Maciej Ziętek [1], Małgorzata Szczuko [2] and Tomasz Machałowski [1,*]

[1] Department of Perinatology, Obstetrics and Gynecology Pomeranian Medical University in Szczecin, 70-204 Szczecin, Poland; maciejzietek@tlen.pl

[2] Department of Human Nutrition and Metabolomics, Pomeranian Medical University in Szczecin, 70-204 Szczecin, Poland; malgorzata.szczuko@pum.edu.pl

* Correspondence: tomasz.machalowski@poczta.onet.pl; Tel.: +48-502-195-645

Abstract: Background: Functional gastrointestinal disorders are very common condition. The aim of this study is to evaluate the implications of the mode of pregnancy termination and early infant feeding on the incidence of gastrointestinal disorders and atopic dermatitis at birth and 3, 6, and 12 months of age. **Methods:** This study included 82 pregnant women and their newborns born at term. All newborns were examined at birth and 3, 6, and 12 months of age according to the ROME IV criteria. **Results:** In children born after cesarean section, the incidence of regurgitation was significantly higher. In children fed mostly or exclusively with formula, dry skin with allergic features was observed more often compared to breastfed children, but this relation was statistically significant only at the age of 12 months. The use of antibiotic therapy increased the risk of allergic skin lesions by almost seven times at 3 months of life. Gastrointestinal disorders in the form of regurgitation, colic, and constipation occur within the period of up to 12 months of the child's life and may be related to the mode of the termination of pregnancy via cesarean section and the use of artificial feeding or antibiotic therapy. The occurrence of atopic dermatitis in infants at 12 months of life is correlated with the mode of the termination of pregnancy after cesarean section. **Conclusions:** One of the risk factors for the occurrence of atopic dermatitis and gastrointestinal disorders in the period up to 12 months of the child's life may be a cesarean section and the use of formula feeding or antibiotic therapy.

Keywords: cesarean section; functional gastrointestinal disorders; nutrition

Citation: Ziętek, M.; Szczuko, M.; Machałowski, T. Gastrointestinal Disorders and Atopic Dermatitis in Infants in the First Year of Life According to ROME IV Criteria—A Possible Association with the Mode of Delivery and Early Life Nutrition. *J. Clin. Med.* **2024**, *13*, 927. https://doi.org/10.3390/jcm13040927

Academic Editors: Ioannis Tsakiridis and Apostolos Mamopoulos

Received: 15 January 2024
Revised: 3 February 2024
Accepted: 4 February 2024
Published: 6 February 2024

Copyright: © 2024 by the authors. Licensee MDPI, Basel, Switzerland. This article is an open access article distributed under the terms and conditions of the Creative Commons Attribution (CC BY) license (https://creativecommons.org/licenses/by/4.0/).

1. Introduction

Functional gastrointestinal disorders (FGIDs) comprise a diverse combination of chronic or recurrent symptoms, the presence of which is not associated with the structural or biochemical abnormalities of a child. They occur with an incidence of 15–30%, and their severity and nature depend on a number of factors, including age and physiological, autonomic, emotional, and intellectual development [1–3]. The symptoms of gastrointestinal disorders are most commonly caused by the immaturity of the gastrointestinal tract, the nervous system, and abnormalities in the gut microbiome of infants. FGIDs may occur in normally developing children or be a consequence of abnormal behavioral responses to internal or external stimuli. Despite the precise classification of the above disorders within the framework of the Rome IV criteria [4], their pathophysiology and importance for the further development of the child are still poorly understood. We should, therefore, treat FGIDs as disorders of the brain–gut axis, for just as the central nervous system influences the functioning of the gut, the gut exerts an influence on the brain [5–7]. In regulating gut–brain interactions, neurogenic, endocrine, and immunological mechanisms are involved, which may be modified by the gut microbiota intestinal microbiota. The microbiome, through secreted metabolites, can exert both salutary and harmful effects on the intestinal mucosa. Factors disrupting normal gut colonization, leading to dysbiosis, can have a significant impact on the occurrence of FGIDs. Since the association of FGIDs, according to the Rome IV Criteria, with the mode of delivery and child feeding has not been studied and published before, in this work, we conducted such an analysis, which is a novel scientific endeavor. The occurrence of FGID is not an indication to discontinue breastfeeding, which should, in fact, be actively encouraged. In infants fed modified milk, special formulas may be considered if reassurance and nutritional recommendations based on adequate milk volume and frequency do not lead to sufficient improvement. In cases of the absence of organic disease, any pharmacologic intervention is unlikely to be helpful or effective. Furthermore, medications may cause side effects and unnecessarily expose the child to additional stress. The occurrence of FGIDs often leads to a vicious circle: the newborn's symptoms make the parents anxious, which leads to the implementation of drugs available at the pharmacy without consulting a doctor. Consequently, the symptoms persist, and diagnosis is delayed. Environmental factors and the type of food consumed by the infant in the early postnatal period play a significant role in the development of the infant's immune system, and it is suspected that they may also be involved in the development of not only FGIDs but also atopic diseases in children. There is also medical evidence that there may be a link between FGIDs and the way pregnancy is terminated. Numerous epidemiological studies have shown an association between cesarean section and an increased risk of developing immunological diseases, including early and persistent wheezing and bronchial asthma [4,8,9], allergic rhinitis, ulcerative colitis, type 1 diabetes, celiac disease, being overweight, and obesity [4,10]. The disturbed composition of the neonatal gut microbiome, resulting from limited contact with maternal rectal and vaginal flora and leading to dysbiosis, may be an initiating factor in the onset of FGIDs. Given that there is an association between the early composition of the neonatal gut microbiota and the occurrence of chronic diseases later in childhood, it is reasonable to assume that impaired intestinal colonization due to cesarean delivery may play an important role in the etiology and pathogenesis of childhood FGIDs. Some symptoms of FGIDs, such as colic, show an association with the presence of more colonies of proteobacteria, including Escherichia, Klebsiella, and Pseudomonas, while Firmicutes and Actinobacteria are more prevalent in infants without colic [11]. The modification of the composition and activity of the child's intestinal microbiota through dietary interventions using probiotics may be one of the directions for the prevention and treatment of infants with FGIDs and allergic diseases. It has been proven that selected probiotic strains from the genus Lactobacillus can alleviate IBS symptoms. The relative risk (RR) value for symptom improvement was 7.69, which means that clinical improvement is more than seven times more likely in those taking the probiotic compared to those not taking such supplementation [12–14]. The gut microbiota occupies a prominent position in the structure and function of the brain–gut axis, which is a bidirectional pathway for the exchange of neural and biochemical signals between the central nervous system and the gastrointestinal tract. The intestinal barrier, which includes the microbiota, is, therefore, a point of interest for potential therapeutic interventions in FGIDs [13–16].

Objectives

The aim of this study is to evaluate the implications of the mode of pregnancy termination and early infant feeding on the incidence of gastrointestinal disorders and atopic dermatitis at birth and 3, 6, and 12 months of age, according to the ROME IV criteria.

2. Material and Methods

This was a prospective cross-sectional study with a group of similar patients that had a regular follow-up at the same time point. The study included 82 randomly selected pregnant women and their newborns born near the term of gestation at the Department of Perinatology, Obstetrics, and Gynecology in Szczecin, Poland. The data were collected between October 2020 and September 2022. The study group was randomly selected from a population list of woman–infant pairs, meaning that random chance decided which woman–infant pair entered the sample. A simple draw (non-return) type of random selection was used for this purpose. The inclusion criteria included a pregnancy terminated between 37 + 0 and 41 + 6 weeks of a singleton pregnancy, maternal consent for the study, the physiological course of the pregnancy and childbirth, a minimum of 8 points with respect to the 5-min Apgar score, and no developmental birth defects. The exclusion criteria included pregnancies terminated before 37 weeks of gestation, comorbidities complicating pregnancy, severe birth status of the newborn, multifetal pregnancy, and a lack of written maternal consent for the study. In pregnant women, anthropometric data, the method of termination of pregnancy, and other medical data, including the course of the current pregnancy and family history of allergy, were considered (Table 1). A Detecto PD200 medical scale (DETECTO Cardinal Scale Manufacturing Co., 203 E. Daugherty, Webb City, MO 64870, USA) has been used for the digital weight, height, and BMI measurements. All infants were examined by a pediatrician at birth and at 3, 6, and 12 months of age consecutively (Table 2). The neonatal clinical examination of the babies was performed at home in their place of residence by a specialist physician. The same doctor carried out examinations during all visits, as it helps the avoidance of methodological errors and differences in diagnoses, especially, since the doctor has many years of experience. At each medical visit, a functional gastrointestinal disorders questionnaire according to the Rome IV: The Rome IV Diagnostic Questionnaire for Functional Gastrointestinal Disorders (R4PDQ—A parent report form for neonates and toddlers 0–3 years old) was completed, and data were collected with respect to the presence of atopic dermatitis and how the children were fed (breastfeeding, formula feeding, supplemental feeding, and supplemental feeding with probiotics). Atopic dermatitis was diagnosed on the basis of clinical signs such as the following: a rash with eczema on the cheeks, forehead, or scalp, which was associated with dry and itchy patches of skin. In some cases, the lesions spread to the knees, elbows, and trunk. The experts on FGIDs and parents reviewed the questionnaire for content, understandability, and completeness. The content's validity was established by comparing the neonatologist and questionnaire diagnoses in the studied group of children. The validation of the questionnaire met the guidelines on how to translate and validate questionnaires, which are included in the document defining the principles of translation and its adaptation to the conditions of the Polish Caucasian population. The high repeatability of the results obtained with the use of the R4PDQ questionnaire allows us to consider the evaluated questionnaire as an accurate measurement tool that may be a source of reliable information with respect to the clinical symptoms of intestinal disorders. In the diagnosis of the functional disorders of the gastrointestinal tract, data obtained from the history and physical examination are of great importance, taking into account alarm signals, which include chronic pain in the right upper or right lower quadrant; pain when waking the child from sleep; swallowing disorders; prolonged vomiting; gastrointestinal bleeding; diarrhea occurring at night; positive family history of inflammatory bowel disease, coeliac disease, or peptic ulcer disease; arthralgia; perianal lesions; weight loss; slowed growth rate; and unexplained fevers. During the examination, weight, height, and head and abdomen circumferences were recorded, and centile grids of the Polish population, according to the WHO's growth standards for children aged 0–3 years, were used [8]. During this period of life, children cannot voice complaints, such as nausea or pain. Therefore, the clinician must rely on the parents' interpretations, which, combined with his knowledge, skills, and experience, allow him to differentiate between health and disease in the first instance.

Table 1. Anthropometric data of the studied pregnant women.

Gestation/Delivery (n = 82)	Mean	SD
Age (years)	31.22	4.49
Body weight before pregnancy (kg)	68.28	17.59
Birth weight during delivery (kg)	82.20	16.55
BMI before pregnancy	24.56	6.05
BMI during delivery	29.57	5.62
Weight gain (kg)	14.24	7.01
Week of gestation completion	38.44	1.30
Natural childbirth n (%)	35 (42.7)	-
Cesarean section n (%)	47 (57.3)	-

Table 2. Anthropometric data of infants on the day of birth and at 3, 6, and 12 months of age.

Parameters	Mean	SD
Male n (%)	38 (46.3)	-
Female n (%)	44 (53.7)	
Neonatal birth weight (g)	3286	395
Neonatal birth weight (g) at 3 MOA (n = 82)	6340	651
Neonatal weight (g) at 6 MOA (n = 82)	8020	900
Neonatal weight (g) at 12 MOA (n = 42)	10,560	1040

MOA—months of age.

Statistical analysis was performed using STATA 11 statistical software (StataCorp LLC, 4905 Lakeway Drive, College Station, TX 77845-4512, USA), license number 30110532736. The Kolmogorov–Smirnov test for normality of distributions was used. If $p < 0.05$, then the Mann–Whitney U or Kruskal–Wallis test was used. For normal distributions, the Student's t-test or ANOVA was used. Correlations were calculated using Spearman's rank test.

3. Results

The study included 82 randomly selected pregnant women and their newborns born near the term of gestation at the Department of Perinatology, Obstetrics, and Gynecology in Szczecin, Poland. Of the infants in the study, 42% were born from nulligravidae. An allergy history was found in 26% of the mothers in the study. Allergies relative to grass pollen (23%) and house dust mites (19%) were the most common. In the fathers of the examined infants, 29% were allergic, and the most common allergen in this group was grass pollen (62%). The median APGAR score was 9.0 (8.0–10.0 IQR) at the fifth minute.

3.1. Functional Gastrointestinal Disorders

In all infants, the process of postpartum adaptation was normal during the first 2 days of life. All infants were discharged home in good condition and breastfed. On the basis of clinical examination and the diagnostics of functional gastrointestinal disorders according to the Rome IV criteria carried out during 3, 6, and 12 months of life, differences in the occurrence of the particular examined parameters were demonstrated (Figure 1). At 3 months of life, the most frequently observed functional gastrointestinal disorder was neonatal regurgitation (56.10%), which gradually decreased to 32.93% and 7.14% at 6 and 12 months of life, respectively. The second most frequently observed symptom was infantile colic, which, although present in 18.29% of infants at 3 months of age, did not appear thereafter. Constipation was also observed in all studied infants, which occurred in 15.85%, 7.32%, and 7.14% consecutively at 3, 6, and 12 months of life (Figure 1). Considering the cumulative incidence of gastrointestinal disorders, it was observed that the most frequent gastrointestinal disorders occurred at 3 months of life in 86.59% of infants, gradually decreasing to 56.10% and 19.05% at 6 and 12 months of life, and these differences were statistically significant ($p < 0.00001$) (Figure 2).

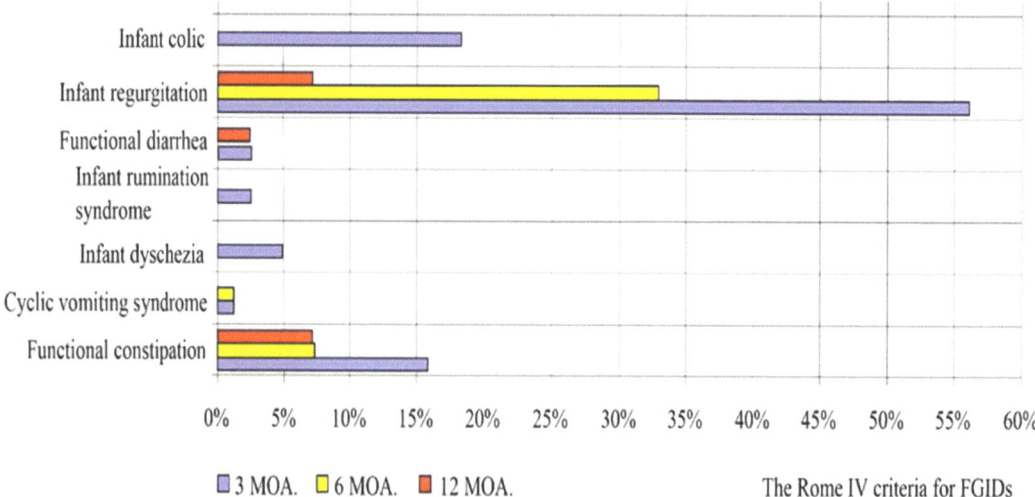

Figure 1. Functional gastrointestinal disorders according to Rome IV criteria.

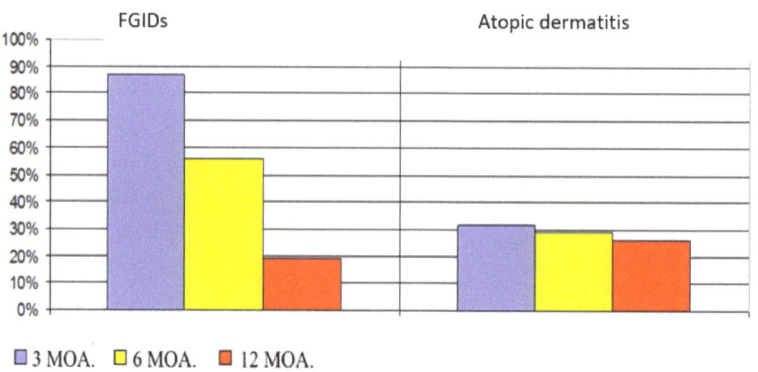

Figure 2. Incidence of gastrointestinal disorders (FGIDs) and atopic dermatitis in infants at 3, 6, and 12 months of age.

3.2. Atopic Dermatitis

Symptoms of atopic dermatitis were observed in 31.71%, 29.27%, and 26.19% of the infants at 3, 6, and 12 months of life, respectively, and these differences were not statistically significant. However, a statistically significant positive correlation ($p = 0.0042$; $r = 0.31$) between the occurrence of gastrointestinal disorders and allergy at 3 months of life was found. Atopic dermatitis was more frequent in female newborns, and this correlation was statistically significant ($p = 0.048$). No similar correlation was found at 6 and 12 months of life (Figure 2).

3.3. Mode of Delivery

The analysis of the mode of delivery revealed that cesarean section is associated with a higher incidence of allergy in infants at the age of 12 months (38.46% vs. 6.25%), and this relation was statistically significant ($p < 0.005$) (Figure 3). The overall risk of allergy at

12 months of life was over nine times higher in children born after cesarean section (OD 9.37; $p = 0.044$). There was no significant increase in allergy in 3 and 6 months of life in infants born after cesarean section. The surgical termination of pregnancy via cesarean section did not show a significant association with most gastrointestinal disorders in infants in any of the analyzed periods of neonatal studies. Only in the group of children born after a cesarean section was regurgitation more frequent, and this relation was statistically significant ($p = 0.0434$). Infants with normal postpartum adaptation in the majority of cases (80%) did not show any gastrointestinal disorders at a later stage. In 20% of infants with normal adaptation, bloating, gas, and colic were observed. However, this relation was statistically significant ($p = 0.00544$) only in the third month of life. The Spearman's rank correlation test showed that the occurrence of both gastrointestinal disorders and allergies significantly correlated with gender only at 6 months of life ($p = 0.0019$). There was no correlation between the birth weight and the occurrence of gastrointestinal disorders and atopic dermatitis; however, a significant correlation was found for pregnant women's body weights and BMIs, but only at 12 months of age.

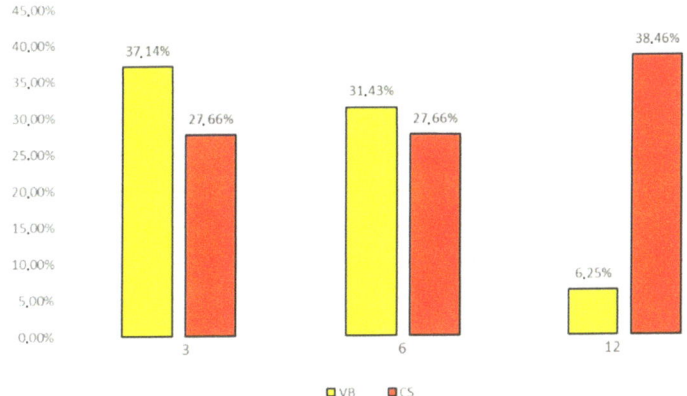

Figure 3. Incidence of atopic dermatitis in infants at 3, 6, and 12 months of age depending on the mode of delivery: vaginal birth (VB) and cesarean section (CS).

3.4. Nutrition

According to the study, the majority of infants were breastfed at 3 months of life (65.85%), and with the passage of time, their percentage was gradually reduced at 6 and 12 months of life, respectively, to 51.22% and 26.19% (Figure 4). This relationship is statistically significant. The use of probiotics in the diet of newborns showed a similar trend. The highest number of infants received probiotic supplementation at 3 months of life (50.00%) and, respectively, at 6 and 12 months of life, 23.17% and 16.67%. As the infant grew older, an expansion of the diet to include solid foods and an increasing use of various types of baby formula milk at the expense of natural breastfeeding were observed. On the other hand, with the passage of time, a more frequent introduction of nutritional supplementation was observed at the expense of natural feeding. The results of the study showed that, at 12 months of age, 73.81% of infants with a recommended properly expanded diet of solid foods in place of maternal milk were fed exclusively with formula nutrition (Figure 4). In order to check which variables influence gastrointestinal complaints and skin lesions, a multivariate discriminant analysis was performed. It was shown that neonatal constipation was more frequently observed when a probiotic was introduced into the diet, and this relationship was statistically significant ($p = 0.0045$). When both the time function of using a given feeding method and the probiotic were eliminated, it was shown that bloating and gas were more common in breastfed babies ($p = 0.0490$). In this group, the symptoms of atopic dermatitis and rash were also more frequent. In more than 50% of artificially fed children and only artificially fed children, dry skin with allergic features was observed more often, but this relationship was statistically significant only at 12 months of age. The presence of colic tended to be more common in infants who were treated with the probiotic and those who were fed formula, but this relationship was at the border of statistical significance. A logistic regression model was used to estimate the risk of various digestive ailments and skin allergic symptoms. The use of a probiotic increases the risk of constipation in the third month of life ($p = 0.045$) fourfold. On the other hand, bloating and gas occur almost four times more often in the third month of life when the child is artificially fed or formula-fed. When a child is fed formula, the overall risk of PP complaints increases over six times more often at 12 months of age ($p = 0.028$). The use of antibiotic therapy increases the risk of skin lesions of an allergic nature during 3 months of life by almost seven times.

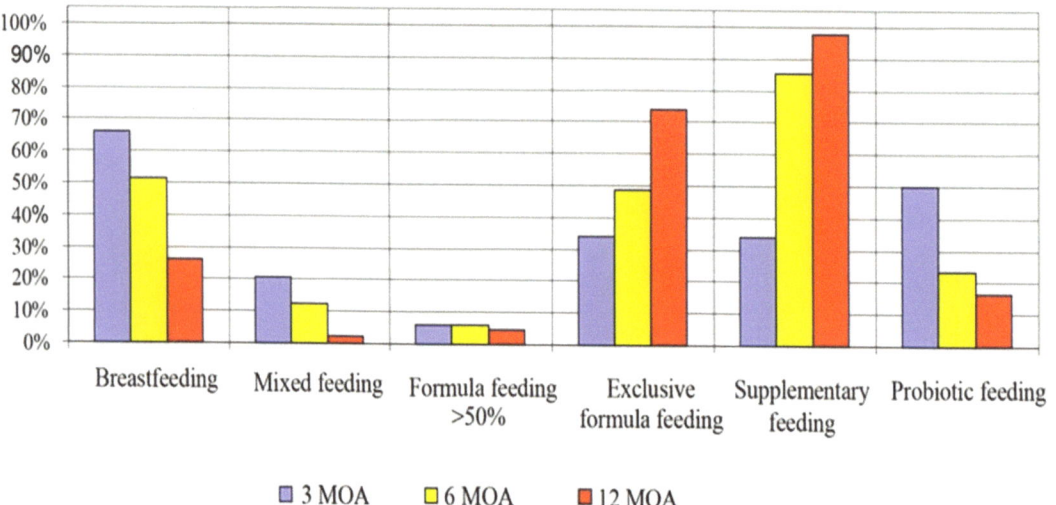

Figure 4. Infants feeding at 3, 6, and 12 months of age.

4. Discussion

FGIDs are common in newborns and infants and concern about 26–60% of them [8–10]. Our study found a statistically significant phenomenon, decreasing with the age of the infant: the frequency of disorders in the FGID spectrum. The frequency of disorders at 3 months of age was 86.59%, 6–56.1% at 6 months of age, and 19.05% at 12 months of age. This phenomenon may be influenced by the adaptation process of the infant to the environment, particularly by developing tolerance to food allergens, increasing the maturity of neurological and digestive systems and the brain–gut axis that underlies the disorders [17]. In the presented study, the most common symptoms of FGIDs were regurgitation at 56.1% during the third month of life, with a subsequent downward trend—32.9% in the sixth month and 7.14% in the twelfth month of life. Similarly, regurgitation, as the most common symptom in the FGID spectrum, is reported to be present in 40% [18,19] and 30% of infants [20]. Kee Seang Chew et al. found regurgitation to appear in only 10.5% of subjects, but the study was conducted in Asia, where the overall frequency of FGID symptoms is low, occurring in 14.6% of infants [21]. Intestinal colic is indicated in many studies as the most common disorder from the FGID spectrum, where it affects up to 57.6% of infants with FGIDs [4]. In our study, it was ranked second and concerned 18.28% of infants. Colic occurs only at 3 months of age, which is typical for this disorder and results from the diagnostic criteria. According to the Rome IV criteria, this disorder appears and disappears by the fifth month of life, and if the parents' care is conscientious and constant, functional gastrointestinal disorders do not pose a danger to the child [18]. The third most common symptom—constipation—occurred in all newborns, with 15.85% of infants at

3 months of age; then, its incidence decreased with the infant's age. These results are consistent with many analyses [18,20]. However, Chogle et al., while studying the infant population in Colombia, assessed constipation as the most common FGID disorder, with a frequency of 16.1% [11]. The incidence of atopic dermatitis did not differ significantly depending on the age of the infant, ranging from 26 to 31%. There is a general upward trend in the incidence of skin allergies worldwide. Symptoms most often appear from early infancy to the age of 1. It is believed that environmental factors trigger an effect in neonates with a genetic predisposition [22]. Our study found a positive correlation between FGID symptoms and the occurrence of allergies, but only at 3 months of age. The source of this phenomenon may be a common etiological factor when the immunologically immature organism reacts to the allergen with both skin and gastrointestinal symptoms. The appearance of the above-described symptoms prompts parents to look for and exclude potential allergens, e.g., a nursing mother's elimination diet, change from natural to artificial feeding, change in the type of milk formula, introduction of probiotics, and change in care cosmetics. Effectively eliminating the allergen could have contributed to the lack of persistence of the correlation between skin lesions and gastrointestinal symptoms after 3 months of age. The development of immunological tolerance, along with the exposure time, may also play an important role [23]. FGIDs are considered to be transient, self-limiting disorders that disappear with the infant's age due to the maturation of the physiological mechanisms responsible for their formation [17,24]. It could also have contributed to the lack of persistence of the positive correlation between FGID and allergies after 3 months of age. The correlation between allergic disorders and FGID was more common in girls. The results vary from study to study. In Campeotto's study, the above symptoms mainly occurred in boys [18]. In our study, a positive correlation was observed between the occurrence of colic and constipation (the latter only at 3 months of age) and the supply of a probiotic. One of the postulated etiological factors of colic is the dysbiosis of the intestinal flora. The supply of Lactobacillus reuteri to breastfed infants with symptoms of colic has proven therapeutic efficacy [12,25]. The correlation obtained may result from the fact that in the event of the appearance of FGID symptoms, probiotic therapy is implemented. Gastrointestinal symptoms, such as bloating and gas, were more frequently observed in breastfed newborns and infants. Allergic dermatitis and rash were also more common. Similar results were obtained in the Danish study [22]. The diet may have influenced this correlation. Formula-fed babies were given a constant formula, while breastfed babies could have been exposed to a variety of ingredients, including allergens, depending on the mother's diet. Currently, elimination diets are not recommended for mothers who are breastfeeding healthy infants; therefore, they could also contain gas or products that are considered to be allergenic. Exclusive breastfeeding until the age of 3–4 months and mainly breastfeeding until the age of 6 months is of prophylactic importance in the development of allergies [26,27]. The described mechanisms include a passive mechanism—reducing the exposure to exogenous allergens—and an active mechanism—secretion into the milk of substances protecting against infections, stimulating the maturation of intestinal mucosa, stimulating the development of normal intestinal flora, and secreting a number of anti-inflammatory and immunomodulatory factors [28,29]. In our study, feeding with a milk mixture was associated with a 6-fold increase in gastrointestinal complaints; moreover, when only formula is used, or formula is used in >50% of feeding, skin allergies were observed, but only at 12 months of age. The fact that the percentage of naturally fed children decreased with age (3 months at 65.85% and 12 months at 26.19%) may account for the statistical significance in the appearance of allergy symptoms at 12 months of age. Moreover, after 6 months of age, expanding the child's diet with solid foods is recommended. Some of them could have an allergenic effect, and in the absence of the protective role of breast milk, skin symptoms could be more strongly expressed with formula feeding. In the present study, the termination of pregnancy via cesarean section was nine times more likely to increase the risk of skin allergy at 12 months of age. Moreover, the need for antibiotic therapy was associated with a 7-fold risk of allergic skin lesions. The adaptation and development of the

immune system are undoubtedly influenced by the intestinal flora of newborns. It differs depending on the pregnancy termination method. After a vaginal birth, the intestinal flora of newborns comprises more bacteria from the mother's intestinal and vaginal flora; after a cesarean section, it comprises skin bacteria. Newborns born after cesarean section have a later maturation of the intestinal flora and a different cytokine profile [30–33]. Selma-Royo et al. found a stronger epithelial barrier function, a higher immune response associated with TL4 pathway activation, and the production of proinflammatory cytokines in neonates born after cesarean section [33,34]. Thus, the mode of delivery seems to be an important factor in the development of the immune system and, consequently, the occurrence of allergies. The implementation of antibiotic therapy in the mother, both in the perinatal period (as prophylaxis)—when the pregnancy is terminated via cesarean section—and in the infant at different stages of life significantly disrupts the composition of the intestinal flora, the function of enterocytes, and the activity of the local immune system, which may have contributed to an increased risk of skin allergies. However, studies are not consistent; Maeda et al. did not find a higher incidence of skin lesions in infants after cesarean section deliveries [30]. The presented study has limitations. It should be taken into account that the diagnosis of FGIDs, based on the Rome IV criteria, took place on the basis of an interview carried out with parents [28]. Their perception of the infant's gastrointestinal physiology, emotional attitude, personal experiences, character traits, and family situation may have reduced the objectivity of the opinion. Some reports emphasize the higher incidence of FGIDs in children or firstborns and with divorced parents [15]. In this study, these factors were not investigated.

5. Limitations of the Study

This study has several limitations. Firstly, our results are based on the diagnosis of FGID symptoms in children, which was carried out in an interview with the parents; despite the use of an objective questionnaire, subjective information arose from the parents' emotional attitudes and experiences. We cannot exclude inconsistencies and missed data. Secondly, the study group only comprised 82 pregnant women and their newborns, and some conclusions may not be confirmed in such a group of people, but the statistical significance of the obtained results encourages carrying out the above analysis in a larger group of women and their children. Third, the group is homogeneous; thus, the results can only refer to this population, and conclusions cannot be drawn about the entire population.

6. Conclusions

Summarizing, regurgitation, infant colic, and functional constipation are common FGIDs that often contribute to a visit to physicians during the first 3 months of an infant's life. Atopic dermatitis and gastrointestinal tract disorders may be associated with a common mechanism triggering these reactions. One of the risk factors for the occurrence of these symptoms in the period up to 12 months of a child's life may be the termination of pregnancy via cesarean section, the use of formula feeding, or antibiotic therapy.

The above observations have proven to be an important clinical application for family doctors, pediatricians, and GPs because they show the probable relationship between the occurrence of gastroenterological disorders, the method of delivery, and the overuse of antibiotics and formula feeding. The results are important, especially in the field of obstetrics in the Polish population, where the percentage of cesarean sections in 2022 was 48%, and in the previous year (2023), it exceeded 50% (according to WHO, this percentage should be about 15%). If the results of this work reach a wider population, perhaps the rate of elective cesarean sections could be reduced. The above relationship concerns the overuse of antibiotics in the Polish population, forcing doctors to prescribe them during viral infections, and the rapid abandonment of breastfeeding among patients after childbirth (exclusive breastfeeding reached 30% in the fourth month and in the sixth month, it went from 4 to 14% depending on the study). Patient awareness is the basis for improving population health.

Author Contributions: Methodology, M.Z., M.S. and T.M.; Validation, M.Z.; Formal analysis, M.Z. and T.M.; Investigation, M.Z., M.S. and T.M.; Writing—original draft, M.Z. and T.M.; Writing—review & editing, M.Z. and M.S. All authors have read and agreed to the published version of the manuscript.

Funding: This research received no external funding.

Institutional Review Board Statement: This study was conducted in accordance with the Declaration of Helsinki and approved by the Pomeranian Medical University Ethics Committee (protocol code KB-0012/70/18 and date of approval 18 June 2018).

Informed Consent Statement: Informed consent was obtained from all subjects involved in the study.

Data Availability Statement: The data presented in this study are availabe on request from the corresponding author (Tomasz Machałowski).

Conflicts of Interest: The authors declare no conflict of interest.

References

1. Bellù, R.; Condò, M. Functional gastrointestinal disorders in newborns: Nutritional perspectives. *Pediatr. Med. Chir.* **2018**, *40*, 23. [CrossRef] [PubMed]
2. Fiori, N.; Serra, M.; Cenni, S.; Pacella, D.; Martinelli, M.; Miele, E.; Staiano, A.; Tolone, C.; Auricchio, R.; Strisciuglio, C. Prevalence of functional gastrointestinal disorders in children with celiac disease on different types of gluten-free diets. *World J. Gastroenterol.* **2022**, *28*, 6589–6598. [CrossRef]
3. Basnayake, C.; Kamm, M.; Stanley, A.; Wilson-O'brien, A.; Burrell, K.; Lees-Trinca, I.; Khera, A.; Kantidakis, J.; Wong, O.; Fox, K.; et al. Long-Term Outcome of Multidisciplinary Versus Standard Gastroenterologist Care for Functional Gastrointestinal Disorders: A Randomized Trial. *Clin. Gastroenterol. Hepatol. Off. Clin. Pract. J. Am. Gastroenterol. Assoc.* **2022**, *20*, 2102–2111. [CrossRef] [PubMed]
4. Zeevenhooven, J.; Koppen, I.J.; Benninga, M.A. The New Rome IV Criteria for Functional Gastrointestinal Disorders in Infants and Toddlers. *Pediatr. Gastroenterol. Hepatol. Nutr.* **2017**, *20*, 1–13. [CrossRef] [PubMed]
5. Jacobs, J.; Gupta, A.; Bhatt, R.; Brawer, J.; Gao, K.; Tillisch, K.; Lagishetty, V.; Firth, R.; Gudleski, G.D.; Ellingson, B.M.; et al. Cognitive behavioral therapy for irritable bowel syndrome induces bidirectional alterations in the brain-gut-microbiome axis associated with gastrointestinal symptom improvement. *Microbiome* **2021**, *9*, 236. [CrossRef] [PubMed]
6. Wauters, L.; Li, H.; Talley, N. Disruption of the Microbiota-Gut-Brain Axis in Functional Dyspepsia and Gastroparesis: Mechanisms and Clinical Implications. *Front. Neurosci.* **2022**, *16*, 941810. [CrossRef] [PubMed]
7. Labanski, A.; Langhorst, J.; Engler, H.; Elsenbruch, S. Stress and the brain-gut axis in functional and chronic-inflammatory gastrointestinal diseases: A transdisciplinary challenge. *Psychoneuroendocrinology* **2020**, *111*, 104501. [CrossRef] [PubMed]
8. Kułaga, Z.; Różdżyńska-Świątkowska, A.; Grajda, A. Percentile charts for growth and nutritional status assessment in Polish children and adolescents from birth to 18 year of age. *Stand. Med. Pediatr.* **2015**, *12*, 119–135.
9. Słabuszewska-Jóźwiak, A.; Szymański, J.K.; Ciebiera, M.; Sarecka-Hujar, B.; Jakiel, G. Pediatrics Consequences of Caesarean Section-A Systematic Review and Meta-Analysis. *Int. J. Environ. Res. Public Health* **2020**, *17*, 8031. [CrossRef]
10. van Berkel, A.C.; den Dekker, H.T.; Jaddoe, V.W.; Reiss, I.K.; Gaillard, R.; Hofman, A.; de Jongste, J.C.; Duijts, L. Mode of delivery and childhood fractional exhaled nitric oxide, interrupter resistance and asthma: The Generation R study. *Pediatr. Allergy Immunol.* **2015**, *26*, 330–336. [CrossRef] [PubMed]
11. Li, H.T.; Zhou, Y.B.; Liu, J.M. The impact of cesarean section on offspring overweight and obesity: A systematic review and meta-analysis. *Int. J. Obes.* **2013**, *37*, 893–899. [CrossRef] [PubMed]
12. Pärtty, A.; Rautava, S.; Kalliomäki, M. Probiotics on Pediatric Functional Gastrointestinal Disorders. *Nutrients* **2018**, *10*, 1836. [CrossRef] [PubMed]
13. Tiequn, B.; Guanqun, C.; Shuo, Z. Therapeutic effects of Lactobacillus in treating irritable bowel syndrome: A meta-analysis. *Intern. Med.* **2015**, *54*, 243–249. [CrossRef] [PubMed]
14. Bellaiche, M.; Ategbo, S.; Krumholz, F.; Ludwig, T.; Miqdady, M.; Abkari, A.; Vandenplas, Y. A large-scale study to describe the prevalence, characteristics and management of functional gastrointestinal disorders in African infants. *Acta Paediatr.* **2020**, *109*, 2366–2373. [CrossRef] [PubMed]
15. Chogle, A.; Velasco-Benitez, C.A.; Koppen, I.J.; Moreno, J.E.; Hernández, C.R.R.; Saps, M. A Population-Based Study on the Epidemiology of Functional Gastrointestinal Disorders in Young Children. *J. Pediatr.* **2016**, *179*, 139–143. [CrossRef] [PubMed]
16. Vandenplas, Y.; Benninga, M.; Broekaert, I.; Falconer, J.; Gottrand, F.; Guarino, A.; Lifschitz, C.; Lionetti, P.; Orel, R.; Papadopoulou, A.; et al. Functional gastro-intestinal disorder algorithms focus on early recognition, parental reassurance and nutritional strategies. *Acta Paediatr.* **2016**, *105*, 244–252, Erratum in *Acta Paediatr.* **2016**, *105*, 984. [CrossRef]
17. Baldassarre, M.E.; Di Mauro, A.; Salvatore, S.; Tafuri, S.; Bianchi, F.P.; Dattoli, E.; Morando, L.; Pensabene, L.; Meneghin, F.; Dilillo, D.; et al. Birth Weight and the Development of Functional Gastrointestinal Disorders in Infants. *Pediatr. Gastroenterol. Hepatol. Nutr.* **2020**, *23*, 366–376. [CrossRef]

18. Campeotto, F.; Barbaza, M.O.; Hospital, V. Functional Gastrointestinal Disorders in Outpatients Aged up to 12 Months: A French Non-Interventional Study. *Int. J. Environ. Res. Public Health* **2020**, *17*, 4031. [CrossRef]
19. Robin, S.G.; Keller, C.; Zwiener, R.; Hyman, P.E.; Nurko, S.; Saps, M.; Di Lorenzo, C.; Shulman, R.J.; Hyams, J.S.; Palsson, O.; et al. Prevalence of Pediatric Functional Gastrointestinal Disorders Utilizing the Rome IV Criteria. *J. Pediatr.* **2018**, *195*, 134–139. [CrossRef] [PubMed]
20. Vandenplas, Y.; Abkari, A.; Bellaiche, M.; Benninga, M.; Chouraqui, J.P.; Çokura, F.; Harb, T.; Hegar, B.; Lifschitz, C.; Ludwig, T.; et al. Prevalence and health outcomes of functional gastrointestinal symptoms in infants from birth to 12 months of age. *J. Pediatr. Gastroenterol. Nutr.* **2015**, *61*, 531–537. [CrossRef] [PubMed]
21. Chew, K.S.; Em, J.M.; Koay, Z.L.; Jalaludin, M.Y.; Ng, R.T.; Lum, L.C.S.; Lee, W.S. Low prevalence of infantile functional gastrointestinal disorders (FGIDs) in a multi-ethnic Asian population. *Pediatr. Neonatol.* **2021**, *62*, 49–54. [CrossRef]
22. Bisgaard, H.; Halkjaer, L.B.; Hinge, R.; Giwercman, C.; Palmer, C.; Silveira, L.; Strand, M. Risk analysis of early childhood eczema. *J. Allergy Clin. Immunol.* **2009**, *123*, 1355–1360. [CrossRef]
23. Woon, F.C.; Chin, Y.S.; Ismail, I.H.; Chan, Y.M.; Batterham, M.; Latiff, A.H.A.; Gan, W.Y.; Appannah, G. Contribution of early nutrition on the development of malnutrition and allergic diseases in the first year of life: A study protocol for the Mother and Infant Cohort Study (MICOS). *BMC Pediatr.* **2018**, *18*, 233. [CrossRef]
24. Salvatore, S.; Barberi, S.; Borrelli, O.; Castellazzi, A.; Di Mauro, D.; Di Mauro, G.; Doria, M.; Francavilla, R.; Landi, M.; Miniello, V.L.; et al. Pharmacological interventions on early functional gastrointestinal disorders. *Ital. J. Pediatr.* **2016**, *42*, 68. [CrossRef]
25. Hojsak, I. Probiotics in Functional Gastrointestinal Disorders. *Adv. Exp. Med. Biol.* **2019**, *1125*, 121–137. [CrossRef]
26. Greer, F.R.; Sicherer, S.H.; Burks, A.W.; Committee On Nutrition; Section on Allergy and Immunology. The Effects of Early Nutritional Interventions on the Development of Atopic Disease in Infants and Children: The Role of Maternal Dietary Restriction, Breastfeeding, Hydrolyzed Formulas, and Timing of Introduction of Allergenic Complementary Foods. *Pediatrics* **2019**, *143*, e20190281. [CrossRef]
27. Lodge, C.J.; Tan, D.J.; Lau, M.X.; Dai, X.; Tham, R.; Lowe, A.J.; Bowatte, G.; Allen, K.J.; Dharmage, S.C. Breastfeeding and asthma and allergies: A systematic review and meta-analysis. *Acta Paediatr.* **2015**, *104*, 38–53. [CrossRef]
28. Ferrante, G.; Carta, M.; Montante, C.; Notarbartolo, V.; Corsello, G.; Giuffrè, M. Current Insights on Early Life Nutrition and Prevention of Allergy. *Front. Pediatr.* **2020**, *6*, 448. [CrossRef]
29. Lifschitz, C.; Szajewska, H. Cow's milk allergy: Evidence-based diagnosis and management for the practitioner. *Eur. J. Pediatr.* **2015**, *174*, 141–150. [CrossRef]
30. Maeda, H.; Hashimoto, K.; Iwasa, H.; Kyozuka, H.; Go, H.; Sato, A.; Ogata, Y.; Murata, T.; Fujimori, K.; Shinoki, K.; et al. Association of cesarean section and allergic outcomes among infants at 1 year of age: Logistics regression analysis using data of 104,065 fetal and children's records from the Japan Environment and Children's Study. *Authorea* **2021**, *118*, 636–638. [CrossRef]
31. Selma-Royo, M.; Calatayud Arroyo, M.; García-Mantrana, I.; Parra-Llorca, A.; Escuriet, R.; Martínez-Costa, C.; Collado, M.C. Perinatal environment shapes microbiota colonization and infant growth: Impact on host response and intestinal function. *Mikrobiom* **2020**, *8*, 167. [CrossRef]
32. Dominguez-Bello, M.G.; Costello, E.K.; Contreras, M.; Magris, M.; Hidalgo, G.; Fierer, N.; Knight, R. Delivery mode shapes the acquisition and structure of the initial microbiota across multiple body habitats in newborns. *Proc. Natl. Acad. Sci. USA* **2010**, *107*, 11971–11975. [CrossRef]
33. Jakobsson, H.E.; Abrahamsson, T.R.; Jenmalm, M.C.; Harris, K.; Quince, C.; Jernberg, C.; Björkstén, B.; Engstrand, L.; Andersson, A.F. Decreased gut microbiota diversity, delayed Bacteroidetes colonisation and reduced Th1 responses in infants delivered by Caesarean section. *Gut* **2014**, *63*, 559–566. [CrossRef] [PubMed]
34. Drossman, D.A. Functional Gastrointestinal Disorders: History, Pathophysiology, Clinical Features and Rome IV. *Gastroenterology* **2016**, *150*, 1262–1279.e2. [CrossRef]

Disclaimer/Publisher's Note: The statements, opinions and data contained in all publications are solely those of the individual author(s) and contributor(s) and not of MDPI and/or the editor(s). MDPI and/or the editor(s) disclaim responsibility for any injury to people or property resulting from any ideas, methods, instructions or products referred to in the content.

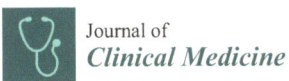 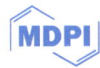

Article

Ultrasonographic Evaluation of the Second Stage of Labor according to the Mode of Delivery: A Prospective Study in Greece

Kyriaki Mitta, Ioannis Tsakiridis *, Themistoklis Dagklis, Ioannis Kalogiannidis, Apostolos Mamopoulos, Georgios Michos, Andriana Virgiliou and Apostolos Athanasiadis

Third Department of Obstetrics and Gynecology, School of Medicine, Faculty of Health Sciences, Aristotle University of Thessaloniki, 54642 Thessaloniki, Greece; kmittb@auth.gr (K.M.); dagklis@auth.gr (T.D.); ikalogia@auth.gr (I.K.); amamop@auth.gr (A.M.); gmichos@auth.gr (G.M.); anvirgiliou@hotmail.com (A.V.); apathana@auth.gr (A.A.)
* Correspondence: iotsakir@gmail.com; Tel.: +30-2313312120; Fax: +30-2310-992950

Abstract: Background and Objectives: Accurate diagnosis of labor progress is crucial for making well-informed decisions regarding timely and appropriate interventions to optimize outcomes for both the mother and the fetus. The aim of this study was to assess the progress of the second stage of labor using intrapartum ultrasound. Material and methods: This was a prospective study (December 2022–December 2023) conducted at the Third Department of Obstetrics and Gynecology, School of Medicine, Faculty of Health Sciences, Aristotle University of Thessaloniki, Greece. Maternal–fetal and labor characteristics were recorded, and two ultrasound parameters were measured: the angle of progression (AoP) and the head–perineum distance (HPD). The correlation between the two ultrasonographic values and the maternal–fetal characteristics was investigated. Multinomial regression analysis was also conducted to investigate any potential predictors of the mode of delivery. Results: A total of 82 women at the second stage of labor were clinically and sonographically assessed. The mean duration of the second stage of labor differed between vaginal and cesarean deliveries (65.3 vs. 160 min; p-value < 0.001) and between cesarean and operative vaginal deliveries (160 vs. 88.6 min; p-value = 0.015). The occiput anterior position was associated with an increased likelihood of vaginal delivery (OR: 24.167; 95% CI: 3.8–152.5; p-value < 0.001). No significant differences were identified in the AoP among the three different modes of delivery (vaginal: 145.7° vs. operative vaginal: 139.9° vs. cesarean: 132.1°; p-value = 0.289). The mean HPD differed significantly between vaginal and cesarean deliveries (28.6 vs. 41.4 mm; p-value < 0.001) and between cesarean and operative vaginal deliveries (41.4 vs. 26.9 mm; p-value = 0.002); it was correlated significantly with maternal BMI (r = 0.268; p-value = 0.024) and the duration of the second stage of labor (r = 0.256; p-value = 0.031). Low parity (OR: 12.024; 95% CI: 6.320–22.876; p-value < 0.001) and high HPD (OR: 1.23; 95% CI: 1.05–1.43; p-value = 0.007) were found to be significant predictors of cesarean delivery. Conclusions: The use of intrapartum ultrasound as an adjunctive technique to the standard clinical evaluation may enhance the diagnostic approach to an abnormal labor progress and predict the need for operative vaginal or cesarean delivery.

Keywords: intrapartum ultrasound; ultrasound in labor; second stage; predictor; mode of delivery

Citation: Mitta, K.; Tsakiridis, I.; Dagklis, T.; Kalogiannidis, I.; Mamopoulos, A.; Michos, G.; Virgiliou, A.; Athanasiadis, A. Ultrasonographic Evaluation of the Second Stage of Labor according to the Mode of Delivery: A Prospective Study in Greece. *J. Clin. Med.* **2024**, *13*, 1068. https://doi.org/10.3390/jcm13041068

Academic Editor: Ferdinando Antonio Gulino

Received: 10 January 2024
Revised: 7 February 2024
Accepted: 12 February 2024
Published: 13 February 2024

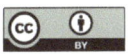

Copyright: © 2024 by the authors. Licensee MDPI, Basel, Switzerland. This article is an open access article distributed under the terms and conditions of the Creative Commons Attribution (CC BY) license (https://creativecommons.org/licenses/by/4.0/).

1. Introduction

For women undergoing labor without neuraxial anesthesia, the second stage usually lasts fewer than three hours for nulliparous individuals and fewer than two hours for multiparous ones; in cases with neuraxial anesthesia, this may be extended by one hour [1,2]. If the duration exceeds these timeframes, it is defined as prolonged; various factors, including fetal size and position, maternal pelvic shape, expulsive efforts, maternal age, obstetric history, and comorbidities such as hypertension or diabetes, may affect the length of the second stage of labor [3].

Traditionally, the assessment and management of the progress of labor are based on clinical assessment [4–6]. The diagnosis of labor arrest and decisions regarding the timing or type of intervention rely mostly on digital evaluation of cervical dilatation and fetal head station/position [7,8]. However, clinical examination of the head station and position may be inaccurate and subjective, especially when caput succedaneum impairs palpation of the sutures and fontanels. The use of ultrasound has been suggested as a valuable tool in labor management; numerous studies have highlighted the superiority of ultrasound examination compared to clinical assessment in diagnosing fetal head position and station and predicting labor arrest [9–15]. Ultrasound examinations can, to some degree, differentiate between women likely to have a spontaneous vaginal delivery and those who may require an operative vaginal delivery [10,15–20]. Intrapartum ultrasound can be conducted through a transabdominal approach, primarily for determining head and spine position, or a transperineal approach to assess the head station and position at lower stations; the most common quantitative sonographic parameters are the angle of progression (AoP) and the head–perineum distance (HPD) [21].

Currently, there is no consensus on the appropriate timing of intrapartum ultrasound use, which specific parameters should be obtained, or how the sonographic findings should be integrated into clinical practice to enhance patient management. Nevertheless, achieving a precise diagnosis of labor progress is essential for making informed decisions about interventions while also ensuring that appropriate measures are taken at the right time to optimize outcomes for both the mother and the fetus.

Thus, the aim of this study was to evaluate the use of intrapartum ultrasound during the second stage of labor.

2. Material and Methods

2.1. Study Design/Parameters

This was a prospective study (December 2022–December 2023) conducted at the Third Department of Obstetrics and Gynecology, School of Medicine, Faculty of Health Sciences, Aristotle University of Thessaloniki, Greece. This study was approved by the Ethics Committee of the Aristotle University of Thessaloniki (3–13 December 2022). Informed consent was obtained before the procedure, and no incentives were provided for participation in the study.

Maternal (age, BMI, parity), fetal/neonatal (fetal head position, birth weight), and labor characteristics (total duration of labor, duration of the second stage of labor, epidural and oxytocin use, spontaneous onset of labor or induction of labor) were recorded, and the AoP and the HPD were measured.

In cases of induction of labor, the Bishop score was calculated to choose the method of induction; if the Bishop score was favorable (≥ 6), rupture of membranes with or without oxytocin was the preferable method of labor induction, whereas when the Bishop score was unfavorable (<6), cervical ripening agents were used first [22]. Induction of labor was performed according to the guidelines of the Hellenic Society of Obstetrics and Gynecology. Regarding cervical ripening agents, either PGE2 (dinoprostone) or PGE1 (misoprostol) was administered if Bishop score was unfavorable; a PGE2 suppository of 3 mg was administered vaginally, with a minimum safe time interval between prostaglandin administration and oxytocin initiation of at least 6 h, or 25–50 mcg of PGE1 was administered as an initial dose for cervical ripening and induction of labor, and oxytocin was administered at least 4 h after the last misoprostol dose. If there was inadequate cervical change with minimal uterine activity after one dose of either intracervical dinoprostone or misoprostol, a second dose was given 6 h later [22].

Operative vaginal delivery (OVD) was attempted when the fetal head station was below +1 level, the AoP was more than 130° (+1), or the HPD was less than 35 mm (mid-cavity), or if the second stage of labor lasted for more than 4 h in primiparous patients with epidural, more than 3 h in primiparous patients without epidural, more than 3 h in multiparous patients with epidural, or more than 2 h in multiparous patients without epidural [23].

2.2. Technique

The sonographic assessment of fetal head station is performed by transperineal ultrasound in the midsagittal or axial plane. The probe is placed between the two labia majora, at the level of the fourchette, with the woman in a semi-recumbent position [21]. The AoP is the angle between the long axis of the pubic bone and a line drawn from the lowest edge of the pubis tangential to the deepest bony part of the fetal skull. It is an accurate and reproducible parameter for the assessment of fetal head descent [20,24]. An angle of progression of 106° has been found to correspond to fetal head station 0 (zero) [20]. The HPD is measured by placing the probe between the labia majora, and the soft tissue is compressed completely against the pubic bone. The transducer should be angled until the skull contour is as clear as possible, indicating that the ultrasound beam is perpendicular to the fetal skull. HPD is measured in a frontal transperineal scan as the shortest distance from the outer bony limit of the fetal skull to the perineum [21,25].

2.3. Statistical Analysis

Ordinal or qualitative data were described as n (%), and quantitative data as the mean (SD). A one-way ANOVA test was conducted to compare the means of the quantitative variables. Post hoc analysis was conducted for significant values. The association between the mode of delivery (cesarean section—CS, vaginal delivery—VD, OVD) and the head position (occiput anterior vs. occiput posterior), as assessed by transabdominal ultrasound, was investigated by means of multinomial regression analysis. The correlation between the two ultrasonographic values (AoP, HPD) and the different maternal–fetal characteristics was investigated with Pearson's (r) correlation coefficient. Additionally, multinomial regression analysis was conducted to investigate any potential predictors of the mode of delivery and any association between epidural, oxytocin use, and the onset of labor (spontaneous vs. induced) with the mode of delivery (VD, OVD, CS). The means of the ultrasonographic parameters (AoP, HPD) were compared between the parturients with normal duration of the second stage and those with a prolonged one using Student's t-test. The level of statistical significance was defined as $p = 0.05$. The statistical package IBM SPSS Statistics 29.0 was used.

3. Results

A total of 82 women at the second stage of labor were assessed both clinically and sonographically. The mean maternal age was 28 years (SD: 6.5), the mean gestational age was 39 weeks (SD: 1.4), the mean parity was 1.3 (IQR: 0.7), and the mean body mass index (BMI) was 29.6 kg/m^2 (SD: 5). The onset of labor was spontaneous in 35 cases (42.7%), while 47 (57.3%) women underwent induction of labor. During labor, 41 women received epidurals (50%) and 59 oxytocin (71.9%). Moreover, 60 women (73.2%) delivered via VD, 11 (13.4%) underwent OVD, and 11 (13.4%) delivered via CS. The mean total duration of labor was 10.5 h (SD: 6.2), whereas the mean duration of the second stage of labor was 81 min (SD: 67). The mean birth weight was 3252 g (SD: 492).

In total, out of 32 women who underwent induction of labor and delivered vaginally, 15 had a favorable Bishop score ($\geq$6), whereas 17 had an unfavorable Bishop score (<6). Out of six women who underwent induction of labor and delivered via CS, all of them had unfavorable Bishop scores before induction of labor. Out of nine parturients who underwent induction and delivered via OVD, all had unfavorable Bishop scores. In total, out of 47 inductions of labor, 15 had favorable Bishop scores, whereas 32 had unfavorable ones. Following the analyses, we found a significant difference in the Bishop scores between the VD and CS (p-value < 0.001) groups and between VD and OVD (p-value = 0.012), but not between CS and OVD (p-value = 0.288).

Maternal and fetal characteristics were analyzed according to the three modes of delivery (VD, OVD, CS) (Table 1). The mean total duration of labor differed between VD and CS (8.8 vs. 16.1 h, p-value < 0.001) and between VD and OVD (8.8 vs. 14.2 h, p-value = 0.011); however, it did not differ significantly between CS and OVD. Moreover, the mean duration of the second stage of labor differed between VD and CS (65.3 vs. 160 min, p-value < 0.001) and OVD and CS (88.6 vs. 160 min, p-value = 0.015). The mean birth weight differed significantly between neonates born vaginally and those via CS (3161 vs. 3572 g, p-value = 0.026).

Table 1. Baseline characteristics according to the mode of delivery.

Characteristics	Mode of Delivery			p-Value
	Vaginal Delivery (VD) $n = 60$ (73.2%)	Operative Vaginal Delivery (OVD) $n = 11$ (13.4%)	Cesarean Section (CS) $n = 11$ (13.4%)	
Maternal age (years)	27.7 (6.9)	29.1 (4.3)	28.9 (6.7)	0.736
Maternal BMI (kg/m^2)	29.5 (5.3)	29.6 (4.4)	30.4 (4.6)	0.876
Gestational age at delivery (weeks)	39 (1.4)	39.3 (1.2)	39.4 (0.9)	0.053
Parity	1.3 (0.6)	1.3 (1.2)	1 (0.3)	0.545
Birth weight (g)	3161 (508)	3429 (249)	3572 (416)	0.015
Duration of second stage of labor (minutes)	65.3 (57.6)	88.6 (67.6)	160 (61.2)	<0.001
Total duration of labor (hours)	8.8 (4.9)	14.2 (5.8)	16.1 (8.3)	<0.001

Data are given as n (%), mean (SD) for parametric values. One-way ANOVA was used for parametric values; SD: standard deviation; IQR: interquartile range; BMI: body mass index.

The association between the mode of delivery and fetal head position (occiput posterior vs. anterior) was also assessed. The occiput anterior position was associated with increased odds of VD compared to CS (OR: 24.167, 95% CI: 3.8–152.5, p-value < 0.001) (Table 2). The mean AoP did not differ significantly among the three groups (145.7° for VD vs. 139.9° for OVD vs. 132.1° for CS, p-value = 0.289). On the contrary, the mean HPD was significantly higher in the CS cases (28.6 vs. 26.9 vs. 41.4, p-value < 0.001) (Table 3). Moreover, post hoc analysis revealed that the mean HPD differed between VD and CS (p-value < 0.001) and CS and OVD (p-value = 0.002), but not between VD and OVD (Figures 1 and 2).

Table 2. Mode of delivery according to fetal head position.

Mode of Delivery	Head Position		ORs	95% CI	p-Value
	Occiput Anterior	Occiput Posterior			
Vaginal delivery	58 (96.7%)	2 (3.3%)	24.167	3.8–152.5	<0.001
Operative vaginal delivery	10 (90.9%)	1 (9.1%)	8.333	0.7–89.4	0.080
Cesarean section	6 (54.5%)	5 (45.5%)		Reference	

Data are given as n (%), multinomial regression analysis was used. ORs: odds ratios, 95% CI: 95% confidence interval.

Table 3. Ultrasonographic characteristics at the second stage of labor, according to the mode of delivery.

Ultrasonographic Characteristics	Mode of Delivery			p-Value
	Vaginal Delivery	Operative Vaginal Delivery	Cesarean Section	
HPD (mm)	28.6 (10.1)	26.9 (6.84)	41.4 (5.3)	<0.001
AoP (°)	145.7 (24.9)	139.9 (23.8)	132.1 (26.2)	0.289

One-way ANOVA, AoP: angle of progression, HPD: head–perineum distance.

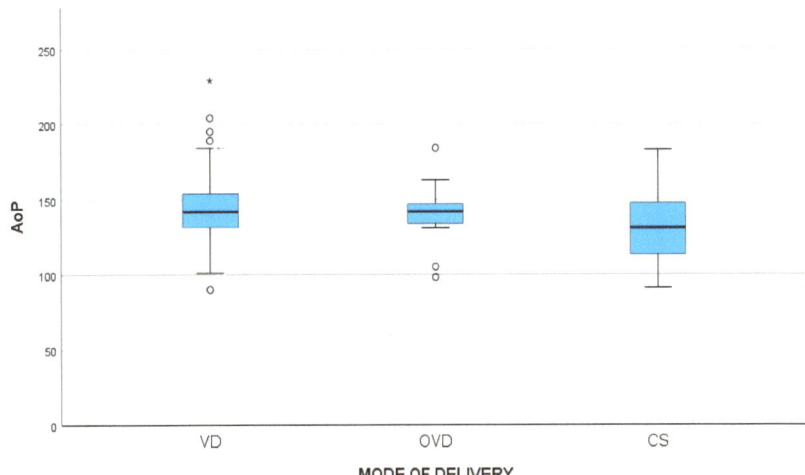

Figure 1. Comparisons of means of angle of progression (AoP) between different modes of delivery (p-value = 0.289). The dots "○" in the figure are the outliers; the values that fall above or below the expected variation and the asterisk "*" is the extreme outlier.

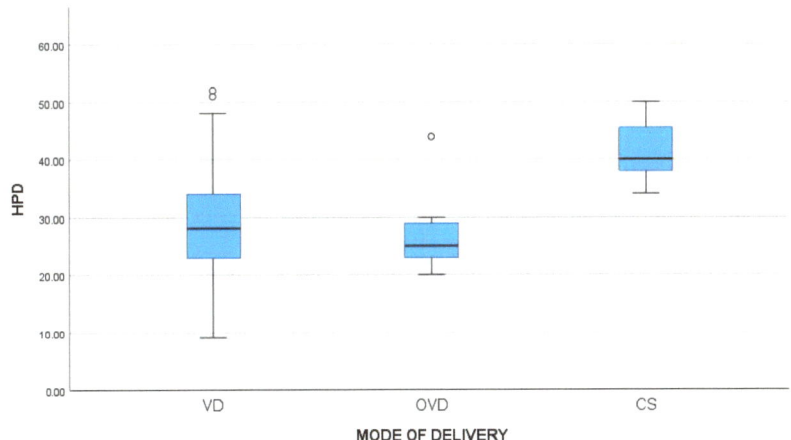

Figure 2. Comparisons of means of head–perineum distance (HPD) between different modes of delivery (p-value < 0.001). The dots "○" in the figure are the outliers; the values that fall above or below the expected variation.

The correlation of AoP with maternal–fetal characteristics was investigated, and we identified a negative association between parity and AoP (Pearson correlation coefficient r = −0.221, p-value = 0.047). In addition, a positive association was identified between HPD and BMI (Pearson correlation coefficient r = 0.268, *p*-value = 0.024), as well as the duration of the second stage of labor (Pearson correlation coefficient r = 0.256, *p*-value = 0.031) (Table 4).

Table 4. Correlation of head–perineum distance (HPD) with maternal–fetal characteristics.

Fetal–Maternal Characteristics	HPD		AoP	
	Pearson r Correlation Coefficient	*p*-Value	Pearson r Correlation Coefficient	*p*-Value
Age (years)	0.084	0.484	0.045	0.686
Gestational age (weeks)	0.128	0.288	−0.187	0.093
Parity	0.226	0.060	−0.221	0.047
BMI (kg/m^2)	0.268	0.024	0.011	0.921
Birth weight (grams)	−0.002	0.985	0.013	0.909
Duration of the second stage of labor (min)	0.256	0.031	−0.186	0.095
Total duration of labor (hours)	0.098	0.418	0.012	0.918

Pearson's correlation coefficient r was used for the parametric values.

Multinomial regression analysis was conducted to investigate any potential predictors of the mode of delivery. Low parity (OR: 12.024, 95% CI: 6.320–22.876, *p*-value < 0.001) and increased HPD (OR: 1.23, 95% CI: 1.05–1.43, *p*-value = 0.007) were found to be significant predictors of CS. The total duration of labor was found to be a significant predictor of OVD (OR: 1.24, 95% CI: 1.05–1.46, *p*-value = 0.007) (Table 5).

Table 5. Predictors of mode of delivery.

Mode of Delivery	Predictor	ORs	95% CI	*p*-Value
Cesarean section vs. Vaginal delivery (Ref)	Age	1.2	0.003–0.003	0.451
	Gestational age	0.68	0.42–1.12	0.133
	Low parity	12.024	6.320–22.876	<0.001
	BMI	0.903	0.700–1.164	0.432
	Birth weight	1	0.99–1	0.079
	Duration of the second stage of labor	1	0.99–1.03	0.208
	Total duration of labor	1.1	0.94–1.34	0.178
	High AoP	1	0.9–1.06	0.655
	High HPD	1.23	1.05–1.43	0.007
Operative vaginal delivery vs. Vaginal delivery (Ref)	Age	1.06	0.942–1.202	0.312
	Gestational age	1.29	0.96–1.73	0.086
	Low parity	1.99	0.55–7.166	0.292
	BMI	1.04	0.86–1.2	0.645
	Birth weight	1	0.99–1	0.292
	Duration of the second stage of labor	1	0.98–1.01	0.821
	Total duration of labor	1.24	1.05–1.46	0.009
	High AoP	0.98	0.94–1.02	0.421
	High HPD	0.91	0.78–1.06	0.244

Vaginal delivery: reference (Ref), ORs: odds ratios, 95% CI: 95% confidence interval, BMI: body mass index, multinomial regression analysis.

Multinomial regression analysis was conducted to investigate any associations between epidural (yes/no), oxytocin (yes/no), or onset of labor (spontaneous/induction of labor) and the mode of delivery (VD, OVD, or CS). Neither epidural nor oxytocin, nor onset of labor could predict the mode of delivery (Table 6).

Table 6. Association of oxytocin, epidural, and spontaneous onset of labor versus induction of labor with the mode of delivery.

Mode of Delivery	Labor Characteristics		ORs	95% CI	p-Value
	Oxytocin		4.603	0.547–38.76	0.160
	Yes	10 (16.9%)			
	No	1 (4.3%)			
	Epidural		1.121	0.286–4.390	0.870
Cesarean section	Yes	6 (14.6%)			
	No	5 (12.2%)			
	Onset of labor		1.051	0.248–4.124	0.943
	Spontaneous	5 (14.3%)			
	Induction	6 (12.8%)			
	Oxytocin		1.168	0.267–5.107	0.837
	Yes	8 (13.6%)			
	No	3 (13.0%)			
	Epidural		0.572	0.147–2.233	0.422
Operative Vaginal Delivery	Yes	5 (12.2%)			
	No	6 (14.6%)			
	Onset of labor		0.219	0.041–1.159	0.074
	Spontaneous	2 (5.7%)			
	Induction	9 (19.1%)			
	Oxytocin			Reference	
	Yes	41 (69.5%)			
	No	19 (82.6%)			
	Epidural				
Vaginal Delivery	Yes	30 (73.2%)			
	No	30 (73.2%)			
	Onset of labor				
	Spontaneous	28 (80.0%)			
	Induction	32 (68.1%)			

ORs: odds ratios, 95% CI: 95% confidence interval, vaginal delivery: reference; multinomial regression analysis was used.

In 11 (13.4%) cases, there was prolongation of the second stage, according to the criteria defined by Zhang et al. [6]. In 2 of these 11 (18.2%) cases, there was an occiput posterior head position; a successful OVD was performed in 1 case, whereas a CS was performed in the other one. The mean AoP did not differ significantly between the groups with prolonged and normal second stages of labor (136.8° vs. 143.8°, p-value = 0.458), whereas the HPD differed significantly between the two groups (39.6 vs. 29.1, p = 0.005) (Figures 3 and 4).

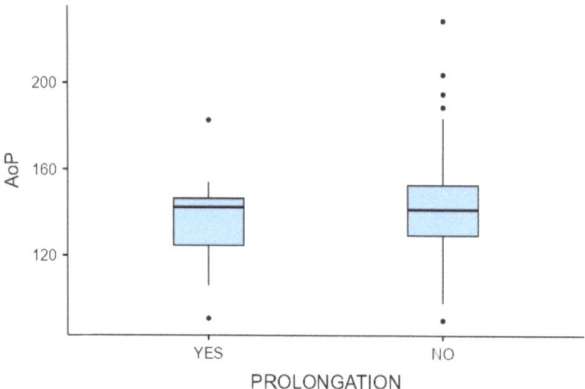

Figure 3. Comparisons of means of angle of progression (AoP) between normal and prolonged second stage of labor (p-value = 0.485). The dots "°" in the figure are the outliers; the values that fall above or below the expected variation.

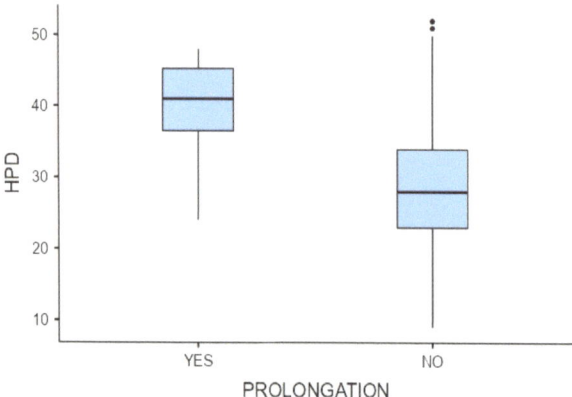

Figure 4. Comparisons of means of head–perineum distance (HPD) between normal and prolonged second stage of labor (p-value = 0.005).

4. Discussion

The main findings of this study were (i) the mean total duration of labor was lower in the VD compared to the CS group; (ii) the mean duration of the second stage of labor was lower in the VD and OVD compared to the CS group; (iii) the occiput anterior position was associated with an increased likelihood of VD; (iv) the mean HPD was lower in the VD compared to the CS group and was associated with increasing maternal BMI and a prolonged second stage of labor; (v) low parity and high HPD were found to be significant predictors of CS; and (vi) increased total duration of labor was a significant predictor of OVD.

A study examining the mode of delivery and outcomes according to birth weight revealed that birth weight is a significant determinant of the mode of delivery; CS rates were increased with increasing birth weight [26], which was in accordance with the findings of our study. Additionally, published data support that longer durations of both the first and the second stages of labor have been associated with higher odds of OVD [27]. Our study revealed a significant difference in the total duration of labor and the duration of the second stage of labor between the delivery modes. Moreover, according to the literature, only 34% of cases with occiput posterior head position do not require any operative intervention, whereas 82% of cases with occiput anterior head position do not require any operative intervention [28,29], which is in agreement with the findings of our study.

Regarding the prediction of the mode of delivery following the measurement of the AoP, the current literature supports that this sonographic parameter can predict the duration of labor, the progress, and the mode of delivery [30]; a larger angle at the beginning of the second stage of labor has been significantly associated with shorter time to delivery [31]. More specifically, one study suggested that an AoP $\geq 113°$ at the second stage of labor was associated with 90% probability of VD [31]. In another study, the odds of OVD were 2.6 times higher for women with an AoP $< 153°$, and the odds of CS were almost six times higher when compared with women with AoP $\geq 153°$ (aOR: 5.8, 95% CI: 1.2–28.3, $p = 0.03$) [32]. According to the results of our study, the mean AoP differed among the three groups (VD, OVD, CS), but not significantly; therefore, it could not predict the mode of delivery in our sample. This could be attributed to the small sample and/or to the fact that a single value of AoP was measured at the beginning of the second stage, without serial measurements unless there was a prolonged second stage.

Regarding HPD, according to published data, VD has been associated with a lower HDP in comparison with those who required OVD or CS (33.2 mm vs. 40.1, p-value = 0.001) [29]; this is in accordance to the findings of our study. High parity, along with low HPD, have been previously identified as significant predictors of VD, which is also in agreement with our findings [17]. In case of a prolonged second stage of labor, the literature supports that both the AoP and the HPD can predict VD [29]. We found that HPD was significantly higher in cases of prolonged second stages of labor. It has been shown that multiparous women maintain a higher station for a longer time before delivery, but often proceed rapidly to delivery once full dilation is reached [33]. Moreover, we found that AoP was correlated negatively with parity; the first measurement of AoP was lower in multiparous than nulliparous patients, despite the shorter durations of their second stages.

This study's main strength lies in its comprehensive approach, integrating both ultrasound and clinical parameters to assess labor progression, particularly during the second stage. Moreover, its prospective nature adds to the strengths of the study. However, it is essential to acknowledge the study's limitations, especially the limited sample size. Another limitation includes the single measurement of the AoP and HDP during the second stage of labor; serial measurements were conducted only in cases of prolonged second stage duration.

5. Conclusions

According to the results of this study, the use of intrapartum ultrasound as an adjunctive technique to the standard clinical evaluation may predict the need for OVD or CS. The optimal mode of delivery remains a prominent concern in modern obstetrics. Over recent years, there has been a progressive increase in the rates of CS, surpassing the recommended limit set by medical societies. Obstetricians often face a challenge, as they lack the requisite technology to assist in determining the appropriateness of a CS based on intrapartum conditions. Integrating intrapartum ultrasound in the assessment of the progress of labor, along with all the clinical parameters, may enhance the diagnostic approach to an abnormal labor progress.

Author Contributions: Conceptualization, K.M. and I.T.; methodology, K.M. and I.T.; validation, T.D., A.V. and G.M.; investigation, I.K.; resources, A.A.; data curation, K.M.; writing—original draft preparation, K.M.; writing—review and editing, I.T. and T.D; visualization, I.K. and A.M.; supervision, T.D. and A.A.; project administration, A.V. and G.M. All authors have read and agreed to the published version of the manuscript.

Funding: This research received no external funding.

Institutional Review Board Statement: This study was approved by the Ethics Committee of the Aristotle University of Thessaloniki (3–13 December 2022).

Informed Consent Statement: Informed consent was obtained before the procedure, and no incentives were provided for participation in the study.

Data Availability Statement: Data are available upon request.

Conflicts of Interest: The authors declare no conflicts of interest.

References

1. Liao, J.B.; Buhimschi, C.S.; Norwitz, E.R. Normal labor: Mechanism and duration. *Obstet. Gynecol. Clin. N. Am.* **2005**, *32*, 145–164. [CrossRef] [PubMed]
2. Wright, A.; Nassar, A.H.; Visser, G.; Ramasauskaite, D.; Theron, G.; Motherhood, F.S.; Newborn Health, C. FIGO good clinical practice paper: Management of the second stage of labor. *Int. J. Gynaecol. Obstet.* **2021**, *152*, 172–181. [CrossRef] [PubMed]
3. Cheng, Y.W.; Caughey, A.B. Defining and Managing Normal and Abnormal Second Stage of Labor. *Obstet. Gynecol. Clin. N. Am.* **2017**, *44*, 547–566. [CrossRef] [PubMed]
4. Hamilton, E.F.; Simoneau, G.; Ciampi, A.; Warrick, P.; Collins, K.; Smith, S.; Garite, T.J. Descent of the fetal head (station) during the first stage of labor. *Am. J. Obstet. Gynecol.* **2016**, *214*, 360.e1–360.e6. [CrossRef] [PubMed]
5. Zhang, J.; Landy, H.J.; Ware Branch, D.; Burkman, R.; Haberman, S.; Gregory, K.D.; Hatjis, C.G.; Ramirez, M.M.; Bailit, J.L.; Gonzalez-Quintero, V.H.; et al. Contemporary patterns of spontaneous labor with normal neonatal outcomes. *Obstet. Gynecol.* **2010**, *116*, 1281–1287. [CrossRef] [PubMed]
6. Zhang, J.; Troendle, J.F.; Yancey, M.K. Reassessing the labor curve in nulliparous women. *Am. J. Obstet. Gynecol.* **2002**, *187*, 824–828. [CrossRef] [PubMed]
7. Caughey, A.B.; Cahill, A.G.; Guise, J.M.; Rouse, D.J.; American College of Obstetricians and Gynecologists and Society for Maternal–Fetal Medicine. Safe prevention of the primary cesarean delivery. *Am. J. Obstet. Gynecol.* **2014**, *210*, 179–193. [CrossRef]
8. Oboro, V.O.; Tabowei, T.O.; Bosah, J.O. Fetal station at the time of labour arrest and risk of caesarean delivery. *J. Obstet. Gynaecol.* **2005**, *25*, 20–22. [CrossRef]
9. Akmal, S.; Kametas, N.; Tsoi, E.; Hargreaves, C.; Nicolaides, K.H. Comparison of transvaginal digital examination with intrapartum sonography to determine fetal head position before instrumental delivery. *Ultrasound Obstet. Gynecol.* **2003**, *21*, 437–440. [CrossRef]
10. Dietz, H.P.; Lanzarone, V. Measuring engagement of the fetal head: Validity and reproducibility of a new ultrasound technique. *Ultrasound Obstet. Gynecol.* **2005**, *25*, 165–168. [CrossRef]
11. Dupuis, O.; Ruimark, S.; Corinne, D.; Simone, T.; Andre, D.; Rene-Charles, R. Fetal head position during the second stage of labor: Comparison of digital vaginal examination and transabdominal ultrasonographic examination. *Eur. J. Obstet. Gynecol. Reprod. Biol.* **2005**, *123*, 193–197. [CrossRef] [PubMed]
12. Ghi, T.; Farina, A.; Pedrazzi, A.; Rizzo, N.; Pelusi, G.; Pilu, G. Diagnosis of station and rotation of the fetal head in the second stage of labor with intrapartum translabial ultrasound. *Ultrasound Obstet. Gynecol.* **2009**, *33*, 331–336. [CrossRef] [PubMed]
13. Sherer, D.M.; Miodovnik, M.; Bradley, K.S.; Langer, O. Intrapartum fetal head position I: Comparison between transvaginal digital examination and transabdominal ultrasound assessment during the active stage of labor. *Ultrasound Obstet. Gynecol.* **2002**, *19*, 258–263. [CrossRef] [PubMed]
14. Sherer, D.M.; Miodovnik, M.; Bradley, K.S.; Langer, O. Intrapartum fetal head position II: Comparison between transvaginal digital examination and transabdominal ultrasound assessment during the second stage of labor. *Ultrasound Obstet. Gynecol.* **2002**, *19*, 264–268. [CrossRef] [PubMed]
15. Tutschek, B.; Torkildsen, E.A.; Eggebo, T.M. Comparison between ultrasound parameters and clinical examination to assess fetal head station in labor. *Ultrasound Obstet. Gynecol.* **2013**, *41*, 425–429. [CrossRef] [PubMed]
16. Eggebo, T.M.; Hassan, W.A.; Salvesen, K.A.; Torkildsen, E.A.; Ostborg, T.B.; Lees, C.C. Prediction of delivery mode by ultrasound-assessed fetal position in nulliparous women with prolonged first stage of labor. *Ultrasound Obstet. Gynecol.* **2015**, *46*, 606–610. [CrossRef] [PubMed]
17. Eggebo, T.M.; Heien, C.; Okland, I.; Gjessing, L.K.; Romundstad, P.; Salvesen, K.A. Ultrasound assessment of fetal head-perineum distance before induction of labor. *Ultrasound Obstet. Gynecol.* **2008**, *32*, 199–204. [CrossRef]
18. Kalache, K.D.; Duckelmann, A.M.; Michaelis, S.A.; Lange, J.; Cichon, G.; Dudenhausen, J.W. Transperineal ultrasound imaging in prolonged second stage of labor with occipitoanterior presenting fetuses: How well does the 'angle of progression' predict the mode of delivery? *Ultrasound Obstet. Gynecol.* **2009**, *33*, 326–330. [CrossRef]
19. Torkildsen, E.A.; Salvesen, K.A.; Eggebo, T.M. Prediction of delivery mode with transperineal ultrasound in women with prolonged first stage of labor. *Ultrasound Obstet. Gynecol.* **2011**, *37*, 702–708. [CrossRef]
20. Tutschek, B.; Braun, T.; Chantraine, F.; Henrich, W. A study of progress of labour using intrapartum translabial ultrasound, assessing head station, direction, and angle of descent. *BJOG Int. J. Obstet. Gynaecol.* **2011**, *118*, 62–69. [CrossRef]
21. Ghi, T.; Eggebo, T.; Lees, C.; Kalache, K.; Rozenberg, P.; Youssef, A.; Salomon, L.J.; Tutschek, B. ISUOG Practice Guidelines: Intrapartum ultrasound. *Ultrasound Obstet. Gynecol.* **2018**, *52*, 128–139. [CrossRef]
22. Tsakiridis, I.; Mamopoulos, A.; Athanasiadis, A.; Dagklis, T. Induction of Labor: An Overview of Guidelines. *Obstet. Gynecol. Surv.* **2020**, *75*, 61–72. [CrossRef] [PubMed]

23. Tsakiridis, I.; Giouleka, S.; Mamopoulos, A.; Athanasiadis, A.; Daniilidis, A.; Dagklis, T. Operative vaginal delivery: A review of four national guidelines. *J. Perinat. Med.* **2020**, *48*, 189–198. [CrossRef] [PubMed]
24. Barbera, A.F.; Pombar, X.; Perugino, G.; Lezotte, D.C.; Hobbins, J.C. A new method to assess fetal head descent in labor with transperineal ultrasound. *Ultrasound Obstet. Gynecol.* **2009**, *33*, 313–319. [CrossRef] [PubMed]
25. Eggebo, T.M.; Gjessing, L.K.; Heien, C.; Smedvig, E.; Okland, I.; Romundstad, P.; Salvesen, K.A. Prediction of labor and delivery by transperineal ultrasound in pregnancies with prelabor rupture of membranes at term. *Ultrasound Obstet. Gynecol.* **2006**, *27*, 387–391. [CrossRef] [PubMed]
26. Walsh, J.M.; Hehir, M.P.; Robson, M.S.; Mahony, R.M. Mode of delivery and outcomes by birth weight among spontaneous and induced singleton cephalic nulliparous labors. *Int. J. Gynaecol. Obstet.* **2015**, *129*, 22–25. [CrossRef] [PubMed]
27. Lundborg, L.; Aberg, K.; Sandstrom, A.; Liu, X.; Tilden, E.; Stephansson, O.; Ahlberg, M. Association between first and second stage of labour duration and mode of delivery: A population-based cohort study. *Paediatr. Perinat. Epidemiol.* **2022**, *36*, 358–367. [CrossRef]
28. Gardberg, M.; Tuppurainen, M. Effects of persistent occiput posterior presentation on mode of delivery. *Z. Geburtshilfe Perinatol.* **1994**, *198*, 117–119.
29. Dall'Asta, A.; Angeli, L.; Masturzo, B.; Volpe, N.; Schera, G.B.L.; Di Pasquo, E.; Girlando, F.; Attini, R.; Menato, G.; Frusca, T.; et al. Prediction of spontaneous vaginal delivery in nulliparous women with a prolonged second stage of labor: The value of intrapartum ultrasound. *Am. J. Obstet. Gynecol.* **2019**, *221*, 642.e1–642.e13. [CrossRef]
30. Jung, J.E.; Lee, Y.J. Intrapartum transperineal ultrasound: Angle of progression to evaluate and predict the mode of delivery and labor progression. *Obstet. Gynecol. Sci.* **2023**, *67*, 1–16. [CrossRef]
31. Marsoosi, V.; Pirjani, R.; Mansouri, B.; Eslamian, L.; Jamal, A.; Heidari, R.; Rahimi-Foroushani, A. Role of 'angle of progression' in prediction of delivery mode. *J. Obstet. Gynaecol. Res.* **2015**, *41*, 1693–1699. [CrossRef]
32. Bibbo, C.; Rouse, C.E.; Cantonwine, D.E.; Little, S.E.; McElrath, T.F.; Robinson, J.N. Angle of Progression on Ultrasound in the Second Stage of Labor and Spontaneous Vaginal Delivery. *Am. J. Perinatol.* **2018**, *35*, 413–420. [CrossRef]
33. Gurewitsch, E.D.; Johnson, E.; Allen, R.H.; Diament, P.; Fong, J.; Weinstein, D.; Chervenak, F.A. The descent curve of the grand multiparous woman. *Am. J. Obstet. Gynecol.* **2003**, *189*, 1036–1041. [CrossRef]

Disclaimer/Publisher's Note: The statements, opinions and data contained in all publications are solely those of the individual author(s) and contributor(s) and not of MDPI and/or the editor(s). MDPI and/or the editor(s) disclaim responsibility for any injury to people or property resulting from any ideas, methods, instructions or products referred to in the content.

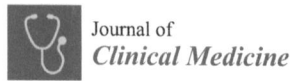

Systematic Review

Genetic and Epigenetic Factors Associated with Postpartum Psychosis: A 5-Year Systematic Review

Sophia Tsokkou [1,2], Dimitrios Kavvadas [1,2], Maria-Nefeli Georgaki [1,3], Kyriaki Papadopoulou [1,2,4], Theodora Papamitsou [1,2] and Sofia Karachrysafi [1,2,*]

[1] Research Team "Histologistas", Interinstitutional Postgraduate Program "Health and Environmental Factors", Department of Medicine, Faculty of Health Sciences, Aristotle University of Thessaloniki, 54124 Thessaloniki, Greece; stsokkou@auth.gr (S.T.); kavvadas@auth.gr (D.K.); mgeorgaki@cheng.auth.gr (M.-N.G.); kyriakinp@auth.gr (K.P.); thpapami@auth.gr (T.P.)
[2] Laboratory of Histology-Embryology, Department of Medicine, Faculty of Health Sciences, Aristotle University of Thessaloniki, 54124 Thessaloniki, Greece
[3] Environmental Engineering Laboratory, Department of Chemical Engineering, Aristotle University of Thessaloniki, 54124 Thessaloniki, Greece
[4] A' Neurosurgery University Clinic, Aristotle University of Thessaloniki, AHEPA General Hospital of Thessaloniki, 54636 Thessaloniki, Greece
* Correspondence: skarachry@auth.gr; Tel.: +30-6949414452

Abstract: Purpose: Postpartum psychosis (PPP) is a serious mental health illness affecting women post-parturition. Around 1 in 1000 women are affected by postpartum psychosis, and the symptoms usually appear within 2 weeks after birth. Postpartum mental disorders are classified into 3 main categories starting from the least to most severe types, including baby blues, postpartum depression, and postpartum psychosis. **Materials and Methods:** In this systematic review, genetic and epigenetic factors associated with postpartum psychosis are discussed. A PRISMA flow diagram was followed, and the following databases were used as main sources: PubMed, ScienceDirect, and Scopus. Additional information was retrieved from external sources and organizations. The time period for the articles extracted was 5 years. **Results:** Initially, a total of 2379 articled were found. After the stated criteria were applied, 58 articles were identified along with 20 articles from additional sources, which were then narrowed down to a final total of 29 articles. **Conclusions:** It can be concluded that there is an association between PPP and genetic and epigenetic risk factors. However, based on the data retrieved and examined, the association was found to be greater for genetic factors. Additionally, the presence of bipolar disorder and disruption of the circadian cycle played a crucial role in the development of PPP.

Keywords: postpartum psychosis; genetic risk factors; epigenetic risk factors

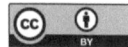

1. Introduction

Postpartum mental disorders refer to a spectrum of mental health conditions affecting women post-parturition [1]. During the postpartum period, it is estimated that around 85% of women are affected by mood disturbances. The symptoms can either be mild or severe, appearing in the form of depression or anxiety. The postpartum mental illness women experience is divided into 3 main categories, including baby blues, which is also known as postpartum blues; postpartum depression; and postpartum psychosis [2]. Baby blues affect around 50–85% of new mothers [3], and it is a temporary episode that settles when hormone levels return to their original state at approximately 2 weeks [4]. Postpartum depression occurs within 6 weeks post-delivery and affects around 6.5–20% of women, especially adolescent women with premature infants, with symptoms lasting up to 1 year [5]. Moreover, postpartum psychosis is a severe but reversible mental health condition affecting women post-parturition [6]. It is a rarer but a more serious form of postpartum mental depression, affecting only 0.089–2.6% of women every 1000 births. Worldwide, postpartum psychosis occurs in around 12 million to 352.3 million women giving birth [7]. Severe postpartum mental disorders raise concerns regarding both clinical and public health, and urgent medical care must be provided in order to secure the safety of both the mother and infant. However, in some cases, the outcomes are unfortunate. For instance, poor fetal development as well as infant death and maternal suicide are among the most severe outcomes that can occur [8]. One important piece of information that must be thoroughly examined is the mechanism involved in the development of postpartum psychosis along with the degree of association to both genetic and epigenetic factors. This information is necessary to successfully manage the symptoms and protect the health of those directly involved, namely, the mother and the child.

1.1. Symptoms of Postpartum Psychosis

The symptoms of PPP usually appear unexpectedly within hours or a few days during the 2 initial weeks after birth. The symptoms include hallucinations, such as auditory, visual, and olfactory sensations, as well as physical sensations that do not exist. Women with PPP tend to be suspicious with fears, thoughts, and beliefs that are not rational and tend to have manic episodes where they feel high and overactive; they tend to excessively and rapidly talk and lack normal inhibitions due to restlessness [6,7]. In contrast, the manic and overactive episodes are accompanied by low mood episodes characterized by signs of depression, withdrawing from social events, a lack of energy, loss of appetite, anxiety, and insomnia. Thus, these women are in a constant fluctuation of manic and hypomanic feelings. Furthermore, they tend to be in a state of confusion [6,7]. In more alarming cases, women tend to have suicidal thoughts and even act poorly with the motive of harming their child [7].

1.1.1. Classifications of Symptoms

Symptoms can be classified into 3 main categories: depressive, manic, and atypical, which is also known as mixed symptoms.

1.1.2. Depressive Symptoms

The depressive category is the most common and most dangerous classification that comprises up to 41% of PPP cases. Evidence reveals that PPP accompanied by depressive symptoms is always a risk factor in women with a tendency to harm themselves and even their child especially during episodes of hallucinations and delusions that "command" them to cause harm [7]. Statistically speaking, the percentage of women causing harm to a child is around 4.5%, which is 5 times greater in comparison to the other 2 classifications. Suicidal rates of up to 5% have been reported for the depressive classification. The symptoms included in the depressive category are hallucinations and delusions; anxiety and panic attacks; loss of appetite; anhedonia, which is loss of enjoyment in things that the individual usually finds pleasant; depression; and thoughts of self-harm and harming their child.

1.1.3. Manic Symptoms

The second most common subtype is the manic category, affecting around 34% of women. Compared with the depressive category, the percentage of women causing self-harm and harming the child is lower, representing 1% of cases. The symptoms of this subcategory include agitation, irritability, aggressive behavior, lack of sleep, constant and rapid talking, and an increased tendency for delusional thoughts [7].

1.1.4. Atypical—Mixed Symptoms

The third category with the lowest percentage of cases compared with the depressive and manic categories is the atypical category, which is also known as the mixed category, with an approximately 25% chance of occurrence. In this category, women tend to be less aware about their environment. They tend to have disorganized behaviors, exhibit unstructured speech, and appear disorientated. They are in a state of confusion and lack the ability to be alerted by situations taking place around them. In certain cases, they are in a state of catatonia [7], which is described as a lack of stimulation to actions occurring in their surroundings; people with catatonia tend to behave strangely and poorly, leading to life-threatening complications [9].

1.2. Risk Factors

PPP is considered to have a multifactorial origin, as various risk factors can trigger its development, including a history of PPP in previous pregnancies, a personal or family history of psychosis or bipolar disorder (BD), a history of schizoaffective disorder, and stopping psychiatric medications during pregnancy [10]. Genetic and epigenetic alterations, conditions during childbirth, and sleep deprivation are considered risk factors for the development of PPP.

1.2.1. Genetic Risk Factors

Genetics, epigenetics, neuroactive molecules, psychiatric history, social support, heath history, use of substances, and adverse life events belong under this branch. Regarding genetics, DNA is an essential baseline for the possible development of diseases [11]. Recent research has shown that 49% of individuals diagnosed with PPP have a history of BD [11]. In cases of full blood siblings where one sister developed PPP, which was triggered during childbirth, higher chances of PPP development are noted for the other sister compared with the rate of occurrence in non-related individuals [12].

1.2.2. Epigenetic Risk Factors

Epigenetics is an alteration in gene function that does not affect the DNA sequence. The main type of alteration that takes place is DNA methylation, which is the addition of a methyl group to the DNA responsible for gene transcription and the specificity of the cell [13]. DNA methylation (DNAm) is a chemical modification found on cytosine phosphate-guanine sites (CpG). DNAm is an influencer of gene expression, genomic stability, and the conformation of chromatin [13]. DNAm biomarkers are used for the identification of any possible alterations in individuals with postpartum mental disorders [13].

1.2.3. Childbirth and Sleep Deprivation as a Risk Factor

Childbirth is a strong biological trigger for the development PPP. Sleep deprivation during labor and the period after childbirth is a risk factor for the development of PPP, especially in women who have previously experienced mania as a result of sleep deprivation. Primiparity is the main obstetric risk factor for the development of PPP in contrast with age, which showed no correlation with PPP [3].

1.3. Mother–Infant Bonding among Mothers Suffering from PPP

PPP has unfavorable consequences for both the mother and infant. Mothers with PPP tend to have delusional thoughts related to the infant, leading to extreme behaviors. On the one hand, the mother may appear to be overprotective of her child. In contrast, she may be abusive and neglect the care of the child. However, studies have suggested that the degree of severity can exhibit sociocultural differences. An Indian study reviled that 43% of women suffering from PPP had infanticidal thoughts and 36% reported infanticidal behavior compared with a rate of 8% among Dutch women [3].

Although PPP is a more severe form of postpartum mental disorder, PPD has a higher rate of disturbed mother–infant bonding at approximately 57.1% and only affects 1 in 5 women (17.6%) suffering from PPP [14]. Evidence suggests that children born to mothers who suffer from PPD have high risks of developing socioemotional and cognitive problems. Infants participate in daily interactive routines with their mothers, but maternal depression can influence those daily activities in 2 main ways: intrusiveness or withdrawal.

Intrusive mothers usually create a hostile environment that disrupts the infant's activities. The infant as a result experiences feelings of anger, which then develop into internalized anger and further into a coping mechanism to prevent its mother intrusive behavior [15].

Withdrawn mothers show a lack of interest in their child, which makes it difficult for them to pay attention and understand when their child is unwell. They are disengage with minimal support of the infant's activities and are mostly unresponsive when it comes to their child's needs. As a result, children are unable to self-regulate this negative attitude and develop self-regulatory behaviors [15].

1.3.1. Effects on the Time Scale from Embryonic Life to Adulthood

Regarding a time scale starting from the prenatal stages, infants tend to have poor nutritional levels, higher chances of being born prematurely, and have a low birth weight and inadequate prenatal care. The inadequate prenatal care is a result of the lack of maternal care and an inability of expression of maternal affection from mothers suffering from postpartum mental disorders.

1.3.2. Infancy

During the infancy period, infants reveal both cognitive and behavioral issues, such as low cognitive performance; this develops as a result of the mother being restrictive towards her child and not allowing it to participate in the everyday life activities as it normally should [16]. This will lead to negative behavioral outcomes, including anger outburst and passivity as a protective coping mechanism as well as withdrawal and self-regulatory behaviors due to the lack of infant–maternal bonding. The infant does not develop the appropriate arousals and regulated attention required for its proper development leading to future problems in its third phase of development, the toddler stage.

1.3.3. Toddler

The toddler tends to have a passive and non-compliance behaviors; it tends to ignore authority figures, such as parents or teachers at pre-school, and acts as if commands and rules are non-existent [17]. The child finds it difficult to develop a form of autonomy resulting in less social interactions and tends to be isolated from the rest of its peers. Its ability to socialize shows a lack of cognitive performance as well as lack of creativity in comparison with the rest of the children its age.

1.3.4. Childhood

When the child reaches a school-appropriate age, certain new traits develop including attention deficit and hyperactivity disorder (ADHD) and the verbal as well as the full IQ scores are found to be lower compared to the average children of its age with non-depressed mothers. Children of depressed mothers have impaired adaptive functioning as well as affective problems, meaning a set of psychiatric disorders, such as depression or bipolar disorder with different extents of severity. Additionally, anxiety disorders and conduct disorders, with disregard to third parties and an inability to properly behave in a socially acceptable manner, are noted [17].

1.3.5. Adolescents

Lastly, during the adolescent years of their lives, teenagers reveal great academic challenges due to ADHD, learning disorders, and affective disorders, such as depression, anxiety disorders, phobias, and panic disorders involving frequent and unexpected panic attacks [16]. These children even end up experiencing alcohol and substance abuse. Other studies have shown that children born to mothers who suffer from PPD are at higher risk of poor health compared to the rest of the population, including shorter gestation periods, impaired cardiovascular function, increased gastrointestinal infections, reduced weight gain, and lower respiratory tract infections [17,18].

1.4. Epidemiology of Postpartum Psychosis

The postpartum period, which is also known as puerperium, is the period post-parturition up to around 6–8 weeks after delivery where the female body goes through certain physiologic changes to bring the body back to its original state before pregnancy was initiated [19]. This stage is considered a high-risk time for the development of psychiatric disorders due to certain triggers taking place during childbirth [7,16]. A UK study revealed that the chances of a psychiatric disorder development was 22 times more likely in the first month post-delivery compared to during and prior to pregnancy. The likelihood of the development of PPP was greater among women who were primiparous, those bearing a child for the first time [7,16]. It is estimated that around 60% of women suffering from PPP have a history of mental disorders that were either managed in the past and have a recurrent effect due to the triggers caused by the pregnancy or were still present during conception as well as during and post-delivery [8,20].

1.5. Evaluation and Diagnosis of Postpartum Psychosis

1.5.1. Medical and Social History

When a patient who has recently given birth presents with psychotic symptoms, a thorough medical history as well as a neuropsychiatric evaluation must take place to obtain a correct diagnosis and treatment [21]. Personal as well as family histories of psychiatric illnesses must be taken into account or excluded. Both prenatal and postpartum records must be thoroughly examined to narrow down any possible medical comorbidities, organic causes, and gynecological and obstetric complications, such as pre-eclampsia, eclampsia, previous negative birth outcomes, and current birth complications [21]. It is important to note whether the patient suffered from past psychotic episodes and whether she continued her medication throughout her pregnancy and or resumed it post-delivery. Any history of substance abuse or current stressors, such as financial difficulties, and social as well as support circles should be taken into consideration when it comes to the evaluation of PPP.

1.5.2. Diagnostic and Statistical Manual of Mental Disorders 5th Edition (DSM5)

The Diagnostic and Statistical Manual of Mental Disorders 5th Edition (DSM5) states that severe depressions are diagnosed based on the presence of 5 out of 9 stated symptoms within 2 weeks that the symptoms appear. The possibility that the symptoms are associated with another condition must be overruled in order to have a clearer diagnosis [22].

1.5.3. Lab Examinations

Lab examinations, including a complete blood count (CBC), electrolytes, blood urea nitrogen (BUM), creatinine levels, glucose, vitamin B12, folate, thyroid function tests (TPO and free T4), calcium, urinalysis, urine culture, urine drug screen, liver function tests (LFTs), CT and brain MRI, can be performed to rule out any medical conditions and organic substances that might interfere and appear as psychotic conditions [7,23]. Conditions that might present as psychosis are hyponatremia; hypernatremia; hypoglycemia; and hyperglycemia, including insulin shock and diabetic ketoacidosis. LFTs will help to exclude hepatic encephalopathy, and thyroid function tests for hypothyroidism and hyperthyroidism should be performed. Urine analysis will be used to identify any possible infections, and CT and MRI examinations are used to evaluate the possibility of a stroke, which is a risk factor for women with pregnancy-induced hypertension, preeclampsia, and eclampsia [21,24].

1.5.4. Edinburgh Postnatal Depression Scale (EPDS)

During prenatal care visits, physicians must provide a screening test also known as the Edinburgh Postnatal Depression Scale (EPDS). The 10-question EPDS includes specific questions that help in the determination and diagnosis of PND. The EPDS is used to evaluate and assess the possible existence of PPP. The EPDS consist of 10 multiple-choice questions provided to the mothers to assess the existence and severity of postpartum depression (PPD) and PPP. The scale is used at 6 to 8 weeks post-delivery and should be fully completed by the mother herself. A score greater than 13 is considered positive for depression [25].

2. Methodology

This is a systematic review study that followed a PRISMA flow diagram (Figure 1) to study targeted papers on the association of PPP with genetic and epigenetic risk factors. A table was then prepared to simplify the main articles found.

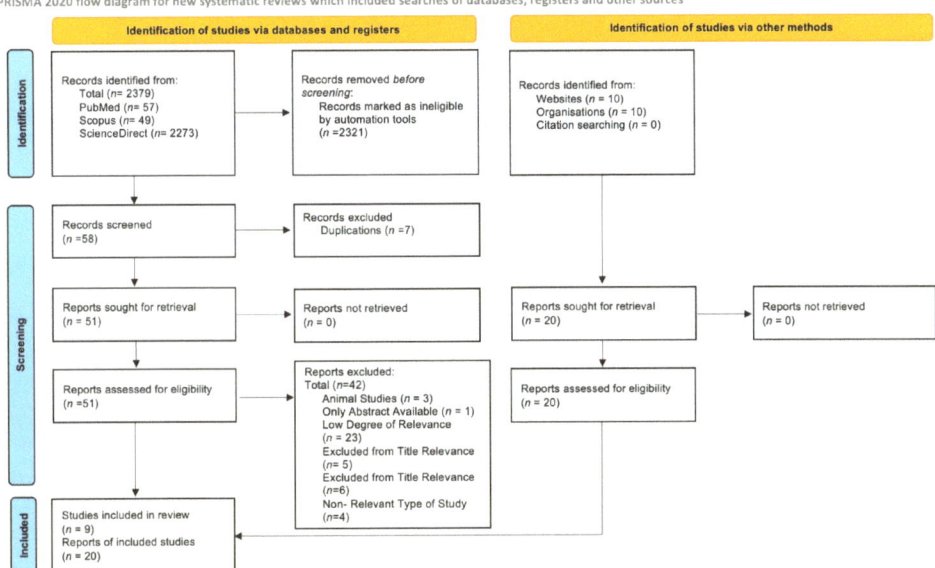

Figure 1. PRISMA Flow Diagram for Postpartum Psychosis and Genetic and Epigenetic Risk Factors. The main databases used include PubMed, ScienceDirect, and Scopus. Studies published during a 5-year period were identified [26].

Materials and Method

A PRISMA flow diagram was followed to narrow down articles based on the following criteria: articles published within a 5-year range between 2019 and 2024 and the type of articles included were either systematic reviews, literature reviews, or meta-analyses. Case reports and trial studies were excluded. The keywords used included postpartum psychosis (PPP), genetic factors, and epigenetic factors. The main databases used were PubMed, Scopus, and ScienceDirect. Additional sources include websites and organizations, such as the NHS, John Hopkins Medicine, American Pregnancy Society, Cleveland Clinic, Frontier, Springer, etc. Any duplicates were removed, and the information found was narrowed based on certain criteria.

3. Results

Initially, before the adjustments for advanced settings were made when searching the keywords stated above in the main databases, 2397 records were identified, including 57 records from PubMed, 49 from Scopus, and 2273 from ScienceDirect. After the application of criteria, 2321 records were excluded automatically. The remaining 58 were screened, and 7 duplicates were removed. Thus, a total of 51 studies remained. From those 51 records, 42 were excluded for the following reasons: 3 were animal studies, 1 was only available as an abstract, 23 papers had low relevance to the current study after the whole article was examined, 5 were excluded due low relevance based on the abstracts examined, 6 were excluded due to low relevance based on the title, and 4 studies were excluded based on study type. Thus, 9 studies remained. In addition, 20 studies were found from additional sources, leading to a total of 29 studies when combined with those identified from the main databases.

After examination of the 9 articles obtained from the main databases, a table (Table 1) was generated using Microsoft Word 2023. The table includes the following categories: Study, Genes and Chromosomal Location—Genetic and Epigenetic Factors, Clinical Aspects, and Treatment. The additional 20 articles found from other sources were used as complementary data to support the main articles. After examination and extraction of data from the 9 main articles, the following observations were made.

Table 1. Data Collected from the PRISMA Flow Diagram.

Study	Genes and Chromosomal Location-Genetic and Epigenetic Factors	Clinical Aspects	Treatment
Perry A, 2021 [8]	Chromosomal locations 16p13 and 8q24 Methyl transferase-like 13 Variations in the 5-HTTT serotonin transporter gene STin2.12 allele	PPP BD	Lithium
Thippeswamy H, 2021 [27]	Deletion of the STS gene	High risk of developmental disorders and associated traits Increased self-reported irritability Psychological distress Manic symptoms Fatigue and altered sleeping patterns Weight changes—rare cases with paranoid schizophrenia	-
Friedman SH, 2023 [20]	PRS folate metabolism (MTHFR C677T)	PPP Major depression BD	Pharmacological intervention for PPP (Lithium) Antipsychotics (Benzodiazepines) ECT
Davies W, 2019 [28]	CCN gene family (elevated CCN2 and CCN3 levels) Chromosomal locations 16p13 and 8q24	PPP BD Sleep deprivation Manic symptoms Depressive symptoms	-
Sharma V, 2022 [29]	-	BD PPP Major Depressive Episodes Manic Symptoms	Neuroleptics (Haloperidol) Lithium Antipsychotics ECT
Alshaya DS, 2022 [30]	SLC6A4 COMT TPH2 FKBP5 MDD1 HTR2A MDD2 Methylation in BDNF, NR3C1, and OXTR genes	PPP Depression	Antidepressants Selective serotonin reuptake inactivators Serotonin/norepinephrine reuptake inhibitors ECT CBT MBC IPT
Walton NL, 2023 [31]	mRNA expression of 5α-reductase type I	PPP Anxiety disorder PPD BD Schizophrenia	ZULRESSO (Brexanolone) Antidepressants Antipsychotics Mood stabilizers
Silveira PP, 2023 [32]	Serotonin transporter gene polymorphism SNPs	Depression	-
Bhatnagar A, 2023 [33]	CCGs	Depressive-like behavior Mood deficits Manic behavior BD	Lithium Light therapy Melatonin supplements Awake-promoting medications

Abbreviations: Postpartum psychosis (PPP), postpartum depression (PPD), bipolar disorder (BD), clock-controlled genes (CCGS), electroconvulsive therapy (ECT), cognitive-behavioral therapy (CBT), mindfulness-based cognitive therapy (MBCT), interpersonal therapy (IPT), single nucleotide polymorphisms (SNPs).

4. Discussion

When the extraction of information from the articles was completed, the following observations were made with regards to the genetic and epigenetic factors, clinical aspects, and methods of treatment.

4.1. Genes and Chromosomal Location—Genetic and Epigenetic Factors

First, a number of genes are associated with depressive disorders, such as variations in the 5-HTT serotonin transporter gene and polymorphisms in the STin2.12 allele [8]; SNPs [9]; clock-controlled genes (CCGs) driven by endogenous molecular clocks that regulate rhythmic expression [31]; SLC6A4, COMT, TPH2, FKBP5, MDD1, HTR2A, and MDD2 as well as methylation in genes BDNF, NR3C1, and OXTR [30]; the CCN gene family with elevated CCN2 and CCN3 expression [28]; deletion of the STS gene [27]; methyl transferase-like 13; chromosomal locations 16p13 and 8q24 [8]; mRNA expression of 5α-reductase type I [25], and PRS folate metabolism (MTHFR C677T) [20]. These genes were found to be mainly associated with PPP, BP, manic symptoms, and major depressive episodes. The 5-HTT serotonin transporter gene, linkage of chromosomal locations 16q13 and 8q24 with CCN2 and CCN3, MTHFR C677T variations and methylation in BDNF, NR3C1, and OXTR genes will be discussed further.

4.1.1. Variations in the 5-HTT Serotonin Transporter Gene

Two studies reported that 5-HTT serotonin transporter gene variations are highly associated with PPP, especially in women with bipolar disorder (BD) [8,32]. Specifically, 5 HTTLPR-VNTR is a variant form of the SLC6A4 gene that is located at the human chromosome 17q11.2 [34]. The polymorphism in this location is biallelic with a 44 bp insertion/deletion leading to the formation of two different alleles: the short (S) allele contains deletions and the long (L) allele contains insertions [35]. Studies have revealed that the presence of allele S decreases the transcriptional efficiency of the 5 HTT promoter, leading to lower levels of serotonin transporter binding and uptake. Thus, a greater risk of susceptibility to psychiatric disorders and major depressive episodes, such as PPD and PPP, is observed [35,36].

4.1.2. Linkage of Chromosomal Locations 16q13 and 8q24 with CCN2 and CCN3

Two studies [8,28] discussed the linkage between PPP and the chromosomal locations 16q13 and 8q24. The CCN gene family comprises of 6 members of which CNN2 and CNN3 are included. Elevated CCN2 and CCN3 gene expression in the brain and abnormal maternal behavioral phenotypes have been indicated [28]. More specifically, it has been associated with PPP, BD, sleep deprivation, manic symptoms, and depressive symptoms. Since the CCN3 gene is located at a distance of 138 cm from 16q13 and 8q24, a signal association can be potentially explained regarding the maternal phenotypic behavior [8,28].

4.1.3. MTHFR C677T Variation

Additionally, two studies discussed SNPs [20,32]. In one of the two studies [16], SNPs of the MTHFR gene are discussed. Specifically, the C677T genetic variant is highlighted [20]. The methylenetetrahydrofolate reductase (MTHFR) gene is located in human chromosomal region 1p36.3. The C677T variant is due to the replacement of a cytosine nucleotide base with thymine, leading to the conversion of the valine to alanine at codon 222 [11]. C677T has been found to be associated with PPP, BD, and major depressive episodes [36].

4.1.4. Methylation in the BDNF and NR3C1 Genes

Epigenetics refers to the science that studies external changes in DNA without any alterations in the nucleotide sequences of the DNA, resulting in functional and behavioral changes in the genes and subsequent alterations in protein function. A study identified from the main database [30] states that degree of methylation, which involves the addition of a methyl group, in the BDNF and NR3C1 genes has a positive association with PPP.

4.1.5. DNA Methylation in the OXTR Gene

DNA methylation (DNAm) was found in oxytocin gene receptors (OXTR), reflecting changes in inflammatory cells. Oxytocin (OT) affects the cell by interacting with the oxytocin receptor gene (OXTR), a G-protein coupled receptor that promotes G-protein signal transduction to the nucleus of the cell upon ligand binding. OXTR transcription is regulated by DNA methylation (DNAm) at a group of sites, such as CpGs, which are present within the OXTR exon. Methylation at these sites can result in various conditions, such as autism spectrum disorder, individual variability, unsocial perception, and callous-unemotional traits. In mice for instance deletion of the OXTR led to deficits in maternal behaviors. Thus, OXTR is consider a risk factor for the development of PPD. Studies support interactions between the OXTR genotype at rs53576 and increased risk for comorbid depressive and disruptive behavior disorders, and OXTR DNAm was associated with women with euthymic moods becoming depressed during postpartum periods [33]. Studies have shown evidence of significant interactions among the rs53576 genotype, the degree of methylation at CpG-934 in OXTR, and the presence of prenatal depression in women with PPD. Moreover, women who do not show any signs of depression throughout pregnancy but who carry the rs53576_GG genotype and display high methylation levels in OXTR are three times as likely to develop PPD in comparison to women with lower methylation levels or carrying the rs53576 A allele [37].

4.2. Management and Treatment Options

4.2.1. Pharmacological Interventions

When it comes to treatment options, second-generation antipsychotics (SGA) are more favorable compared with first-generation antipsychotics (FGA) due to lower rates of extrapyramidal symptoms and a reduced likelihood of tardive dyskinesia [38].

4.2.2. Lithium

The advisable treatments include pharmacological interventions, such as lithium, which is an FGA, as a treatment option or for prophylaxis. Lithium is used as a standard treatment for BD and psychotic disorders, such as PPP. Lithium reduces excitation of dopamine and glutamate and increases inhibitory GABA neurotransmission. In more severe cases where psychosis is present prior to delivery, lithium is advisable despite being considered harmful to the embryo's development, especially in extreme cases where the mother is capable of harming herself and the infant and the benefit of taking the medication outweighs the costs [8,33,38,39]. However, it must be noted that lithium comes with high risk factors; thus, certain examinations must be performed before the administration of lithium, such as renal disease screening and thyroid disease analysis, and an electrocardiogram (ECG) should be performed for individuals with coronary risk factors, hypertension, dyslipidemia, and smoking habits [38]. Additionally, if the woman wants to breastfeed her child, lithium might not be the best option. Lithium crosses into breast milk in large quantities and thus may affect the infant [10].

4.2.3. Benzodiazepines and Brexanolone—GABA Inhibitory Neurotransmitter

Another form of medication is antipsychotics, specifically benzodiazepines falling under the FGA category. These drugs are favorable, especially in cases of women suffering from insomnia [21] as they increase inhibitory GABA neurotransmission [40,41]. Additionally, ZULRESSO (Brexanolone) is another medication prescribed for moderate to severe forms of PPD and PPP. Brexanolone is a neurosteroid like allopregnanolone; these drugs are neuroactive GABA inhibitory neurotransmitters that act as receptor modulators [42].

4.2.4. Antidepressants

Antidepressants, such as selective serotonin reuptake inhibitors (SSRIs) as well as norepinephrine reuptake inhibitors, have been suggested as effective treatments for PPD and show favorable results in women suffering from BD [29–31].

4.2.5. Neuroleptics

Neuroleptics, such as haloperidol, have been used as treatment options for PPP and BD. However, as haloperidol is an FGA, it is more likely to cause adverse effects; thus, SGA medications are more favorable as a treatment method [31].

4.2.6. SGA Antipsychotics

As stated above, SGA antipsychotics are more favorable than FGA. When it comes to the best choice for use, the patient's additional health issues and psychiatric symptoms must be taken into account. For patients who cannot take lithium as a treatment option, SGAs are used as an alternative monotherapy. SGAs include olanzapine, quetiapine, risperidone, and clozapine. It has been suggested that both olanzapine and quetiapine are the best options for women who want to breastfeed their children [10,38,43]. Clozapine is considered unsafe while breastfeeding.

4.2.7. Hypnotics

Zopiclone is another treatment option; however, it is important that breast-fed infants are monitored for sedation, hypotonia, and respiratory distress, especially with regular use of large doses of hypnotics [10].

4.2.8. Alternative Forms of Treatment—Non-Pharmacological Agents

Cognitive-behavioral therapy (CBT) involves efforts to change thinking and mindset [44]. Mindfulness-based cognitive therapy (MBCT) prevents relapse of recurring episodes of depression or deep unhappiness [45]. Interpersonal therapy (IPT) is a form of psychotherapy that focuses on relieving symptoms by improving interpersonal functioning [17]. These therapies have been suggested as methods of treatments, but the most common treatment found in 3 of the 9 articles [20,29,30] is electroconvulsive therapy (ECT).

4.2.9. Electroconvulsive Therapy (ECT)

ECT is an alternative form of treatment and is usually performed in patients who do not respond to antipsychotic medication and mood stabilizers [46]. ECT is procedure performed under anesthesia, and it involves the use of small electric currents passing through the brain and causing minor and brief seizures, with the aim of altering the chemical wiring of the brain and thus reversing the symptoms of PPP [47]. It is mostly used to treat depressive episodes, but it is also used for the treatment of schizophrenia. There is a 77% rate of success in schizophrenic patients. Strong evidence was found for improvements in women with PPP after undergoing ECT [39,47]. However, side effects include temporary memory loss of current events, headaches, nausea and brief confusion that does not last longer than a few hours [39,47].

5. Conclusions

The aim of this study was to assess the genetic and epigenetic factors associated with PPP. After reviewing the articles, it was found that genetic factors play a more dominant role compared with epigenetic alterations. Genes found to play a significant role include the 5-HTT serotonin transporter gene. Methylation was noted in the following genes: OXTR, the CCN gene family with elevated CCN2 and CCN3 expression, and PRS folate metabolism (MTHFR C677T). Throughout the examination of the articles, high linkage between PPP of BD was observed. Women with a history of BD had a much higher risk of developing PPP, which was triggered during and after childbirth, in comparison with women with no history of BD. The disruption of the circadian rhythm was seen to play an equally important role as clock-controlled genes (CCGs) have been found to affect mood-regulating brain regions, leading to the development of mood disorders [33]. Thus, further investigations are needed to assess the relationship among the 3 factors as well as existing and additional genes that are linked with PPP, BD, and circadian rhythms. ECT might be the last treatment option. However, it is considered as an early option in severe cases to minimize the risk of unwanted outcomes regarding the well-being of the mother and the child [10]. Lastly, lithium is a commonly used approach for both BD and PPP. However, because it is a FGA antipsychotic, evidence suggests that the use of SGA antipsychotics might be a more favorable option as there are lower rates of extrapyramidal symptoms and a reduced likelihood of tardive dyskinesia. In addition, SGA antipsychotics, such as olanzapine and quetiapine, have been suggested as best treatment options while breastfeeding due to lower transmission to the maternal milk compared with lithium [10].

Author Contributions: Conceptualization, S.T., S.K. and M.-N.G.; methodology, S.T. and S.K.; software, S.T.; validation, S.T., S.K., D.K. and M.-N.G.; formal analysis, S.T., S.K., D.K., M.-N.G., K.P. and T.P.; investigation, S.T.; resources, S.T.; data curation, S.T. and S.K.; writing—original draft preparation, S.T., S.K., D.K., M.-N.G. and K.P.; writing—review and editing, S.T., S.K. and T.P.; visualization, S.T.; supervision, S.K.; project administration, S.K. All authors have read and agreed to the published version of the manuscript.

Funding: This research received no external funding.

Data Availability Statement: The data presented in this study are available on request from the corresponding author Karachrysafi Sofia (email: skarachry@auth.gr).

Conflicts of Interest: The authors declare no conflicts of interest.

References

1. American Psychiatric Association. What Is Perinatal Depression? 2024. Available online: https://www.psychiatry.org/patients-families/peripartum-depression/what-is-peripartum-depression?fbclid=IwAR3dy4O1cgJpTd-0wUhmRkk51HxS6iQIKz4E1h5Uy4YpQJBVLKPXQYxqDiE (accessed on 30 January 2024).
2. MGH Center for Women's Mental Health. Postpartum Psychiatric Disordes. 2008. Available online: https://womensmentalhealth.org/specialty-clinics-2/postpartum-psychiatric-disorders-2/?fbclid=IwAR216bGFIxrW5ZrF1Ela8CflNnZMQZUcebr43hgHpebrZsSGHwR1ynp-vIQ (accessed on 30 January 2024).
3. Osborne, L. Baby Blues and Postpartum Depression: Mood Disorders and Pregnancy. 2023. Available online: https://www.hopkinsmedicine.org/health/wellness-and-prevention/postpartum-mood-disorders-what-new-moms-need-to-know (accessed on 7 January 2024).
4. American Pregnancy Association. Baby Blues. 2023. Available online: https://americanpregnancy.org/healthy-pregnancy/first-year-of-life/baby-blues/ (accessed on 7 January 2024).
5. Mugha, S.; Azhar, Y.; Siddiqui, W. Postpartum Depression—Statpearls—NCBI Bookshelf. 2022. Available online: https://www.ncbi.nlm.nih.gov/books/NBK519070/ (accessed on 7 January 2024).
6. NHS. Postpartum Psychosis. 2023. Available online: https://www.nhs.uk/mental-health/conditions/post-partum-psychosis/#:~:text=Postpartum%20psychosis%20is%20a%20serious,as%20the%20%22baby%20blues%22 (accessed on 7 January 2024).
7. Professional CC Medical. Postpartum Psychosis: What It Is, Symptoms & Treatment. Available online: https://my.clevelandclinic.org/health/diseases/24152-postpartum-psychosis (accessed on 7 January 2024).
8. Perry, A.; Gordon-Smith, K.; Jones, L.; Jones, I. Phenomenology, Epidemiology and Aetiology of Postpartum Psychosis: A Review. *Brain Sci.* **2021**, *11*, 47. [CrossRef] [PubMed]
9. Cleveland Clinic. Catatonia. Available online: https://my.clevelandclinic.org/health/diseases/23503-catatonia (accessed on 7 January 2024).
10. Jairaj, C.; Seneviratne, G.; Bergink, V.; Sommer, I.E.; Dazzan, P. Postpartum psychosis: A proposed treatment algorithm. *J. Psychopharmacol.* **2023**, *37*, 960–970. [CrossRef] [PubMed]
11. Zhang, Y.X.; Yang, L.P.; Gai, C.; Cheng, C.C.; Guo, Z.Y.; Sun, H.M.; Hu, D. Association between variants of MTHFR genes and psychiatric disorders: A meta-analysis. *Front. Psychiatry* **2022**, *13*, 976428. [CrossRef]
12. Kepinska, A.P.; Robakis, T.; Humphreys, K.; Liu, X.; Kahn, R.S.; Munk-Olsen, T.; Bergink, V.; Mahjani, B. Familial risk of postpartum psychosis. *Eur. Neuropsychopharmacol.* **2023**, *75*, S239–S240. [CrossRef]
13. Guintivano, J.; Manuck, T.; Meltzer-Brody, S. Predictors of Postpartum Depression: A Comprehensive Review of the Last Decade of Evidence. *Clin. Obs. Gynecol.* **2018**, *61*, 591–603. [CrossRef] [PubMed]

14. Gilden, J.; Molenaar, N.M.; Smit, A.K.; Hoogendijk, W.J.; Rommel, A.S.; Kamperman, A.M.; Bergink, V. Mother-to-infant bonding in women with postpartum psychosis and severe postpartum depression: A clinical cohort study. *J. Clin. Med.* **2020**, *9*, 2291. [CrossRef]
15. Bernard-Bonnin, A.-C.; Society, C.P. Maternal depression and child development. *Paediatr. Child Health* **2004**, *9*, 575–598. [CrossRef]
16. Duan, C.; Hare, M.M.; Staring, M.; Deligiannidis, K.M. Examining the relationship between perinatal depression and neurodevelopment in infants and children through structural and functional neuroimaging research. *Int. Rev. Psychiatry* **2019**, *31*, 264–279. [CrossRef]
17. MGH Center for Women's Mental Health. Postpartum Depression and Its Effects on Children's IQ. 2017. Available online: https://womensmentalhealth.org/posts/postpartum-depression-effects-childrens-iq/#:~ (accessed on 7 January 2024).
18. Liu, B.; Du, Q.; Chen, L.; Fu, G.; Li, S.; Fu, L.; Zhang, X.; Ma, C.; Bin, C. CpG methylation patterns of human mitochondrial DNA. *Sci. Rep.* **2016**, *6*, 23421. [CrossRef]
19. Berens, P. Overview of the postpartum period: Normal physiology and routine maternal care. *UptoDate* **2020**, *15*, 1–34.
20. Friedman, S.H.; Reed, E.; Ross, N.E. Postpartum psychosis. *Curr. Psychiatry Rep.* **2023**, *25*, 65–72. [CrossRef]
21. Raza, S.K.; Raza, S. Postpartum psychosis. In *StatPearls*; StatPearls Publishing: Treasure Island, FL, USA, 2019.
22. Tolentino, J.C.; Schmidt, S.L. DSM-5 criteria and depression severity: Implications for clinical practice. *Front. Psychiatry* **2018**, *9*, 450. [CrossRef]
23. Sit, D.; Rothschild, A.J.; Wisner, K.L. A review of postpartum psychosis. *J. Womens Health* **2006**, *15*, 352–368. [CrossRef] [PubMed]
24. Slivinski, N.; Seed, S.; Begum, J. Postpartum Psychosis: Symptoms, Causes, Risks, Treatment, and Recovery. WebMD. 2023. Available online: https://www.webmd.com/parenting/baby/postpartum-psychosis-overview (accessed on 7 January 2024).
25. Edinburgh Postnatal Depression Scale (EPDS)—Stanford Medicine. Available online: https://med.stanford.edu/content/dam/sm/ppc/documents/DBP/EDPS_text_added.pdf (accessed on 7 January 2024).
26. Page, M.J.; McKenzie, J.E.; Bossuyt, P.M.; Boutron, I.; Hoffmann, T.C.; Mulrow, C.D.; Shamseer, L.; Tetzlaff, J.M.; Akl, E.A.; Brennan, S.E.; et al. The PRISMA 2020 statement: An updated guideline for reporting systematic reviews. *BMJ* **2021**, *372*, n71. [CrossRef] [PubMed]
27. Thippeswamy, H.; Davies, W. A new molecular risk pathway for postpartum mood disorders: Clues from steroid sulfatase-deficient individuals. *Arch. Women's Ment. Health* **2021**, *24*, 391–401. [CrossRef] [PubMed]
28. Davies, W. An Analysis of Cellular Communication Network Factor Proteins as Candidate Mediators of Postpartum Psychosis Risk. *Front. Psychiatry* **2019**, *10*, 876. [CrossRef]
29. Sharma, V.; Mazmanian, D.; Palagini, L.; Bramante, A. Postpartum psychosis: Revisiting the phenomenology, nosology, and treatment. *J. Affect. Disord. Rep.* **2022**, *10*, 100378. [CrossRef]
30. Alshaya, D.S. Genetic and epigenetic factors associated with depression: An updated overview. *Saudi J. Biol. Sci.* **2022**, *29*, 103311. [CrossRef]
31. Walton, N.L.; Antonoudiou, P.; Maguire, J.L. Neurosteroid influence on affective tone. *Neurosci. Biobehav. Rev.* **2023**, *152*, 105327. [CrossRef]
32. Silveira, P.P.; Meaney, M.J. Examining the biological mechanisms of human mental disorders resulting from gene-environment interdependence using novel functional genomic approaches. *Neurobiol. Dis.* **2023**, *178*, 106008. [CrossRef]
33. Bhatnagar, A.; Murray, G.; Ray, S. Circadian biology to advance therapeutics for mood disorders. *Trends Pharmacol. Sci.* **2023**, *44*, 689–704. [CrossRef]
34. Hande, S.H.; Krishna, S.M.; Sahote, K.K.; Dev, N.; Erl, T.P.; Ramakrishna, K.; Ravidhran, R.; Das, R. Population genetic variation of SLC6A4 gene, associated with neurophysiological development. *J. Genet.* **2021**, *100*, 16. [CrossRef] [PubMed]
35. Li, J.; Chen, Y.; Xiang, Q.; Xiang, J.; Tang, Y.; Tang, L. 5HTTLPR polymorphism and postpartum depression risk: A meta-analysis. *Medicine* **2020**, *99*, e22319. [CrossRef] [PubMed]
36. Fratelli, C.; Siqueira, J.; Silva, C.; Ferreira, E.; Silva, I. 5HTTLPR Genetic Variant and Major De-pressive Disorder: A Review. *Genes* **2020**, *11*, 1260. [CrossRef] [PubMed]
37. Rodriguez, A.C.I.; Smith, L.; Harris, R.; Nephew, B.C.; Santos, H.P., Jr.; Murgatroyd, C. Oxytocin modulates sensitivity to acculturation and discrimination stress in pregnan-cy. *Psychoneuroendocrinology* **2022**, *141*, 105769. [CrossRef] [PubMed]
38. Payne, J. *Treatment of Postpartum Psychosis*; UpToDate: Waltham, MA, USA, 2019; pp. 1–20.
39. National Center for Biotechnology Information (NCBI) Bookshelf. Lithium. Available online: https://www.ncbi.nlm.nih.gov/books/NBK544304/#:~:text=[15][16%25D%20Lithium,isolated%20episodes%20of%20postpartum%20psychosis (accessed on 7 January 2024).
40. Professional CC Medical. Benzodiazepines: What They Are, Uses, Side Effects & Risks. Available online: https://my.clevelandclinic.org/health/treatments/24570-benzodiazepines-benzos (accessed on 7 January 2024).
41. Pope, C. List of Common Benzodiazepines + Uses & Side Effects. Available online: https://www.drugs.com/drug-class/benzodiazepines.html (accessed on 7 January 2024).
42. Cornett, E.M.; Rando, L.; Labbé, A.M.; Perkins, W.; Kaye, A.M.; Kaye, A.D.; Viswanath, O.; Urits, I. Brexanolone to Treat Postpartum Depression in Adult Women. *Psychopharmacol. Bull.* **2021**, *51*, 115–130.
43. Teodorescu, A.; Dima, L.; Popa, M.A.; Moga, M.A.; Bîgiu, N.F.; Ifteni, P. Antipsychotics in postpartum psychosis. *Am. J. Ther.* **2021**, *28*, e341–e348. [CrossRef]

44. American Psychological Association. What Is Cognitive Behavioral Therapy? Available online: https://www.apa.org/ptsd-guideline/patients-and-families/cognitive-behavioral (accessed on 7 January 2024).
45. CBCT. 2021. Available online: https://www.mbct.com/ (accessed on 7 January 2024).
46. Payne, J.; Marder, S.; Friedman, M. Treatment of Postpartum Psychosis. 2023. Available online: https://www.uptodate.com/contents/treatment-of-postpartum-psychosis/print (accessed on 7 January 2024).
47. Mayo Foundation for Medical Education and Research. Electroconvulsive Therapy (ECT). 2018. Available online: https://www.mayoclinic.org/tests-procedures/electroconvulsive-therapy/about/pac-20393894 (accessed on 7 January 2024).

Disclaimer/Publisher's Note: The statements, opinions and data contained in all publications are solely those of the individual author(s) and contributor(s) and not of MDPI and/or the editor(s). MDPI and/or the editor(s) disclaim responsibility for any injury to people or property resulting from any ideas, methods, instructions or products referred to in the content.

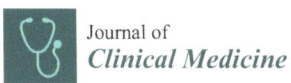

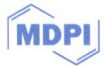

Article

Accuracy and Reliability of Pelvimetry Measures Obtained by Manual or Automatic Labeling of Three-Dimensional Pelvic Models

Johann Hêches [1], Sandra Marcadent [2], Anna Fernandez [3], Stephen Adjahou [3], Jean-Yves Meuwly [4], Jean-Philippe Thiran [2,4], David Desseauve [3] and Julien Favre [1,5,*]

1. Swiss BioMotion Lab, Lausanne University Hospital (CHUV) and University of Lausanne (UNIL), CH-1011 Lausanne, Switzerland; johann.heches@chuv.ch
2. Signal Processing Laboratory 5, École Polytechnique Fédérale de Lausanne (EPFL), CH-1015 Lausanne, Switzerland; sandra.marcadent@epfl.ch (S.M.); jean-philippe.thiran@epfl.ch (J.-P.T.)
3. Women-Mother-Child Department, Lausanne University Hospital (CHUV) and University of Lausanne (UNIL), CH-1011 Lausanne, Switzerland; anna.fernandez@chuv.ch (A.F.); stephen.adjahou@chuv.ch (S.A.); david.desseauve@chuv.ch (D.D.)
4. Department of Radiology, Lausanne University Hospital (CHUV) and University of Lausanne (UNIL), CH-1011 Lausanne, Switzerland; jean-yves.meuwly@chuv.ch
5. The Sense Innovation and Research Center, CH-1007 Lausanne, Switzerland
* Correspondence: julien.favre@chuv.ch

Abstract: (1) **Background**: The morphology of the pelvic cavity is important for decision-making in obstetrics. This study aimed to estimate the accuracy and reliability of pelvimetry measures obtained when radiologists manually label anatomical landmarks on three-dimensional (3D) pelvic models. A second objective was to design an automatic labeling method. (2) **Methods**: Three operators segmented 10 computed tomography scans each. Three radiologists then labeled 12 anatomical landmarks on the pelvic models, which allowed for the calculation of 15 pelvimetry measures. Additionally, an automatic labeling method was developed based on a reference pelvic model, including reference anatomical landmarks, matching the individual pelvic models. (3) **Results**: Heterogeneity among landmarks in radiologists' labeling accuracy was observed, with some landmarks being rarely mislabeled by more than 4 mm and others being frequently mislabeled by 10 mm or more. The propagation to the pelvimetry measures was limited; only one out of the 15 measures reported a median error above 5 mm or 5°, and all measures showed moderate to excellent inter-radiologist reliability. The automatic method outperformed manual labeling. (4) **Conclusions**: This study confirmed the suitability of pelvimetry measures based on manual labeling of 3D pelvic models. Automatic labeling offers promising perspectives to decrease the demand on radiologists, standardize the labeling, and describe the pelvic cavity in more detail.

Keywords: atlas; anatomical landmarks; birth delivery; cephalopelvic disproportion; cesarean section; computed tomography; labeling; pelvimetry; pelvis; segmentation; registration; 3D model

Citation: Hêches, J.; Marcadent, S.; Fernandez, A.; Adjahou, S.; Meuwly, J.-Y.; Thiran, J.-P.; Desseauve, D.; Favre, J. Accuracy and Reliability of Pelvimetry Measures Obtained by Manual or Automatic Labeling of Three-Dimensional Pelvic Models. *J. Clin. Med.* **2024**, *13*, 689. https://doi.org/10.3390/jcm13030689

Academic Editors: Apostolos Mamopoulos and Ioannis Tsakiridis

Received: 12 December 2023
Revised: 19 January 2024
Accepted: 22 January 2024
Published: 25 January 2024

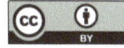

Copyright: © 2024 by the authors. Licensee MDPI, Basel, Switzerland. This article is an open access article distributed under the terms and conditions of the Creative Commons Attribution (CC BY) license (https://creativecommons.org/licenses/by/4.0/).

1. Introduction

A cephalopelvic disproportion (CPD) is a general concept referring to an inadequacy between the size of the fetus's head and the size of the parturient pelvic cavity. It is a serious condition, as a large head with respect to the pelvic cavity could lead to an arrest of the delivery progression [1]. Worldwide, vaginal deliveries with this condition have been estimated to lead to maternal death in 8% of the cases [2]. It is therefore important to detect CPD ahead of time to anticipate possible complications and plan the delivery accordingly. Precise predictions are indeed required, as both underestimating and overestimating the complications could be detrimental. In some situations, vaginal deliveries could be made more difficult by CPD, possibly leading to emergency cesarean sections, and in other situations, elective cesarean sections could be decided, whereas vaginal deliveries would have occurred without complications [3,4].

CPD being particularly dependent on the morphology of the pelvic cavity [5], diverse imaging methods have been proposed to quantify this bony structure, for example using ultrasound [6], X-ray [7], magnetic resonance imaging (MRI) [8], or computed tomography (CT) [9]. Other authors also worked on defining predictors of labor complications associated with CPD based on morphological measures [10–16]. Regrettably, our capacity to predict CPD complications remains insufficient [17,18]. Further efforts are thus necessary, particularly to improve the description of pelvis morphology.

Quantifying the morphology of the pelvic cavity requires identifying anatomical landmarks in pelvis images, and thus the quality of the quantification depends on the labeling accuracy [19]. A few studies assessed the accuracy and reliability of radiologists labeling pelvic landmarks in two-dimensional (2D) images and the impact of these errors on the pelvimetry measures [20,21]. However, to the authors' knowledge, no comparable assessment has been published for 3D imaging where the labeling is carried out using 3D pelvic models [5]. Assessing the labeling errors on 3D models and their propagation to pelvimetry measures is necessary for the proper use of the growing 3D model-based approach.

The anatomical landmarks required to quantify the pelvic cavity are labeled manually most of the time, notably because there is a lack of assistive tools. Indeed, so far, developments in this regard have mainly consisted of methods to label 2D images [22,23] and to derive a 2D pelvic inlet shape from a 3D pelvic model [24]. No method exists to automatically label anatomical landmarks relevant to obstetrics on 3D pelvic models, whereas such options have been proposed in different disciplines for a variety of bones [25,26]. Introducing automatic labeling methods for pelvimetry could be very helpful, as it could allow considering more comprehensive sets of anatomical landmarks, potentially leading to better descriptions of the pelvic cavity and better prediction of complications associated with CPD ahead of labor. Automatic methods could also improve accuracy and reliability while limiting the demand for radiologists. Consequently, there is a need to develop and assess automatic labeling in pelvimetry.

This study first aimed to assess the accuracy and reliability of radiologists manually labeling anatomical landmarks on 3D pelvic models and evaluate the impact of these errors on pelvimetry measures. A second objective was to design an automatic labeling method and compare it with the standard manual approach.

2. Materials and Methods

2.1. Three-Dimensional Pelvic Models

A set of 10 anonymized pelvic CT scans without contrast agents were extracted retrospectively from the institution database for this study, following approval from the local ethics committee. The inclusion criteria were: females aged between 20 and 40 years old, without bone abnormality at the pelvis or spine (e.g., scoliosis or fracture), and who gave their consent to further use of their data for research purposes. All scans were acquired on one of the three following machines: Révolution scanner (General Electric, Boston, MA, USA), Electric Discovery 750HD FREEdom scanner (General Electric, Boston, MA, USA), or INGENUITY 128 interventionnal scanner (Philips, Amsterdam, The Netherlands). Voxel dimensions ranged from $0.57 \times 0.57 \times 0.5$ mm^3 to $1.13 \times 1.13 \times 2.5$ mm^3.

Each of the 10 CT scans was segmented by three operators for a total of 30 segmentations using 3D Slicers software [27] (http://www.slicer.org, version 4.10.2). The segmentation included three segments: the sacrum as well as the left and right hips (Figure 1). The coccyx was not included because of its limited interest in obstetrics and its poor visibility on most of the CT scans. Then, each segment was converted into a 3D voxel-based model, which was subsequently converted into a 3D surface mesh model composed of 25,000 vertices and 50,000 faces with the use of a marching cubes algorithm [28]. A total of 30 pelvic models were thus generated, each including their respective three bones as independent 3D surface mesh models.

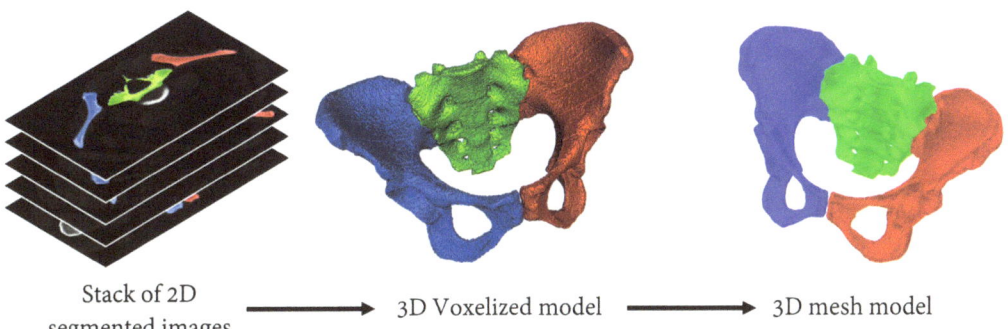

Figure 1. Illustration of the procedure used to obtain the 3D mesh models from the CT scans. Red and blue segments correspond to the left and right hips, respectively. The sacrum, the third segment of the pelvic model, is displayed in green.

The variations among segmentations were assessed by quantifying the spatial overlap of the segments produced by the three operators. Concretely, this was conducted using both the Sørensen-dice index [29,30] and the mesh-to-mesh Hausdorff distance [31].

2.2. Manual Pelvimetry

Twelve anatomical landmarks were selected for this study based on their prevalence in the pelvimetry literature [16,32–34] (Figure 2). Three radiologists from the institution performing pelvimetry analyses routinely labeled these 12 landmarks on the 30 pelvic models using a custom-made graphical interface mimicking the ones of usual radiology software. Ten landmarks are bilateral and were labeled for the left and right sides. For each labeling of each pelvic model, 15 common pelvimetry measures (13 lengths and 2 angles) were calculated based on the anatomical landmarks, as detailed in Figure 3.

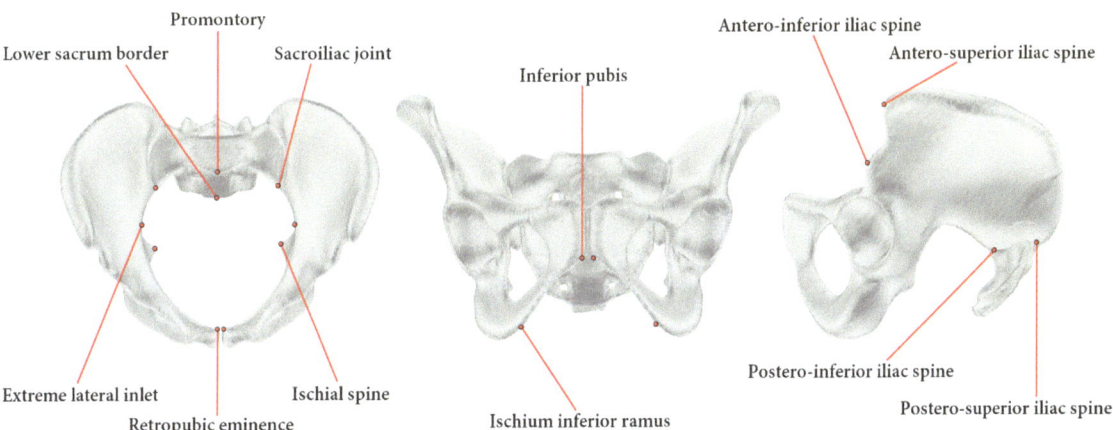

Figure 2. Pelvic model with indication of the 12 anatomical landmarks. To facilitate the reading, the landmarks are presented in either a transverse (**left**), a coronal (**middle**), or a sagittal (**right**) view of the pelvis. Please note that all landmarks except two, the promontory and the lower sacrum border, are bilateral.

	Pelvimetry measures	Landmarks used			Values		
					Mean ± SD	Min	Max
Lengths [mm]	Iliopectineal cord	Left or right sacroiliac joint		Left or right retropubic eminence	117.2 ± 9.3	98.3	134.1
	Inlet anterior space	Left or right retropubic eminence		Left or right extreme lateral inlet	97.1 ± 6.3	85.4	111.4
	Inlet posterior space	Left or right sacroiliac joint		Left or right extreme lateral inlet	36.3 ± 5.1	26.4	44.1
	Inlet sacral breadth	Left sacroiliac joint		Right sacroiliac joint	89.8 ± 5.5	80.0	97.8
	Inter antero-inferior iliac spine	Left antero-inferior iliac spine		Right antero-inferior iliac spine	187.7 ± 11.5	170.7	205.6
	Inter antero-superior iliac spine	Left antero-superior iliac spine		Right antero-superior iliac spine	221.9 ± 19.9	194.5	251.3
	Inter postero-inferior iliac spine	Left postero-inferior iliac spine		Right postero-inferior iliac spine	100.8 ± 7.0	85.8	109.4
	Inter postero-superior iliac spine	Left postero-superior iliac spine		Right postero-superior iliac spine	101.3 ± 7.3	91.9	113.2
	Interspinous	Left ischial spine		Right ischial spine	109.1 ± 8.2	90.8	119.8
	Max transverse	Left extreme lateral inlet		Right extreme lateral inlet	122.4 ± 7.0	110.7	133.5
	Obstetrical conjugate	Center retropubic eminence		Promontory	123.7 ± 13.4	94.4	137.7
	Outlet antero-superior	Center inferior pubis		Lower sacrum border	129.6 ± 8.7	118.6	144.0
	Sacral cord	Lower sacrum border		Promontory	102.0 ± 10.8	81.2	118.7
Angles [deg]	Pectineal	Left extreme lateral inlet	Center retropubic eminence	Right extreme lateral inlet	76.7 ± 5.0	66.3	84.6
	Subpubic	Left ischium inferior ramus	Center inferior pubis	Right ischium inferior ramus	89.6 ± 7.6	75.2	99.3

Figure 3. Definition of the 15 pelvimetric measures. This figure also reports the means and standard deviations (SD) as well as ranges (min and max) of the pelvimetric measures in the study population.

To assess the accuracy, a labeling error was computed for each landmark of the 90 labeled pelvic models (30 pelvic models labeled by 3 radiologists). This was carried out by calculating the distance between the position of the landmark of interest and the average position of the corresponding landmark labeled by the two other radiologists. Pelvimetry measure errors were quantified in a similar manner as the absolute differences between one measure and the average value of the same measure obtained by the two other radiologists. In addition, the reliability of the pelvimetry measures among radiologists was assessed using the intraclass correlation coefficient [35] (ICC (3, k)) as well as the complementary standard error of measurement (SEM) [36]. This inter-radiologist assessment was carried out separately for each measure based on the 30 pelvic models.

Finally, the ICC (3, 1) and the SEM were also used to evaluate the reliability of the pelvimetry measures across segmentations. This evaluation was conducted separately for each measure and radiologist based on the three segmentations of the 10 CT scans. The ICC values were classified [37] as being excellent (ICC $\geq$ 0.9), good (0.9 > ICC $\geq$ 0.75), moderate (0.75 > ICC $\geq$ 0.5), or poor (0.5 > ICC).

2.3. Automatic Labeling

A method was developed to label anatomical landmarks automatically in any pelvic model. It consists of matching a reference pelvic model to a target pelvic model using a 3D shape registration and then projecting embedded anatomical landmarks from the matched reference pelvis onto the pelvis of interest [38].

The reference model was obtained by "averaging" all the models in this study. To this end, a ground truth was determined for each landmark of the 30 pelvic models as the average position of the landmarks labeled by the three radiologists. Then, a spatial correspondence was established among the 30 models using a non-rigid registration algorithm [39]. This allowed us to calculate a reference model, including reference landmarks, by averaging all the models and their landmarks (Figure 2). When automatically labeling a pelvis, the same registration procedure was used to match the reference model to the pelvis of interest.

The accuracy of the automatic labeling and resultant pelvimetry measures was assessed similarly to the manual procedure, with the exception of using the averages of the three radiologists (instead of the averages of the two other radiologists) as comparison values when calculating the errors. The reliability of the pelvimetry measures obtained by automatic labeling with respect to the segmentation was evaluated using exactly the same method as described above.

2.4. Statistical Analyses

The labeling and pelvimetry measure errors were compared between manual and automatic labeling using Wilcoxon signed rank tests [40]. Non-parametric statistics were used after refuting a normal distribution for the data based on D'Agostino's K^2 tests [41].

All software developments and statistical analyses were conducted using Matlab R2019b (The MathWorks Inc., Natick, MA, USA).

3. Results

3.1. Landmarks Labeling Accuracy

The median error of the 12 landmarks varied in the range of 2.3–11.6 mm when the labeling was carried out manually by the radiologists and in the range of 1.9–6.3 mm with the automatic labeling (Figure 4). For six landmarks, the error differed statistically significantly between the radiologists and the automatic method ($p \leq 0.008$). In all these cases, the errors were lower with automatic labeling. The differences in median errors for these six landmarks varied between 0.6 mm for the ischial spine (smallest significant difference between radiologists and automatic labeling) and 7.5 mm for the Ischium Inferior Ramus (largest significant difference between radiologists and automatic labeling).

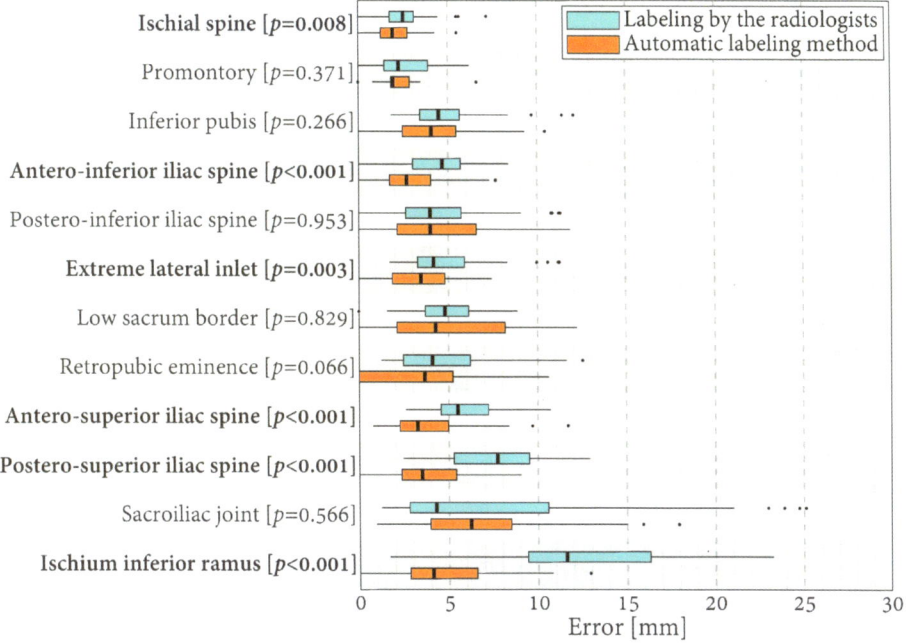

Figure 4. Boxplots of the errors in landmark labeling for the radiologists and the proposed automatic method. Labels in bold indicate landmarks with statistically significantly different errors between the radiologists and the automatic method ($p < 0.05$).

3.2. Pelvimetry Measures Accuracy and Inter-Radiologist Reliability

The mean, standard deviation, and range of the pelvimetry measures in this study are reported in Figure 3.

Regarding the pelvimetry length measures, the median errors varied in the range of 0.7–5.5 mm for the labeling carried out by the radiologists and in the range of 0.6–4.1 mm for the automatic labeling (Figure 5). Relative to the lengths, they corresponded to errors of 3.1–26.9% for the radiologists and errors of 1.9–23.1% for the automatic method. For six of the 13 length measures, the errors differed statistically significantly between the evaluations conducted by the radiologists and the automatic method ($p \leq 0.048$). For these six lengths, lower errors were always obtained using automatic labeling. Specifically, the differences in median errors varied between 0.6 mm for the obstetric conjugate (smallest significant difference between the evaluations performed by the radiologists and the automatic method) and 3.3 mm for the inter postero-superior iliac spine (largest significant difference between the evaluations performed by the radiologists and the automatic method).

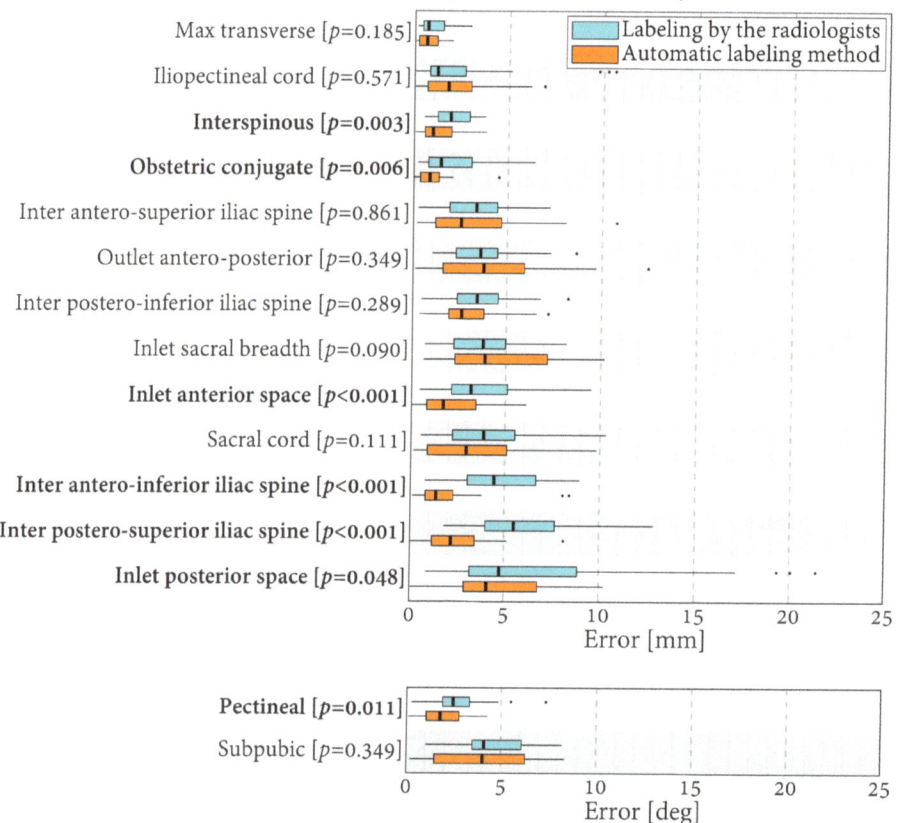

Figure 5. Boxplots of the errors in pelvimetry measures for the radiologists and the proposed automatic labeling method. Labels in bold indicate measures with statistically significantly different errors between the radiologists and the automatic method ($p < 0.05$).

Concerning the pelvimetry angle measures obtained by the radiologists, the median errors were 2.5° for the pectineal and 4.1° for the subpubic. This corresponds to relative errors of 13.5% and 17.0%, respectively. In comparison, the errors with the automatic labeling were 1.8° (9.7%) and 4.0° (16.7%), respectively. For the pectineal, the errors differed statistically significantly, with better results observed using the automatic method (difference of medians of 0.7°, $p = 0.011$).

The ICC quantifying the inter-radiologist reliability of the pelvimetry measures varied in the range of 0.63–0.99 (Figure 6). These values indicated excellent reliability for 10 measures, good reliability for four measures, and moderate reliability for one measure. No measure reported poor inter-radiologist reliability. The SEM were between 0.6 and 5.6 mm for the length measures and between 1.8° and 2.7° for the angular measures.

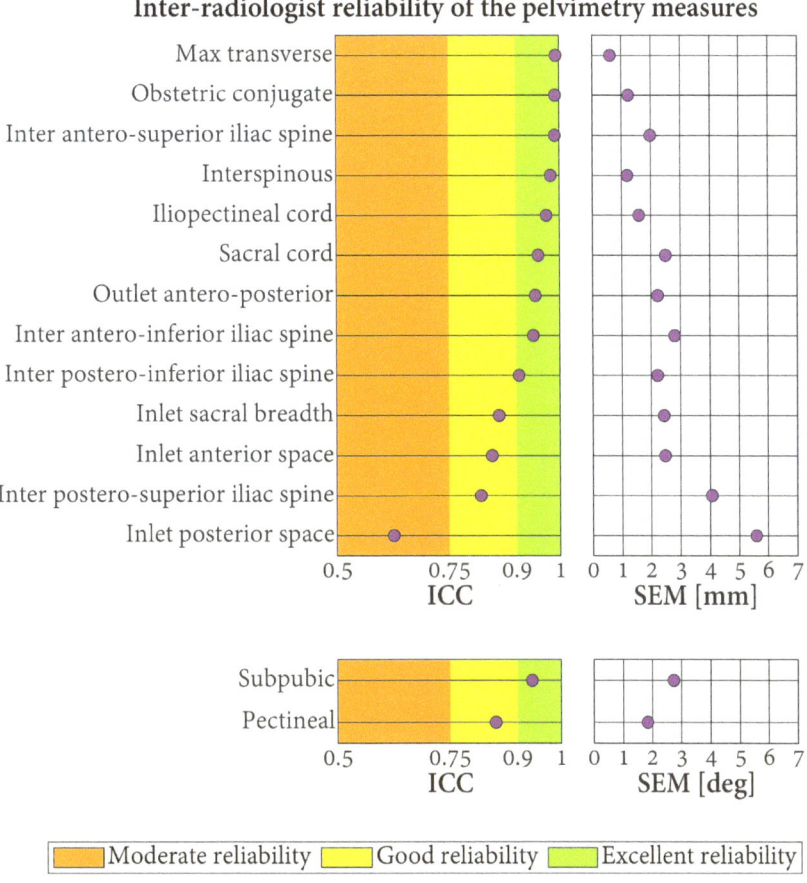

Figure 6. Inter-radiologist reliability of the pelvimetry measures based on three radiologists labeling 30 pelvic models. ICC: intraclass correlation coefficient. SEM: standard error of measurement.

3.3. Pelvimetry Measures Reliability across Segmentations

The three operators segmented the pelves with median Sørensen-dice scores of 94.3% (interquartile range: 93.6–95.6%) for the sacrum and 95.6% (interquartile range: 95.0–96.9%) for the hips. The median model-to-model Hausdorff distances were 0.40 mm (interquartile range: 0.32–0.47 mm) for the sacrum and 0.34 mm (interquartile range: 0.28–0.39 mm) for the hips.

The ICC for the reliability of the pelvimetry measures when the segmentations of the CT scans were repeated by different operators and the labeling was conducted by the radiologists varied between 0.68 and 0.99 (Figure 7). Approximately 64.4% of these results corresponded to excellent reliability, 33.3% to good reliability, and 2.2% to moderate reliability. The associated SEM were in the range of 0.7–6.4 mm for the length measures and in the range of 1.3–2.1° for the angle measures. For all the measures, better reliability was obtained when the segmentation repeats were labeled automatically (all ICC indicating excellent reliability (range of 0.95–1.0; SEM of length measures between 0.2 and 1.6 mm; SEM of angle measures between 0.4° and 0.6°).

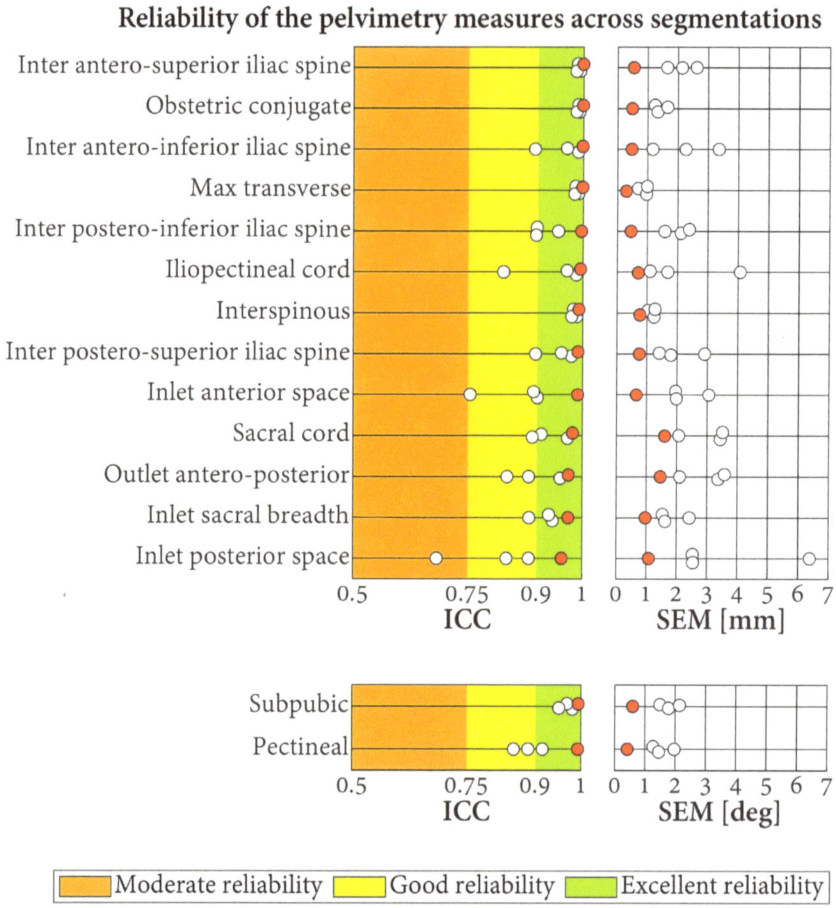

Figure 7. Reliability of the pelvimetry measures across segmentations. Each result is based on 10 CT scans, segmented three times by different operators. Results for the labeling conducted by the three radiologists and the automatic labeling method are displayed with white and red dots, respectively. ICC: intraclass correlation coefficient. SEM: standard error of measurement.

4. Discussion

This study showed heterogeneity among landmarks in radiologists' labeling accuracy, from some landmarks being rarely mislabeled by more than 4 mm to others being frequently mislabeled by 10 mm or more. Interestingly, the propagation of the labeling errors to the pelvimetry measures was limited, with only one out of the 15 measures reporting a median error above 5 mm or 5°. While a threshold has not been firmly established for pelvimetry measures in obstetrics, errors up to 5 mm were considered acceptable clinically [21]. The inter-radiologist reliability corroborated the accuracy results, with two-thirds of the measures reporting excellent reliability and all being at least moderately reliable. A rigorous performance comparison between the present pelvimetry measures obtained from 3D pelvic models and those in prior studies derived from 2D pelvic images is difficult because experimental conditions are too different across studies [20,21]. Nevertheless, the reliability ranges appear similar, and prior studies also reported heterogeneity among measures. Therefore, the present study supports the use of 3D pelvic models to quantify the morphology of the pelvic cavity manually by radiologists.

A second major finding was to demonstrate the possibility of automating the labeling. Indeed, an automatic method was developed and shown to achieve comparable to better accuracy and reliability across segmentation to the labeling conducted by the radiologists. Even though some accuracy and reliability results were better with the automatic labeling, the improvements remained generally limited and, on their own, did not strongly recommend using an automatic approach. That being said, the possibility of saving radiologists time and labeling a larger number of anatomical landmarks without prejudicing their accuracy and reliability is a compelling motivation for the use of automatic labeling in the future. Although introducing more specific labeling guidelines could certainly improve consistency among radiologists, automating the labeling could be an easier solution to uniformize the labeling and facilitate the establishment of multi-center databases that appear essential to improving our understanding of the role of pelvic morphology in childbirth.

Indirectly, this study further highlighted the carefulness required when using pelvimetry measures in clinics. Specifically, in view of the possible errors, developing effective indices to predict complications associated with CPD based on simple combinations of a few pelvimetry measures seems unlikely [21]. While reducing the complex morphology of the pelvic cavity to a few features, which are also not free of error, is certainly not the single cause of the feeble prediction capacity of such indices [17,18], it is probably an important contributor. The possibility offered by automatic labeling to consider new anatomical landmarks and pelvimetry measures while diminishing the demand on radiologists is extremely promising. Indeed, it could allow analyzing big datasets of pelvis images and childbirth clinical outcomes to identify the most pertinent landmarks and pelvimetry measures and hopefully also suggest more effective indices of CPD complications. An effort in this direction based on a hundred pelves labeled manually was recently presented and confirmed the potential of the approach [16]. Upscaling the effort by automating the labeling and using artificial intelligence to combine the measures could significantly improve the prediction of childbirth complications associated with pelvic morphology. Since the fetal head has also been reported to play a role in childbirth complications, including CPD [1,42], extending the automatic labeling to the fetal head could be of further benefit in clinical practice.

This study was motivated by obstetrics. But the need to quantify the morphology of the pelvis is not exclusive to this discipline. Consequently, the results of the present work, particularly the possibilities offered by automatic labeling, could also be important for other fields, such as oncology [8,22,43] and orthopedic surgery [44,45]. Nothing should prevent the use of the methods in this study in other fields, including with men and/or individuals of different age ranges. However, carefulness might be required when interpreting the results from a different perspective than obstetrics, as the patient population and the error expectations in this study corresponded to research questions specific to obstetrics.

This study involved three radiologists and three segmentation operators. While this was appropriate with respect to the present objectives, the results should be considered with care, as they might not be generalizable to any radiologist or operator. For example, it is possible that comparing radiologists from diverse institutions could lead to different results. The relevance of conducting more extensive assessments to understand the causes of variability with manual labeling could, however, be limited in view of the alternative, automatic method proposed in this work. Further studies combining morphological and clinical data remain required to improve the use of pelvimetry measures in obstetrics. This will certainly necessitate large datasets that could benefit from the automatic method proposed in this study. Manually segmenting CT or MRI images to obtain 3D pelvic models is time-consuming and could be perceived as an obstacle to their implementation in clinical routine. In this regard, it is worth mentioning that automatic segmentation methods exist [46,47] and could be combined with the proposed labeling method to offer a fully automatic solution. Currently, 3D pelvimetry requires access to an MRI or CT machine, which limits its widespread use. New developments in ultrasound imaging, particularly with respect to probe tracking, suggest that alternatives could exist in the near future for 3D imaging of the pelvis with simpler instrumentation [48,49]. Extending the possibility of ultrasound imaging in this regard is particularly interesting because this technology is already widely employed in obstetrics.

5. Conclusions

This study showed the suitability of pelvimetry measures based on radiologists manually labeling anatomical landmarks on 3D pelvic models. It also introduced an automatic labeling method that appeared promising to decrease the demand on radiologists, standardize the labeling, and allow a more detailed description of the pelvic cavity. These possibilities could prove pivotal for the creation of large datasets of pelvimetry measures and clinical outcomes necessary to improve our understanding of childbirth complications, particularly with CPD.

Author Contributions: Conceptualization, J.H., D.D. and J.F.; methodology, J.H. and J.F.; software, J.H.; validation, J.H. and J.-Y.M.; formal analysis, J.H.; investigation, J.H.; resources, J.H., S.M., A.F., S.A., J.-Y.M. and D.D.; data curation, J.H., A.F. and S.A.; writing—original draft preparation, J.H. and J.F.; writing—review and editing, all authors; visualization, J.H. and J.F.; supervision, J.-P.T., D.D. and J.F.; project administration, all authors; funding acquisition, J.-P.T., D.D. and J.F.; J.-P.T., D.D. and J.F. supervised this research and should be considered co-authors. All authors have read and agreed to the published version of the manuscript.

Funding: This research was supported by the Leenaards Foundation, Switzerland.

Institutional Review Board Statement: The study was conducted in accordance with the Declaration of Taipei and the Swiss law on human research. The study was authorized by the local ethical committee (CER-VD. 2019-01349).

Informed Consent Statement: Participants gave their consent for the use of the data in this study.

Data Availability Statement: The data are not publicly available due to regulatory provisions.

Acknowledgments: The authors warmly thank the involved radiologists for their assistance in data analysis.

Conflicts of Interest: The authors declare no conflicts of interest.

References

1. Maharaj, D. Assessing cephalopelvic disproportion: Back to the basics. *Obstet. Gynecol. Surv.* **2010**, *65*, 387–395. [CrossRef]
2. WHO. *Make Every Mother and Child Count: The World Health Report*; World Health Organization: Geneva, Switzerland, 2005.
3. Yang, X.-J.; Sun, S.-S. Comparison of maternal and fetal complications in elective and emergency cesarean section: A systematic review and meta-analysis. *Arch. Gynecol. Obstet.* **2017**, *296*, 503–512. [CrossRef]
4. Ryding, E.L.; Wijma, K.; Wijma, B. Psychological impact of emergency cesarean section in comparison with elective cesarean section, instrumental and normal vaginal delivery. *J. Psychosom. Obstet. Gynecol.* **1998**, *19*, 135–144. [CrossRef]
5. Nishikawa, S.; Miki, M.; Chigusa, Y.; Furuta, M.; Kido, A.; Kawamura, Y.; Ueda, Y.; Mandai, M.; Mogami, H. Obstetric pelvimetry by three-dimensional computed tomography in non-pregnant Japanese women: A retrospective single-center study. *J. Matern. Fetal Neonatal Med.* **2023**, *36*, 2190444. [CrossRef]
6. Bian, X.; Zhuang, J.; Cheng, X. Combination of ultrasound pelvimetry and fetal sonography in predicting cephalopelvic disproportion. *Chin. Med. J.* **1997**, *110*, 942–945. [PubMed]
7. Thubisi, M.; Ebrahim, A.; Moodley, J.; Shweni, P. Vaginal delivery after previous caesarean section: Is X-ray pelvimetry necessary? *BJOG Int. J. Obstet. Gynaecol.* **1993**, *100*, 421–424. [CrossRef]
8. Hong, J.-Y.; Brown, K.; Waller, J.; Young, C.; Solomon, M. The role of MRI pelvimetry in predicting technical difficulty and outcomes of open and minimally invasive total mesorectal excision: A systematic review. *Tech. Coloproctol.* **2020**, *24*, 991–1000. [CrossRef] [PubMed]
9. Capelle, C.; Devos, P.; Caudrelier, C.; Verpillat, P.; Fourquet, T.; Puech, P.; Garabedian, C.; Lemaitre, L. How reproducible are classical and new CT-pelvimetry measurements? *Diagn. Interv. Imaging* **2020**, *101*, 79–89. [CrossRef] [PubMed]
10. Fremondiere, P.; Fournie, A. Disproportion fœto-pelvienne et radiopelvimétrie. *Gynécologie Obs. Fertil.* **2011**, *39*, 8–11. [CrossRef] [PubMed]
11. Mengert, W.F. Estimation of pelvic capacity: Chairman's address. *J. Am. Med. Assoc.* **1948**, *138*, 169–174. [CrossRef] [PubMed]
12. Morgan, M.A.; Thurnau, G.R.; Fishburne Jr, J.I. The fetal-pelvic index as an indicator of fetal-pelvic disproportion: A preliminary report. *Am. J. Obstet. Gynecol.* **1986**, *155*, 608–613. [CrossRef]
13. Abitbol, M.; Taylor, U.; Castillo, I.; Rochelson, B. The cephalopelvic disproportion index. Combined fetal sonography and X-ray pelvimetry for early detection of cephalopelvic disproportion. *J. Reprod. Med.* **1991**, *36*, 369–373.

14. Bian, X.; Zhuang, J.; Cheng, X. Prediction of cephalopelvic disproportion by ultrasonographic cephalopelic. *Zhonghua Fu Chan Ke Za Zhi* **1998**, *33*, 533–535.
15. Morganelli, G.; di Pasquo, E.; Dall'Asta, A.; Volpe, N.; Zegarra, R.R.; Corno, E.; Melandri, E.; Abou-Dakn, M.; Ghi, T. OC14. 01: Prediction of cephalopelvic disproportion by evaluating the ratio between the head circumference and the obstetric conjugate. *Ultrasound Obstet. Gynecol.* **2021**, *58*, 40. [CrossRef]
16. Frémondière, P.; Thollon, L.; Adalian, P.; Delotte, J.; Marchal, F. Which foetal-pelvic variables are useful for predicting caesarean section and instrumental assistance. *Med. Princ. Pract.* **2017**, *26*, 359–367. [CrossRef]
17. Korhonen, U.; Taipale, P.; Heinonen, S. Fetal pelvic index to predict cephalopelvic disproportion–a retrospective clinical cohort study. *Acta Obstet. Et Gynecol. Scand.* **2015**, *94*, 615–621. [CrossRef]
18. Roux, N.; Korb, D.; Morin, C.; Sibony, O. Trial of labor after cesarean and contribution of pelvimetry in the prognosis of neonatal morbidity. *J. Gynecol. Obstet. Hum. Reprod.* **2020**, *49*, 101681. [CrossRef]
19. Lenhard, M.S.; Johnson, T.R.; Weckbach, S.; Nikolaou, K.; Friese, K.; Hasbargen, U. Pelvimetry revisited: Analyzing cephalopelvic disproportion. *Eur. J. Radiol.* **2010**, *74*, e107–e111. [CrossRef]
20. Anderson, N.; Humphries, N.; Wells, J. Measurement error in computed tomography pelvimetry. *Australas. Radiol.* **2005**, *49*, 104–107. [CrossRef]
21. Korhonen, U.; Solja, R.; Laitinen, J.; Heinonen, S.; Taipale, P. MR pelvimetry measurements, analysis of inter-and intra-observer variation. *Eur. J. Radiol.* **2010**, *75*, e56–e61. [CrossRef]
22. Atasoy, G.; Arslan, N.C.; Elibol, F.D.; Sagol, O.; Obuz, F.; Sokmen, S. Magnetic resonance-based pelvimetry and tumor volumetry can predict surgical difficulty and oncological outcome in locally advanced mid–low rectal cancer. *Surg. Today* **2018**, *48*, 1040–1051. [CrossRef]
23. Onal, S.; Lai-Yuen, S.; Hart, S.; Bao, P.; Weitzenfeld, A. MRI-based semi-automatic pelvimetry measurement for pelvic organ prolapse diagnosis. In Proceedings of the 2012 11th International Conference on Information Science, Signal Processing and their Applications (ISSPA), Montreal, QC, Canada, 2–5 July 2012; pp. 804–808.
24. Gao, Q.; Ali, S.M.; Edwards, P. Automated atlas-based pelvimetry using hybrid registration. In Proceedings of the 2013 IEEE 10th International Symposium on Biomedical Imaging, San Francisco, CA, USA, 7–11 April 2013; pp. 1292–1295.
25. Yang, D.; Zhang, S.; Yan, Z.; Tan, C.; Li, K.; Metaxas, D. Automated anatomical landmark detection on distal femur surface using convolutional neural network. In Proceedings of the 2015 IEEE 12th International Symposium on Biomedical Imaging (ISBI), Brooklyn, NY, USA, 16–19 April 2015; pp. 17–21.
26. Kai, S.; Sato, T.; Koga, Y.; Omori, G.; Kobayashi, K.; Sakamoto, M.; Tanabe, Y. Automatic construction of an anatomical coordinate system for three-dimensional bone models of the lower extremities–pelvis, femur, and tibia. *J. Biomech.* **2014**, *47*, 1229–1233. [CrossRef]
27. Pieper, S.; Halle, M.; Kikinis, R. 3D Slicer. In Proceedings of the 2004 2nd IEEE International Symposium on Biomedical Imaging: Nano to Macro (IEEE Cat No. 04EX821), Arlington, VA, USA, 18 April 2004; pp. 632–635.
28. Lorensen, W.E.; Cline, H.E. Marching cubes: A high resolution 3D surface construction algorithm. *ACM Siggraph Comput. Graph.* **1987**, *21*, 163–169. [CrossRef]
29. Dice, L.R. Measures of the amount of ecologic association between species. *Ecology* **1945**, *26*, 297–302. [CrossRef]
30. Sørensen, T.J. *A Method of Establishing Groups of Equal Amplitude in Plant Sociology Based on Similarity of Species Content and Its Application to Analyses of the Vegetation on Danish Commons*; I kommission hos E. Munksgaard: Copenhagen, Denmark, 1948.
31. Aspert, N.; Santa-Cruz, D.; Ebrahimi, T. Mesh: Measuring errors between surfaces using the hausdorff distance. In Proceedings of the Proceedings. IEEE International Conference on Multimedia and Expo, Lausanne, Switzerland, 26–29 August 2002; pp. 705–708.
32. Buli, H.C. Pelvimetry in obstetrics. *Postgrad. Med. J.* **1949**, *25*, 310. [CrossRef]
33. Sako, N.; Kaku, N.; Kubota, Y.; Kitahara, Y.; Tagomori, H.; Tsumura, H. Iliac anatomy in women with developmental dysplasia of the hip: Measurements using three-dimensional computed tomography. *J. Orthop.* **2021**, *25*, 1–5. [CrossRef]
34. Terrier, A.; Parvex, V.; Rüdiger, H.A. Impact of individual anatomy on the benefit of cup medialisation in total hip arthroplasty. *Hip Int.* **2016**, *26*, 537–542. [CrossRef]
35. Bartko, J.J. The intraclass correlation coefficient as a measure of reliability. *Psychol. Rep.* **1966**, *19*, 3–11. [CrossRef]
36. Stratford, P.W.; Goldsmith, C.H. Use of the standard error as a reliability index of interest: An applied example using elbow flexor strength data. *Phys. Ther.* **1997**, *77*, 745–750. [CrossRef]
37. Koo, T.K.; Li, M.Y. A guideline of selecting and reporting intraclass correlation coefficients for reliability research. *J. Chiropr. Med.* **2016**, *15*, 155–163. [CrossRef]
38. Castellani, U.; Bartoli, A. 3d shape registration. In *3D Imaging, Analysis and Applications*; Springer: Berlin/Heidelberg, Germany, 2020; pp. 353–411.
39. Meller, S.; Kalender, W.A. Building a statistical shape model of the pelvis. In *International Congress Series*; Elsevier: Amsterdam, The Netherlands, 2004; pp. 561–566.
40. Woolson, R.F. Wilcoxon Signed-Rank Test. In *Wiley Encyclopedia of Clinical Trials*; Wiley: Hoboken, NJ, USA, 2007; pp. 1–3.
41. D'Agostino, R.B. Tests for the normal distribution. In *Goodness-of-Fit Techniques*; Routledge: Abingdon, UK, 2017; pp. 367–420.
42. Mujugira, A.; Osoti, A.; Deya, R.; Hawes, S.E.; Phipps, A.I. Fetal head circumference, operative delivery, and fetal outcomes: A multi-ethnic population-based cohort study. *BMC Pregnancy Childbirth* **2013**, *13*, 106. [CrossRef]

43. Lorenzon, L.; Bini, F.; Landolfi, F.; Quinzi, S.; Balducci, G.; Marinozzi, F.; Biondi, A.; Persiani, R.; D'Ugo, D.; Tirelli, F. 3D pelvimetry and biometric measurements: A surgical perspective for colorectal resections. *Int. J. Color. Dis.* **2021**, *36*, 977–986. [CrossRef]
44. Dandachli, W.; Ul Islam, S.; Tippett, R.; Hall-Craggs, M.A.; Witt, J.D. Analysis of acetabular version in the native hip: Comparison between 2D axial CT and 3D CT measurements. *Skelet. Radiol.* **2011**, *40*, 877–883. [CrossRef]
45. Wang, R.; Xu, W.; Kong, X.; Yang, L.; Yang, S. Measurement of acetabular inclination and anteversion via CT generated 3D pelvic model. *BMC Musculoskelet. Disord.* **2017**, *18*, 373. [CrossRef]
46. Seim, H.; Kainmueller, D.; Heller, M.; Lamecker, H.; Zachow, S.; Hege, H.-C. Automatic Segmentation of the Pelvic Bones from CT Data Based on a Statistical Shape Model. *VCBM* **2008**, *8*, 93–100.
47. Hemke, R.; Buckless, C.G.; Tsao, A.; Wang, B.; Torriani, M. Deep learning for automated segmentation of pelvic muscles, fat, and bone from CT studies for body composition assessment. *Skelet. Radiol.* **2020**, *49*, 387–395. [CrossRef]
48. Barratt, D.C.; Chan, C.S.; Edwards, P.J.; Penney, G.P.; Slomczykowski, M.; Carter, T.J.; Hawkes, D.J. Instantiation and registration of statistical shape models of the femur and pelvis using 3D ultrasound imaging. *Med. Image Anal.* **2008**, *12*, 358–374. [CrossRef]
49. Prevost, R.; Salehi, M.; Jagoda, S.; Kumar, N.; Sprung, J.; Ladikos, A.; Bauer, R.; Zettinig, O.; Wein, W. 3D freehand ultrasound without external tracking using deep learning. *Med. Image Anal.* **2018**, *48*, 187–202. [CrossRef]

Disclaimer/Publisher's Note: The statements, opinions and data contained in all publications are solely those of the individual author(s) and contributor(s) and not of MDPI and/or the editor(s). MDPI and/or the editor(s) disclaim responsibility for any injury to people or property resulting from any ideas, methods, instructions or products referred to in the content.

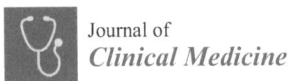

Article

Maternal Stress, Anxiety, Well-Being, and Sleep Quality in Pregnant Women throughout Gestation

Rosalia Pascal [1,2,3,†], Irene Casas [1,4,†], Mariona Genero [1,3,†], Ayako Nakaki [1,4], Lina Youssef [1,4,5], Marta Larroya [1,4], Leticia Benitez [1,4], Yvan Gomez [1], Anabel Martinez-Aran [6], Ivette Morilla [6], Teresa M. Oller-Guzmán [7], Andrés Martín-Asuero [7], Eduard Vieta [6], Fàtima Crispi [1,4,8], Eduard Gratacos [1,3,4,8], María Dolores Gomez-Roig [1,2,3,‡] and Francesca Crovetto [1,2,3,*,‡]

1. BCNatal (Hospital Sant Joan de Déu and Hospital Clínic), University of Barcelona, Passeig Sant Joan de Déu, 2, 08959 Esplugues de Llobregat, Spain; rosalia.pascal@sjd.es (R.P.); irene.casas@sjd.es (I.C.); mariona.genero@sjd.es (M.G.); lyoussef@recerca.clinic.cat (L.Y.); larroya@clinic.cat (M.L.); lbenitez@clinic.cat (L.B.); yvan.gomez@chuv.ch (Y.G.); fcrispi@clinic.cat (F.C.); egratacos@ub.edu (E.G.); lola.gomezroig@sjd.es (M.D.G.-R.)
2. Primary Care Interventions to Prevent Maternal and Child Chronic Diseases of Perinatal and Development Origin, RD21/0012/0003, Instituto de Salud Carlos III, 28040 Barcelona, Spain
3. Institut de Recerca Sant Joan de Déu (IRSJD), 08950 Barcelona, Spain
4. Institut D'investigacions Biomèdiques August Pi Sunyer (IDIBAPS), 08036 Barcelona, Spain
5. Josep Carreras Leukaemia Research Institute, Hospital Clinic/University of Barcelona Campus, 08036 Barcelona, Spain
6. Department of Psychiatry and Psychology, Hospital Clinic, Neuroscience Insititute, IDIBAPS, University of Barcelona CIBERSAM, 08035 Barcelona, Spain; amartiar@clinic.cat (A.M.-A.); imorilla@clinic.cat (I.M.); evieta@clinic.cat (E.V.)
7. Instituto esMindfulness, 08015 Barcelona, Spain; m.teresa@esmindfulness.com (T.M.O.-G.); andres@esmindfulness.com (A.M.-A.)
8. Center for Biomedical Network Research on Rare Diseases, 28029 Madrid, Spain
* Correspondence: francesca.crovetto@sjd.es
† These authors contributed equally to this work.
‡ These authors also contributed equally to this work.

Abstract: Background: Maternal stress, anxiety, well-being, and sleep quality during pregnancy have been described as influencing factors during pregnancy. Aim: We aimed to describe maternal stress, anxiety, well-being, and sleep quality in pregnant women throughout gestation and their related factors. Methods: A prospective study including pregnant women attending BCNatal, in Barcelona, Spain ($n = 630$). Maternal stress and anxiety were assessed by the Perceived Stress Scale (PSS) and State-Trait Anxiety Inventory (STAI)-validated questionnaires. Maternal well-being was assessed using the World Health Organization Well-Being Index Questionnaire (WHO-5), and sleep quality was assessed using the Pittsburgh Sleep Quality Index Questionnaire (PSQI). All questionnaires were obtained twice during the second and third trimester of pregnancy. A multivariate analysis was conducted to assess factors related to higher maternal stress and anxiety and worse well-being and sleep quality. Results: High levels of maternal stress were reported in 23.1% of participants at the end of pregnancy, with maternal age <40 years (OR 2.02; 95% CI 1.08–3.81, $p = 0.03$), non-white ethnicity (OR 2.09; 95% CI 1.19–4.02, $p = 0.01$), and non-university studies (OR 1.86; 95% CI 1.08–3.19, $p = 0.02$) being the parameters mostly associated with it. A total of 20.7% of women had high levels of anxiety in the third trimester and the presence of psychiatric disorders (OR 3.62; 95% CI 1.34–9.78, $p = 0.01$) and non-university studies (OR 1.70; 95% CI 1.11–2.59, $p = 0.01$) provided a significant contribution to high anxiety at multivariate analysis. Poor maternal well-being was observed in 26.5% of women and a significant contribution was provided by the presence of psychiatric disorders (OR 2.96; 95% CI 1.07–8.25, $p = 0.04$) and non-university studies (OR 1.74; 95% CI 1.10–2.74, $p = 0.02$). Finally, less sleep quality was observed at the end of pregnancy ($p < 0.001$), with 81.1% of women reporting poor sleep quality. Conclusion: Maternal stress and anxiety, compromised maternal well-being, and sleep quality disturbances are prevalent throughout pregnancy. Anxiety and compromised sleep quality may increase over gestation. The screening of these conditions at different stages of pregnancy and awareness of the associated risk factors can help to identify women at potential risk.

Citation: Pascal, R.; Casas, I.; Genero, M.; Nakaki, A.; Youssef, L.; Larroya, M.; Benitez, L.; Gomez, Y.; Martinez-Aran, A.; Morilla, I.; et al. Maternal Stress, Anxiety, Well-Being, and Sleep Quality in Pregnant Women throughout Gestation. *J. Clin. Med.* 2023, 12, 7333. https://doi.org/10.3390/jcm12237333

Academic Editors: Apostolos Mamopoulos and Ioannis Tsakiridis

Received: 18 October 2023
Revised: 24 November 2023
Accepted: 24 November 2023
Published: 26 November 2023

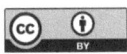

Copyright: © 2023 by the authors. Licensee MDPI, Basel, Switzerland. This article is an open access article distributed under the terms and conditions of the Creative Commons Attribution (CC BY) license (https://creativecommons.org/licenses/by/4.0/).

Keywords: mental stress; anxiety; well-being; sleep quality; pregnancy

1. Introduction

According to the World Health Organization (WHO), health is a "state of complete physical, mental, and social well-being, and not merely the absence of disease or infirmity". Therefore, mental health, defined by the WHO as a "state of mental well-being that enables people to cope with the stresses of life, realize their abilities, learn well and work well, and contribute to their community", is as fundamental as physical health in the achievement of positive overall wellness in an individual [1].

Stress, anxiety, compromised mental well-being, and sleep quality are fundamental and interconnected aspects of mental health. They can impact each other and together contribute to a general state of emotional and mental wellness. Mental stress can be medically understood as the 'individual's perception of a stimulus as overwhelming' which results in a response and a transformed state [2]. Anxiety is defined by the American Psychological Association as "an emotion characterized by feelings of tension, worried thoughts, and physical changes like increased blood pressure." Both stress and anxiety are emotional responses. Stress is usually precipitated by an external factor, whereas anxiety is defined by the persistence of excessive worries even in the absence of a stressor. Well-being is broadly defined as 'the quality and state of a person's life' [3] and consists of two components: feeling healthy and relatively robust and being able to carry out one's job and other tasks satisfactorily [4]. Finally, sleep quality is defined as an individual's level of satisfaction with all aspects of the sleep experience [5]. Sleep quality is highly dependent on the person's general well-being.

Maternal mental stress, anxiety, compromised well-being, and sleep quality have been associated with several adverse pregnancy outcomes such as preterm birth (PTB) [6–12], low birthweight (LBW) [7,13–15], gestational diabetes (GD) [16,17], labor complications [12,18–21], or hypertension and preeclampsia (PE) [22,23]. Moreover, maternal stress has been demonstrated to be a prenatal programming factor that affects the fetal neurodevelopment [24] and could compromise the socioemotional competencies in childhood that are the foundation for future well-being [24].

Mental stress, anxiety, compromised well-being, and sleep disturbances are common during pregnancy. Around 20% of pregnant women could experience excessive concern regarding future events in pregnancy under normal circumstances [4]. Up to 70% of pregnant women report symptoms of stress and anxiety during pregnancy, with between 10% and 16% of them fulfilling the criteria for a major depressive disorder [25,26]. While the real prevalence of antenatal psychosocial stress is still unclear [27], in a 2003 study, Rondó et al. found high stress in 22–25% of pregnant women during the three trimesters of pregnancy [7]. In a meta-analysis of 102 studies involving 221,974 women, Dennis et al. found that the prevalence rate for self-reported anxiety symptoms in the first trimester was 18.2% and 24.6% in the third trimester [28]. These percentages decreased when employing diagnostic interviews: the prevalence rate for any anxiety disorder during the first trimester was 18% and 15% in the final two trimesters of pregnancy [28]. However, we can speculate that the symptoms of depression can overlap with some normal feelings during pregnancy, which could explain such high percentages and the disparity found among studies [26]. There is no clear evidence of the prevalence of compromised well-being during pregnancy. A highly variable prevalence of poor sleep quality in pregnant women has also been reported, ranging from 17% to 76% [29]. This disparity could be due to dissimilar sample compositions and different methods and timings of assessments [30]. Moreover, some authors have even postulated the possibility that the previously validated cut-off values for sleep questionnaires in the general population may not be valid in pregnancy, thus requiring a higher score [30].

Different risk factors for antenatal mood disorders have been postulated in the previously published literature. Sociodemographic variables such as age have been considered in multiple studies with inconsistent findings among them [31,32]. Other sociodemographic variables considered in the previous literature are maternal socioeconomic status and educational level: in a 2010 systematic review, Lancaster et al. found a small association between low educational level and depression symptoms that could not be demonstrated in the multivariate analyses [33]. Later, Biaggi et al. found low maternal educational level to be associated with anxiety and depressive symptoms [32]. As for ethnicity, socioeconomic status, employment, an unfavorable socioeconomic situation, unemployment, and belonging to a minority ethnic group are associated with depression in several studies [31,32,34] but inconsistent results are described in others [32,33]. On the other hand, other factors such as smoking, alcohol intake, and drug abuse showed inconsistent findings in their association with depression and sleep quality [29,32–34]. A personal medical history of anxiety and depression has strongly been associated with perinatal depression [31–34]. Other studies suggest an association between previous obstetric history, like previous abortions or pregnancy complications, with depressive symptoms and poor sleep quality [29,31,32] but also with inconsistent findings [33]. A complex multifactorial origin for the etiology of these conditions could be a possible explanation for such different results reported in the literature [33].

Despite the high prevalence of these antenatal negative affective states and their impact on pregnancy, it is still unclear if they worsened during pregnancy and what the potential risk factors for these conditions are during pregnancy.

The aim of this study was to determine maternal stress, anxiety, well-being, and sleep quality across different stages of pregnancy and to identify related risk factors.

2. Materials and Methods

2.1. Study Design and Participants

A prospective study was carried out at BCNatal (Hospital Clinic and Hospital Sant Joan de Déu), a large referral center for maternal-fetal and neonatal medicine in Barcelona, Spain. Inclusion criteria were pregnant women with a singleton fetus who attended our center for their second trimester scan (19–23 weeks of gestation), and who were able to respond to maternal stress, anxiety, well-being, and sleep quality validated questionnaires. The exclusion criteria for the study are as follows: maternal mental retardation or other mental or psychiatric disorders that raise doubts regarding the patient's real willingness to participate in the study and the impossibility of completing questionnaires or other procedures in the study, congenital infections, fetal anomalies including chromosomal abnormalities or structural malformations detected by ultrasound prenatally, and neonatal abnormalities diagnosed after birth. The study was approved by the hospital ethical committee (HCB-2016-0830 and HCB/2020/0209) and written informed consent was obtained from all participants.

2.2. Study Aims

The main aim of the study was to evaluate maternal stress, anxiety, well-being, and sleep quality at two moments during pregnancy, assessed using four different validated questionnaires: the Perceived Stress Scale (PSS) [35] and State-Trait Anxiety Inventory (STAI) [36] for maternal stress and anxiety, respectively, the World Health Organization Well-Being Index Questionnaire (WHO-5 Index) for maternal well-being [37], and the Pittsburgh Sleep Quality Index (PSQI) [38] for sleep quality.

The secondary aim was to evaluate maternal and pregnancy factors acting as potential risk factors for increased maternal stress and anxiety, poorer maternal well-being status, and poorer sleep quality during gestation.

2.3. Data Collection

All questionnaires were completed twice during pregnancy: at recruitment of the study population in their second trimester of pregnancy (19–23 weeks of gestation) and again at the end of the third trimester of pregnancy (34–36 weeks of gestation).

The Perceived Stress Scale was designed to measure "the degree to which individuals appraise situations in their lives as stressful" [35]. It is a brief scale, consisting of only 14 items evaluating stress within the last 8 weeks. PSS scores are obtained by reversing responses to the 4 positively stated items (items 4, 5, 7, and 8) and then adding across all scale items. It is not a diagnostic instrument; therefore, there are no cut-offs for classification of the stress, but it gives a comparison instrument between people [39]. The higher stress group in this cohort was considered the 75th percentile at the first evaluation (19–23 weeks of gestation).

The STAI questionnaire consists of two subscales: the State Anxiety Scale (STAI-S), which evaluates the current state of anxiety, and the Trait Anxiety Scale (STAI-T), which evaluates individual aspects of "anxiety proneness". The STAI has 40 items, 20 items allocated to each of the S-State and T-Trait subscales. The range of scores for each subtest is 20–80, the higher indicating greater anxiety [40,41]. The higher stress group in this cohort was considered the 75th percentile at the first evaluation (19–23 weeks of gestation).

The WHO-5 consists of a five-item scale and it is used to rate quality of life and psychological well-being, according to the participant's feelings within the last 15 days. The raw score ranges from 0 to 25: 0 representing worst possible and 25 representing best possible quality of life. Following total scores, standardized scores (0–100) are calculated. Women were classified according to their well-being status as with a poor ($\leq$52) or favorable (>52) WHO-5 score [42].

The PSQI assesses sleep quality and disturbances over a monthly interval. It contains 19 self-rated questions which are combined to form 7 component scores: subjective sleep quality, sleep latency, sleep duration, habitual sleep efficiency, sleep disturbances, use of sleeping medication, and daytime dysfunction. Each of these components has a range of 0–3 points (where 0 means no difficulty and 3 indicates severe difficulty). The 7 component scores are added to give a global score, with a range of 0–21 points, 0 indicating no difficulty and 21 indicating severe difficulties in all areas. A global PSQI score greater than 5 defines poor sleep quality [38].

Baseline and socioeconomic characteristics, such as maternal age, ethnicity, educational level, or pre-pregnancy body mass index (BMI) were obtained from a structured questionnaire. Medical and obstetric history were obtained from the medical records at recruitment.

2.4. Statistical Analysis

For the first aim, the analysis was based on the scores of PSS, STAI-S, STAI-T, WHO-5, and PSQI-validated questionnaires. Continuous variables were assessed for normality using the Shapiro–Wilk's test. Normally distributed variables were compared using a t-test and expressed as mean and standard deviation (SD). Non-normally distributed variables were compared using the U–Mann–Whitney test and expressed as the median and interquartile range (IQR). Categorical variables were compared using χ^2 or Fisher's exact test where appropriate. To study the correlation of the different tests, Pearson correlation analyses were performed. For the secondary outcomes, logistic regression analysis with forward stepwise selection was performed to assess the association between maternal higher stress (>p75) (PSS, STAI-S, STAI-T), poor well-being ($\leq$52 WHO-5), and lower sleep quality (>5 PSQI), with potential maternal risk factors at final evaluation (34–36 weeks of gestation). A multivariate analysis was performed for the variables found to have a significant effect in bivariate analyses. The odds ratio (OR) and a 95% confidence interval (95% CI) were calculated. A p-value < 0.05 was considered statistically significant. The analysis was performed using SPSS v26 (New York, NY, USA).

3. Results

3.1. Study Population

A total of 630 women were recruited in the second trimester at a median [IQR] gestational age of 20 weeks [20,21]). The majority of women (n = 497, 79.3%) were of white ethnicity and with university studies (n = 427, 68%). Baseline characteristics of the study population are shown in Table 1. Regarding their medical history, 2.7% of women (n = 17) had psychiatric disorders requiring therapy, 5.6% (n = 35) had thyroid disorders, and 7.8% (n = 49) had a BMI ≥ 30.

Table 1. Baseline characteristics of participants included in the study (n = 630).

Characteristics	Total Cohort n = 630
Age at recruitment (years)	35.8 (32.2–38.7)
Ethnicity	
White	497 (79.3%)
Latin	98 (15.6%)
Afro-American	6 (1%)
Asian	16 (2.6%)
Others	10 (1.6%)
Low socioeconomic status [a]	25 (4%)
Study class	
Primary	25 (4%)
Secondary	176 (28%)
University	427 (68%)
BMI before pregnancy (Kg/m^2)	23.4 (4.1)
Medical history	
Autoimmune disease	64 (10.2%)
Obesity (BMI ≥ 30)	49 (7.8%)
Thyroid disorders	35 (5.6%)
Chronic hypertension	18 (2.9%)
Psychiatric disorders [b]	17 (2.7%)
Diabetes mellitus	14 (2.2%)
Chronic kidney disease	8 (1.3%)
Obstetric history	
Nulliparous	393 (62.4%)
Previous preeclampsia	17 (2.7%)
Previous stillbirth	5 (0.8%)
Use of assisted reproductive technologies	121 (19.2%)
Cigarette smoking during pregnancy	81 (12.9%)
Alcohol intake during pregnancy	14 (2.2%)
Drug consumption during pregnancy	15 (2.4%)
Sports practice during pregnancy	103 (16.3%)
Yoga or Pilates during pregnancy	141 (22.4%)

BMI: body-mass index. Data are expressed as median (IQR) or mean (SD) or n (%). [a] Low socioeconomic status: low (never worked or unemployed >2 years). [b] Psychiatric disorders: requiring therapy for psychiatric disorder.

3.2. Stress, Anxiety, Well-Being, and Sleep Quality throughout Pregnancy

The median [IQR] scores of the PSS at the second trimester evaluation was 16 (11–22), and it did not change during pregnancy, as reported in Table 2 and Figure 1A. No changes during gestation were found for STAI-T and for the well-being evaluation (WHO-5) (see Table 2 and Figure 1B,C). On the contrary, an increasing score during the third trimester was observed for the STAI-S ($p < 0.001$) and PSQI questionnaires ($p < 0.001$) (see Table 2 and Figure 1D,E).

The correlation between the final results of the stress and anxiety tests was calculated by the Pearson correlation coefficient, which showed a significative positive strong correlation between the levels of stress and anxiety (PSS vs. STAI-S, $r = 0.72$, $p < 0.001$; PSS vs. STAI-T, $r = 0.69$, $p < 0.001$; STAI-T vs. STAI-S, $r = 0.75$, $p < 0.001$). A significative negative moderate correlation was observed between WHO-5 and the stress and anxiety tests, highlighting poorer mental well-being in relation to higher levels of anxiety and stress (WHO-5 vs. PSS, r = −0.58, $p < 0.001$; WHO-5 vs. STAI-S, r = −0.63, $p < 0.001$; WHO-5 vs. STAI-T, r = −0.65, $p < 0.001$). Finally, the correlation found between sleep quality and stress, anxiety, and mental well-being was low (PSQI vs. STAI-S, r = 0.31, $p < 0.001$; PSQI vs. STAI-T, r = 0.34, $p < 0.001$; PSQI vs. PSS, r = 0.33, $p < 0.001$; PSQI vs. WHO-5, r = 0.40, $p < 0.001$).

Table 2. Stress, anxiety, and sleep quality of women included in the study at second and third trimester of pregnancy (n = 630).

Characteristics	2nd Trimester n = 630	3rd Trimester n = 630	p Value
Perceived stress scale score	16 (11–22)	16 (12–23)	0.07
State-trait Anxiety Inventory (anxiety)	13 (8–18)	14 (9–20)	<0.001
State-trait Anxiety Inventory (personality)	14 (10–21)	15 (10–21)	0.88
Five well-being Index	68 (56–76)	64 (52–76)	0.81
Pittsburg quality sleep index	7 (5–8.5)	8 (9–10)	<0.001

Data are expressed as median (IQR).

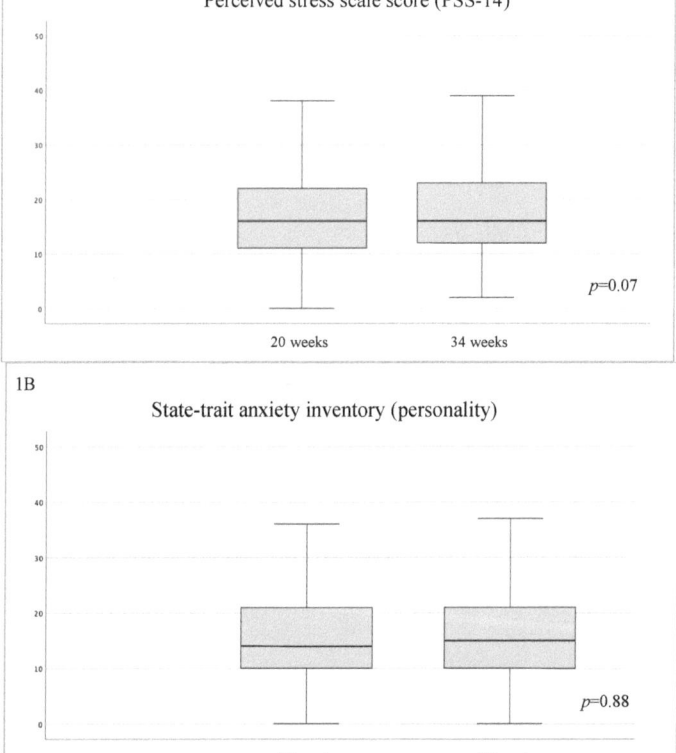

Figure 1. Cont.

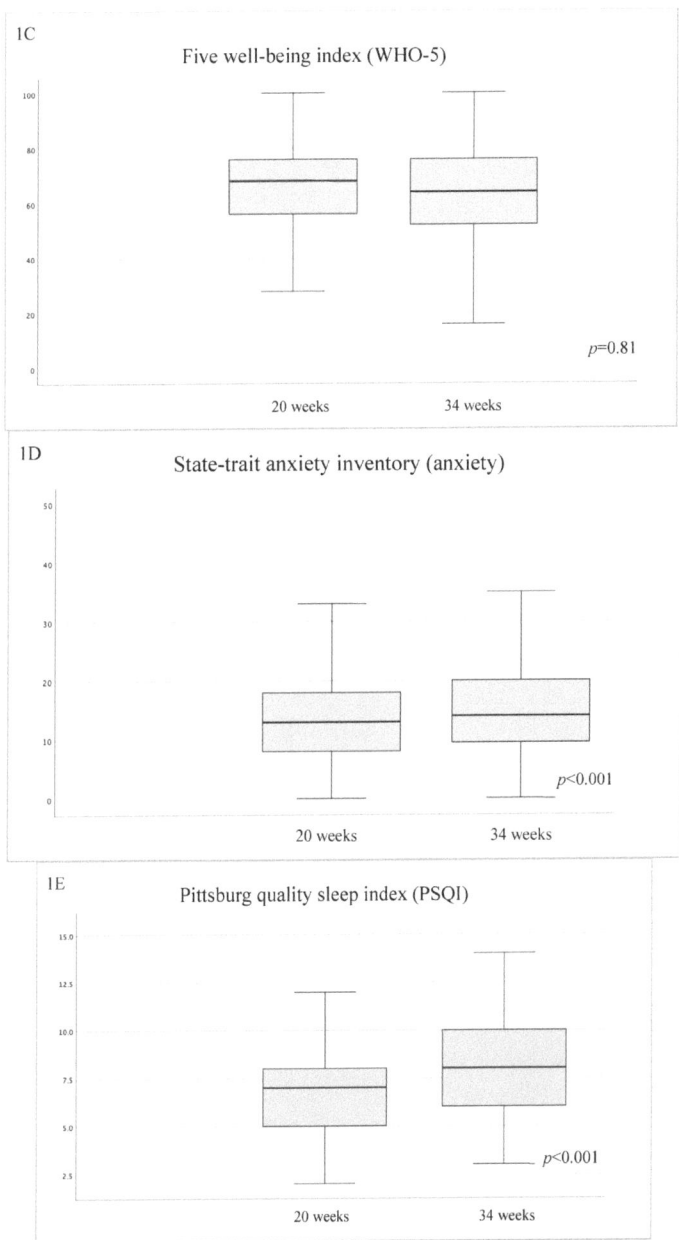

Figure 1. (**A**) Evolution in PSS-14 test score at baseline (20 weeks) and at the end of gestation (34 weeks). The median (IQR) scores of the PSS at second trimester evaluation was 16 (11–22) and it did not change during pregnancy. (**B**) Evolution in STAI-T test score at baseline (20 weeks) and at the end of gestation (34 weeks). No changes during gestation were found. (**C**) Evolution in WHO-5 test score at baseline (20 weeks) and at the end of gestation (34 weeks). No changes during gestation were found. (**D**) Evolution in STAI-S test score at baseline (20 weeks) and at the end of gestation (34 weeks). An increased score during the third trimester was observed. (**E**) Evolution in PSQI test score at baseline (20 weeks) and at the end of gestation (34 weeks). An increased score during the third trimester was observed.

3.3. Maternal Stress and Anxiety

High levels of maternal PSS were reported in 115 women (23.1%) at the end of pregnancy. At multivariate analysis, a significant contribution to this condition was provided by maternal age <40 years (OR 2.02; 95% CI 1.08–3.81, p = 0.03), non-white ethnicity (OR 2.09; 95% CI 1.19–4.02, p = 0.01), and non-university studies (OR 1.86; 95% CI 1.08–3.19, p = 0.02). Details are reported in Table 3.

Table 3. Univariate and multivariate analysis of factors associated with a poor maternal PSS-14 questionnaire.

Characteristics	Univariate Analysis OR (95% CI)	p Value	Multivariate Analysis OR (95% CI)	p Value	Beta Coefficient
Maternal age < 40 years	2.24 (1.21–4.15)	0.01	2.01 (1.08–3.81)	0.03	0.705
Ethnicity					
White	0.42 (0.26–0.69)	<0.001			
Non-white	2.36 (1.45–3.83)	<0.001	2.19 (1.19–4.02)	0.01	0.786
Low socioeconomic status [a]	1.82 (0.75–4.41)	0.18			
Study class					
Primary or secondary	2.19 (1.43–3.39)	<0.001	1.86 (1.08–3.19)	0.02	0.620
University	0.46 (0.30–0.70)	<0.001			
Medical history					
Obesity (BMI ≥ 30)	1.27 (0.633–2.56)	0.5			
Diabetes mellitus	1.34 (0.41–4.35)	1.34			
Autoimmune disease	1.15 (0.63–2.12)	0.65			
Thyroid disorders	0.53 (0.20–1.41)	0.2			
Psychiatric disorders [b]	1.85 (0.67–5.13)	0.233			
Chronic hypertension	0.66 (0.19–2.3)	0.51			
Obstetric history					
Nulliparous	1.11 (0.73–1.71)	0.62			
Previous preeclampsia	3 (1.17–8.22)	0.02	2.7 (0.98–7.46)	0.06	0.993
Use of assisted reproductive technologies	0.58 (0.34–1.01)	0.06			
Cigarette smoking during pregnancy	0.93 (0.52–1.67)	0.81			
Alcohol intake during pregnancy	1.18 (0.74–1.87)	0.5			
Drug consumption during pregnancy	1.89 (0.62–5.75)	0.26			
Yoga or Pilates during pregnancy	0.73 (0.43–1.23)	0.24			
Constant			−2.204		
Data are expressed as n (%)					

PSS: Perceived Stress Scale; OR: Odds Ratio; CI: confidence interval; BMI: body-mass index. [a] Low socioeconomic status: low (never worked or unemployed >2 years). [b] Psychiatric disorders: requiring therapy for psychiatric disorder.

According to the STAI questionnaire (anxiety, STAI-S), 129 women (20.7%) had high levels of anxiety in the third trimester. In these women, a significant contribution to multivariate analysis was provided by the presence of psychiatric disorders (OR 3.62; 95% CI 1.34–9.78, p = 0.01), and non-university studies (OR 1.70; 95% CI 1.11–2.59, p = 0.01). Details are reported in Table 4.

According to the STAI-T personality questionnaire, 116 women (23.6%) ended pregnancy with a high anxiety trait level. In the multivariate analysis, a significant contribution to this condition was provided by maternal age <40 years (OR 2.07; 95% CI 1.11–3.88, p = 0.02) and preeclampsia in a previous pregnancy (OR 2.9; 95% CI 1.03–8.2, p = 0.04). Details are reported in Table 5.

3.4. Maternal Well-Being

Poor maternal well-being (WHO-5 score ≤52) was observed in 131 women (26.5%) in the 3rd trimester assessment. Significant contribution to a low maternal well-being was provided by the presence of psychiatric disorders (OR 2.96; 95% CI 1.07–8.25, p = 0.04), and non-university studies (OR 1.74; 95% CI 1.10–2.74, p = 0.02). Details are reported in Table 6.

Table 4. Univariate and multivariate analysis of factors associated with a poor maternal STAI anxiety questionnaire.

Characteristics	Univariate Analysis OR (95% CI)	p Value	Multivariate Analysis OR (95% CI)	p Value	Beta Coefficient
Maternal age < 40 years	1.69 (0.92–3.12)	0.09			
Ethnicity					
White	0.7 (0.44–1.1)	0.12			
Non-white	1.43 (0.91–2.26)	0.12			
Low socioeconomic status [a]	0.76 (0.26–2.27)	0.63			
Study class					
Primary or secondary	1.75 (1.17–2.61)	0.01	1.70 (1.11–2.59)	0.01	0.529
University	0.57 (0.38–0.85)	0.01			
Medical history					
Obesity (BMI $\geq$ 30)	1.01 (0.49–2.09)	0.97			
Diabetes mellitus	1.05 (0.29–3.8)	0.95			
Autoimmune disease	1.81 (1.02–3.23)	0.04	1.56 (0.84–2.89)	0.16	0.446
Thyroid disorders	2.1 (1.02–4.34)	0.04	1.81 (0.84–3.90)	0.13	0.595
Psychiatric disorders [b]	3.56 (1.35–9.42)	0.01	3.62 (1.34–9.78)	0.01	1288
Chronic hypertension	0.76 (0.22–2.67)	0.67			
Chronic kidney disease	1.28 (0.25–6.42)	0.76			
Obstetric history					
Nulliparous	1.43 (0.96–2.12)	0.07			
Previous preeclampsia	1.77 (0.6–5.19)	0.3			
Previous stillbirth	0.96 (0.11–8.63)	0.97			
Use of assisted reproductive technologies	0.64 (0.37–1.01)	0.11			
Cigarette smoking during pregnancy	1.13 (0.64–2)	0.67			
Alcohol intake during pregnancy	0.92 (0.59–1.43)	0.72			
Drugs consumption during pregnancy	0.96 (0.27–3.47)	0.96			
Yoga or Pilates during pregnancy	0.5 (0.29–0.85)	0.01	0.62 (0.35–1.1)	0.1	−1.059
Constant			−1.586		

Data are expressed as n (%)

STAI: State-Trait Anxiety Inventory; OR: Odds Ratio; CI: confidence interval; BMI: Body-mass index. [a] Low socioeconomic status: low (never worked or unemployed >2 years). [b] Psychiatric disorders: requiring therapy for psychiatric disorder.

Table 5. Univariate and multivariate analysis of factors associated with a poor maternal STAI personality questionnaire.

Characteristics	Univariate Analysis OR (95% CI)	p Value	Multivariate Analysis OR (95% CI)	p Value	Beta Coefficient
Maternal age < 40 years	2.28 (1.23–4.23)	0.01	2.07 (1.11–3.88)	0.02	0.729
Ethnicity					
White	0.54 (0.33–9.86)	0.02			
Non-white	1.85 (1.13–3.03)	0.02	1.55 (0.83–2.92)	0.17	−0.440
Low socioeconomic status [a]	1.22 (0.47–3.19)	0.68			
Study class					
Primary or secondary	2.09 (1.36–3.22)	0.01	1.42 (0.81–2.49)	0.22	0.350
University	0.48 (0.31–7.36)	0.01			
Medical history					
Obesity (BMI $\geq$ 30)	0.95 (0.45–1.98)	0.88			
Diabetes mellitus	1.83 (0.60–5.58)	0.28			
Autoimmune disease	1.26 (0.69–2.3)	0.45			
Thyroid disorders	0.96 (0.42–2.16)	0.91			
Psychiatric disorders [b]	2.34 (0.87–6.30)	0.09			
Chronic hypertension	0.64 (0.18–2.24)	0.48			
Chronic kidney disease	0.46 (0.05–3.75)	0.47			

Table 5. Cont.

Characteristics	Univariate Analysis OR (95% CI)	p Value	Multivariate Analysis OR (95% CI)	p Value	Beta Coefficient
Obstetric history					
Nulliparous	1.16 (0.76–1.77)	0.50			
Previous preeclampsia	3.4 (1.25–9.27)	0.01	2.9 (1.03–8.2)	0.04	1.069
Previous stillbirth	0.81 (0.09–7.29)	0.85			
Use of assisted reproductive technologies	0.79 (0.47–1.33)	0.37			
Cigarette smoking during pregnancy	1.62 (0.95–2.77)	0.08			
Alcohol intake during pregnancy	0.97 (0.6–1.55)	0.89			
Drugs consumption during pregnancy	1.3 (0.4–4.24)	0.66			
Yoga or Pilates during pregnancy	0.53 (0.3–0.92)	0.03	0.92 (0.46–1.84)	0.82	−0.079
Constant			−1.976		

Data are expressed as n (%)

STAI: State-Trait Anxiety Inventory; OR: Odds Ratio; CI: confidence interval; BMI: body-mass index. [a] Low socioeconomic status: low (never worked or unemployed >2 years). [b] Psychiatric disorders: requiring therapy for psychiatric disorder.

Table 6. Univariate and multivariate analysis of factors associated with poor maternal WHO-5 questionnaire.

Characteristics	Univariate Analysis OR (95% CI)	p Value	Multivariate Analysis OR (95% CI)	p Value	Beta Coefficient
Maternal age < 40 years	1.64 (0.95–2.84)	0.07			
Ethnicity					
White	0.76 (0.46–1.25)	0.28			
Non-white	1.31 (0.80–2.15)	0.28			
Low socioeconomic status [a]	1.51 (0.62–3.64)	0.36			
Study class					
Primary or secondary	1.86 (1.23–282)	0.01	1.74 (1.10–2.74)	0.02	0.553
University	0.54 (0.35–0.82)	0.01			
Medical history					
Obesity (BMI ≥ 30)	2.01 (1.07–3.79)	0.03	1.71 (0.88–3.32)	0.11	0.536
Diabetes mellitus	2.13 (0.72–6.26)	0.17			
Autoimmune disease	1.42 (0.81–2.50)	0.22			
Thyroid disorders	1.29 (0.61–2.72)	0.49			
Psychiatric disorders [b]	3.27 (1.24–8.67)	0.02	2.96 (1.07–8.25)	0.04	1.087
Chronic hypertension	2.29 (0.89–5.95)	0.09			
Chronic kidney disease	0.39 (0.05–3.21)	0.38			
Obstetric history					
Nulliparous	1.49 (0.99–2.23)	0.05	1.26 (0.81–1.94)	0.29	0.231
Previous preeclampsia	1.54 (0.56–4.24)	0.41			
Previous stillbirth	0.69 (0.08–6.23)	0.74			
Assisted reproductive technologies	0.95 (0.58–1.54)	0.82			
Cigarette smoking during pregnancy	1.55 (0.92–2.62)	0.10			
Alcohol intake during pregnancy	1.24 (0.79–1.93)	0.34			
Drug consumption during pregnancy	1.56 (0.51–4.74)	0.43			
Yoga or Pilates during pregnancy	0.54 (0.32–0.91)	0.02	0.66 (0.37–1.17)	0.16	−0.413
Constant			−1.339		

Data are expressed as n (%)

WHO-5: World Health Organization Well-Being Index Questionnaire; OR: Odds Ratio; CI: confidence interval; BMI: body-mass index [a] Low socioeconomic status: low (never worked or unemployed >2 years). [b] Psychiatric disorders: requiring therapy for psychiatric disorder.

3.5. Maternal Sleep Quality

Poor maternal sleep quality affected 309 women (81.1%) at 34–36 weeks of gestation. While non-white ethnicity (OR 2.74; 95% CI 1.13–6.61, $p = 0.03$) and obesity (OR 2.01; 95% CI 1.07–3.79, $p = 0.03$) were significant contributors to low maternal sleep quality in the univariate analysis, in the multivariate analysis no significant contributing factors were found, as reported in Table 7.

Table 7. Univariate and multivariate analysis of factors associated with poor maternal Pittsburg questionnaire.

Characteristics	Univariate Analysis		Multivariate Analysis		
	OR (95% CI)	p Value	OR (95% CI)	p Value	Beta Coefficient
Maternal age < 40 years	1.08 (0.56–2.09)	0.81			
Ethnicity					
White	0.36 (0.15–0.88)	0.03			
Non-white	2.74 (1.13–6.61)	0.03	2.13 (0.86–5.30)	0.10	0.758
Low socioeconomic status [a]	1.18 (0.33–4.2)	0.80			
Study class					
Primary or Secondary	1.96 (1.04–3.69)	0.04	1.91 (0.98–3.77)	0.06	0.649
University	0.51 (0.27–0.96)	0.04			
Medical history					
Obesity (BMI ≥ 30)	3.1 (0.73–13.6)	0.13			
Diabetes mellitus	0.93 (0.19–4.48)	0.93			
Autoimmune disease	1.42 (0.61–3.31)	0.42			
Thyroid disorders	0.64 (0.24–1.69)	0.37			
Psychiatric disorders [b]	2.87 (0.37–22.43)	0.32			
Chronic hypertension	2.37 (0.3–18.9)	0.41			
Chronic kidney disease	0.93 (0.1–8.46)	0.95			
Obstetric history					
Nulliparous	1.16 (0.68–2)	0.59			
Use of assisted reproductive technologies	0.95 (0.51–1.8)	0.88			
Cigarette smoking during pregnancy	0.49 (0.25–0.95)	0.03	0.51 (0.25–1.02)	0.06	−0.676
Alcohol intake during pregnancy	0.76 (0.43–1.32)	0.33			
Drug consumption during pregnancy	1.94 (0.24–15.75)	0.54			
Yoga or Pilates during pregnancy	0.88 (0.48–1.58)	0.65			
Constant			1.183		
Data are expressed as n (%)					

OR: Odds Ratio; CI: confidence interval; BMI: body-mass index. [a] Low socioeconomic status: low (never worked or unemployed >2 years). [b] Psychiatric disorders: requiring therapy for psychiatric disorder.

4. Discussion

Our study reveals the potential importance of assessing antenatal negative affective states in a pregnant population. Stress, anxiety, compromised well-being, and sleep disorders have been reported by a significant number of pregnant participants in our cohort. There is a possible underassessment of these conditions by obstetric-care providers in daily clinical practice and our results stress the importance of actively evaluating signs and symptoms of negative affective states and sleep quality throughout gestation.

Perceived stress and STAI-T did not change throughout pregnancy; however, STAI-S increased in the third trimester of pregnancy. Previously published studies have shown that anxiety and depressive symptoms are not homogeneous during the perinatal period [32,43,44]. Thus, nearly one quarter of participants scored as high stress and anxiety in the third trimester of pregnancy. Such percentages of perceived stress and anxiety highlight the importance of targeting these patients with clinically validated questionnaires in routine pregnancy follow-ups, with the aim of offering support interventions to these patients. Moreover, previous evidence has suggested that pregnancy-related anxiety constitutes a different concept from general anxiety. This fact could be a possible explanation for a limited measurement and assessment of anxiety in pregnancies and could also encourage the need for research in pregnancy-adapted measurement tools [45].

To the best of our knowledge, there are no data regarding the prevalence of compromised well-being in the pregnant population with which to compare our results. However, in a study conducted by Sattler et al. in a group of overweight and obese women in Europe, a prevalence of low well-being of 27% before 20 weeks of pregnancy is reported [46]. Similarly, during the COVID-19 pandemic Mortazavi et al. reported a prevalence of compromised wellbeing of 24.4% pregnant women during gestation [4]. Around 26% of our population had compromised well-being, which is a similar percentage. The WHO-5 questionnaire is considered a good screening questionnaire with high sensitivity and specificity for clinical depression [46]. It has the advantage of being a relatively easy and quick instrument to use in daily clinical practice allowing a first detection of women with a negative affective state who could benefit from a further mental health assessment.

The prevalence of sleep disturbances in our cohort was very high: more than 80% of participants were found to have compromised sleep at 34–36 weeks of gestation. Our prevalence results are higher than expected according to the literature, ranging from 17% to 76% [29]. As suggested in previous studies, this fact could highlight the possibility that the validated cut-off for sleep questionnaires in the general population may not be valid in pregnancies, the latter requiring a higher score [30]. Moreover, we found that the results of sleep quality questionnaires worsened in the third-trimester assessment as compared to the results found in the previous weeks of gestation. The worsening of sleep quality throughout gestation identified in our cohort is in line with previous evidence: according to a meta-analysis of 24 studies, it was found that sleep disturbances tend to increase during pregnancy and clinicians should be aware that complaints of very poor sleep could require intervention [30].

Diagnosis and screening of maternal mental health have long been recommended by scientific societies. For instance, the American College of Obstetricians and Gynecologists recommends the use of a validated and standardized tool to screen pregnant women at least once during the perinatal period for symptoms of depression and anxiety [47]. However, the use of multiple questionnaires to assess maternal mental health and sleep quality can be challenging in daily clinical practice, especially in an environment with a high healthcare workload. Therefore, we believe that understanding the associated risk factors may help to target those patients at higher risk and thus facilitate daily clinical practice as they can be identified at the beginning of pregnancy. Various risk factors for antenatal negative mood states have been postulated in the previous literature [29,31–34].

In our cohort, we found that a main risk factor for maternal perceived stress, a higher level of state anxiety, and poorer well-being in the third trimester was non-university studies. In line with these results, some previous research in the pregnant population had already postulated a low educational profile as a risk factor for antenatal depression [31,32]. However, in contrast to our findings, Lancaster et al. described only a small association of lower educational levels with depressive symptoms in a systematic review [33]. In general, among the non-pregnant population, a low educational level has also been associated with anxiety and depression [48]. Our results could be explained by the fact that, as previously suggested in the literature, normally, education is likely to result in good mental health rather than come from good mental health and, in turn, education may also provide success in pursuing personal ends that include emotional well-being [48,49].

For the STAI-T personality questionnaire, we found preeclampsia in a previous pregnancy to be a potential risk factor. In a systematic review, Grigoriadis et al. found that prenatal maternal anxiety was not significantly associated with preeclampsia, although there was a significant heterogeneity across studies [50]. However, we did not find any data regarding the association between previous preeclampsia and compromised mental health in subsequent pregnancies in the previous literature. A prior history of adverse obstetric events has already been related to the symptoms of anxiety and depression [31,32,51], which could be in line with our results regarding the occurrence of preeclampsia in a previous pregnancy.

Perceived stress was also influenced in our cohort by non-white ethnicity and a maternal age of <40 years, and the latter was also found to be a risk factor for a higher score in trait anxiety among our participants. The literature also provides inconsistent findings as far as maternal age and ethnicity are concerned, as reported in the systematic reviews by Lancaster et al. [33] and Biaggi et al. [32]. In their review, Biaggi et al. described 13 studies where young age was posited as a risk factor, in contrast with 10 studies where advanced maternal age was described as a risk factor for antenatal depression and anxiety [32].

A higher level of anxiety in the third trimester and poorer maternal well-being in the third-trimester assessment were provided by the presence of a previous psychiatric disorder. These results are in line with previously published evidence, as previous mental health disorders have been strongly related to higher anxiety in the past, in particular a history of anxiety and depression and a history of psychiatric treatment [32]. Lancaster et al. also reported an association between a personal history of depression and an increased risk of antepartum depressive symptoms [33]. Multiple studies conducted during the COVID-19 pandemic on maternal mental status proposed the presence of a previous psychiatric disorder as a risk factor for negative maternal affective states [52–55].

As for poor maternal sleep quality, no significant contributing factors were found. These findings are in contrast with those found in previous research where some risk factors could be postulated as contributors to sleep disturbances during pregnancy, such as a history of stillbirth, general health-related quality of life, or insufficient physical activity [29]. Christian et al. found that African-Americans' ethnicity and multiparity were related to poor sleep during pregnancy [56]. Other studies reported gestational age [30] or previous maternal BMI to be contributing factors [57]. Our univariate analysis also suggested ethnicity and obesity to be contributing factors; however, we could not demonstrate it in the multivariate analysis.

Finally, previous research has a well-documented association between anxiety, life stress, sleep quality, and maternal mental well-being [29,32,33]. Our results are in line with previous evidence as we found a correlation between anxiety, stress, and poorer mental well-being. In contrast, we found a low correlation between sleep quality and stress, anxiety, and mental well-being.

On the other hand, despite these associations, we believe the use of four validated questionnaires assessing different dimensions of maternal mental health may provide a more integrative approach to overall mental health, as the absence of problems in one dimension does not necessarily guarantee the same results in other aspects of mental health.

The strengths of this study were the use of various validated questionnaires with potential clinical applicability to assess different aspects of mental health: mental stress, anxiety, well-being, and sleep quality; and that they were assessed in the second and third trimester of pregnancy, which allowed an analysis of the experimented changes throughout pregnancy.

Among the study's limitations is the fact that our population was a high socioeconomic cohort, with a high education profile, and most of the participants were between 30 and 40 years of age, with a low level of ethnical variety and a low proportion of obesity and gestational diabetes. This might explain some of the findings, especially in sleep disturbances, where we could not demonstrate the contribution of these factors in multivariate analysis.

We have no data regarding the first trimester of pregnancy nor the influence that these negative affective states had on perinatal results. Moreover, the neurocognitive function was not assessed, despite its potential influence on mental health [58]. In interpreting the results, it is important to understand that the use of self-reporting instruments may potentially overestimate prevalence, but it is also important to state that they also have high clinical applicability in public health and daily obstetric-care practice. Our study confirms the importance of promoting good mental health [59], especially during pregnancy.

5. Conclusions

Maternal stress and anxiety compromised maternal well-being, and sleep quality disturbances are very frequent and not static throughout pregnancy. Screening for these conditions at different stages of pregnancy should be recommended to professionals providing obstetric care. However, in high-pressure healthcare conditions, universal screening could be challenging; therefore, knowing the risk factors associated with these conditions can help clinicians identify pregnant women at potential risk.

Author Contributions: F.C. (Francesca Crovetto), F.C. (Fàtima Crispi), and E.G. conceived and designed the study; F.C. (Francesca Crovetto) and F.C. (Fàtima Crispi) were responsible for the study protocol and ensured the correct execution of the study; F.C. (Francesca Crovetto) and F.C. (Fàtima Crispi) were the supervisors for the day-to-day running of the study, including participant recruitment and data collection; R.P., M.G., M.L., A.N., L.B., Y.G. and I.C. were responsible for medical file revision and data collection; I.C. and L.Y. performed the data analyses; F.C. (Francesca Crovetto) supervised the data analysis; R.P., M.D.G.-R. and F.C. (Francesca Crovetto) drafted the first version of the manuscript; A.M.-A. (Anabel Martinez-Aran), I.M., T.M.O.-G., A.M.-A. (Andrés Martín-Asuero), E.V. and M.D.G.-R. contributed to the final version of the manuscript. None of the authors received any compensation for their contribution. All authors have read and agreed to the published version of the manuscript.

Funding: This study was partially funded by the "LaCaixa" Foundation under grant agreements LCF/PR/GN14/10270005 and LCF/PR/GN18/10310003, the CEREBRA Foundation for the Brain Injured Child (Carmarthen, Wales, UK) and the Departament de Recerca i Universitats de la Generalitat de Catalunya 2021-SGR-01422. LB and FC have received funding from the Instituto de Salud Carlos III (ISCIII) through the projects CM21/00058 and INT21/00027 which are co-funded by the European Union. Funders played no role in the study's design, data collection, data analysis, data interpretation, or the writing of the manuscript.

Institutional Review Board Statement: The study was conducted in accordance with the Declaration of Helsinki and approved by the Ethics Committee of Hospital Clínic (HCB-2016-0830—date of approval: 16 December 2016 and HCB/2020/0209—date of approval: 12 March 2020).

Informed Consent Statement: Informed consent was obtained from all study participants.

Data Availability Statement: Data available subject to previous ethics committee agreement.

Conflicts of Interest: EG reports grants from the "La Caixa" Foundation during the conduct of the study. EV has received grants and served as a consultant, advisor, or CME speaker for the following entities: AB-Biotics, AbbVie, Adamed, Angelini, Biogen, Biohaven, Boehringer-Ingelheim, Celon Pharma, Compass, Dainippon Sumitomo Pharma, Ethypharm, Ferrer, Gedeon Richter, GH Research, Glaxo-Smith Kline, HMNC, Idorsia, Janssen, Lundbeck, Medincell, Merck, Novartis, Orion Corporation, Organon, Otsuka, Roche, Rovi, Sage, Sanofi-Aventis, Sunovion, Takeda, and Viatris, outside the submitted work. The remaining authors have no conflicts of interest to declare. The funders had no role in the design of the study; in the collection, analyses, or interpretation of data; in the writing of the manuscript, or in the decision to publish the results.

References

1. Barry, S. Mental Health. Available online: https://www.who.int/news-room/fact-sheets/detail/mental-health-strengthening-our-response/?gclid=CjwKCAjw3oqoBhAjEiwA_UaLtg3dLdefpMp9F7CLA{-}{-}-TMdtDcnayk4zxWGnbDRZV9h6RTCQb1AjfhoC28wQAvD_BwE (accessed on 15 September 2023).
2. Goodnite, P.M. Stress: A Concept Analysis. *Nurs. Forum* **2014**, *49*, 71–74. [CrossRef] [PubMed]
3. Linton, M.J.; Dieppe, P.; Medina-Lara, A. Review of 99 self-report measures for assessing well-being in adults: Exploring dimensions of well-being and developments over time. *BMJ Open* **2016**, *6*, e010641. [CrossRef] [PubMed]
4. Mortazavi, F.; Mehrabad, M.; KiaeeTabar, R. Pregnant Women's Well-being and Worry During the COVID-19 Pandemic: A Comparative Study. *BMC Pregnancy Childbirth* **2021**, *21*, 59.
5. Nelson, K.L.; Davis, J.E.; Corbett, C.F. Sleep quality: An evolutionary concept analysis. *Nurs. Forum.* **2022**, *57*, 144–151. [CrossRef]
6. Traylor, C.S.; Johnson, J.D.; Kimmel, M.C.; Manuck, T.A. Effects of psychological stress on adverse pregnancy outcomes and nonpharmacologic approaches for reduction: An expert review. *Am. J. Obstet. Gynecol. MFM* **2020**, *2*, 100229. [CrossRef] [PubMed]
7. Rondó, P.H.C.; Ferreira, R.F.; Nogueira, F.; Ribeiro, M.C.N.; Lobert, H.; Artes, R. Maternal psychological stress and distress as predictors of low birth weight, prematurity and intrauterine growth retardation. *Eur. J. Clin. Nutr.* **2003**, *57*, 266–272. Available online: www.nature.com/ejcn (accessed on 23 February 2021). [CrossRef]
8. Zhu, P.; Tao, F.; Hao, J.; Sun, Y.; Jiang, X. Prenatal life events stress: Implications for preterm birth and infant birthweight. *Am. J. Obstet. Gynecol.* **2010**, *203*, 34.e1–34.e8. [CrossRef]
9. Ding, X.-X.; Wu, Y.-L.; Xu, S.-J.; Zhu, R.-P.; Jia, X.-M.; Zhang, S.-F.; Huang, K.; Zhu, P.; Hao, J.-H.; Tao, F.-B. Maternal anxiety during pregnancy and adverse birth outcomes: A systematic review and meta-analysis of prospective cohort studies. *J. Affect. Disord.* **2014**, *159*, 103–110. [CrossRef]
10. Staneva, A.; Bogossian, F.; Pritchard, M.; Wittkowski, A. The effects of maternal depression, anxiety, and perceived stress during pregnancy on preterm birth: A systematic review. *Women Birth* **2015**, *28*, 179–193. [CrossRef]
11. Okun, M.L.; Schetter, C.D.; Glynn, L.M. Poor sleep quality is associated with preterm birth. *Sleep* **2011**, *34*, 1493–1498. [CrossRef]
12. Li, R.; Zhang, J.; Zhou, R.; Liu, J.; Dai, Z.; Liu, D.; Wang, Y.; Zhang, H.; Li, Y.; Zeng, G. Sleep disturbances during pregnancy are associated with cesarean delivery and preterm birth. *J. Matern. Neonatal-Fetal Neonatal Med.* **2017**, *30*, 733–738. [CrossRef]

13. Khashan, A.S.M.; McNamee, R.; Abel, K.M.M.; Pedersen, M.G.M.; Webb, R.T.; Kenny, L.C.P.; Mortensen, P.B.M.; Baker, P.N.D. Reduced infant birthweight consequent upon maternal exposure to severe life events. *Psychosom. Med.* **2008**, *70*, 688–694. [CrossRef] [PubMed]
14. Khashan, A.S.; Everard, C.; McCowan, L.M.E.; Dekker, G.; Moss-Morris, R.; Baker, P.N.; Poston, L.; Walker, J.J.; Kenny, L.C. Second-trimester maternal distress increases the risk of small for gestational age. *Psychol. Med.* **2014**, *44*, 2799–2810. Available online: https://pubmed.ncbi.nlm.nih.gov/25066370/ (accessed on 23 February 2021). [CrossRef] [PubMed]
15. Gilles, M.; Otto, H.; Wolf, I.A.; Scharnholz, B.; Peus, V.; Schredl, M.; Sütterlin, M.W.; Witt, S.H.; Rietschel, M.; Laucht, M.; et al. Maternal hypothalamus-pituitary-adrenal (HPA) system activity and stress during pregnancy: Effects on gestational age and infant's anthropometric measures at birth. *Psychoneuroendocrinology* **2018**, *94*, 152–161. [CrossRef] [PubMed]
16. Cai, S.; Tan, S.; Gluckman, P.D.; Godfrey, K.M.; Saw, S.-M.; Teoh, O.H.; Chong, Y.-S.; Meaney, M.J.; Kramer, M.S.; Gooley, J.J.; et al. Sleep quality and nocturnal sleep duration in pregnancy and risk of gestational diabetes mellitus. *Sleep* **2017**, *40*, 5–12. [CrossRef] [PubMed]
17. Facco, F.L.; Parker, C.B.; Hunter, S.; Reid, K.J.; Zee, P.P.; Silver, R.M.; Pien, G.; Chung, J.H.; Louis, J.M.; Haas, D.M.; et al. Later sleep timing is associated with an increased risk of preterm birth in nulliparous women. *Am. J. Obstet. Gynecol. MFM.* **2019**, *1*, 100040. [CrossRef] [PubMed]
18. Hung, H.M.; Ko, S.H.; Chen, C.H. The association between prenatal sleep quality and obstetric outcome. *J. Nurs. Res.* **2014**, *22*, 146–154. [CrossRef]
19. Slade, P.; Sheen, K.; Weeks, A.; Wray, S.; De Pascalis, L.; Lunt, K.; Bedwell, C.; Thompson, B.; Hill, J.; Sharp, H. Do stress and anxiety in early pregnancy affect the progress of labor: Evidence from the Wirral Child Health and Development Study. *Acta Obstet. Gynecol. Scand.* **2021**, *100*, 1288–1296. [CrossRef]
20. Chen, X.; Hong, F.; Wang, D.; Bai, B.; Xia, Y.; Wang, C. Related Psychosocial Factors and Delivery Mode of Depression and Anxiety in Primipara in Late Pregnancy. *Evid.-Based Complement. Altern. Med.* **2021**, *2021*, 3254707. [CrossRef]
21. Sanni, K.R.; Eeva, E.; Noora, S.M.; Laura, K.S.; Linnea, K.; Hasse, K. The influence of maternal psychological distress on the mode of birth and duration of labor: Findings from the FinnBrain Birth Cohort Study. *Arch. Womens Ment. Health* **2022**, *25*, 463–472. [CrossRef]
22. Yu, Y.; Zhang, S.; Wang, G.; Hong, X.; Mallow, E.B.; Walker, S.O.; Pearson, C.; Heffner, L.; Zuckerman, B.; Wang, X. The combined association of psychosocial stress and chronic hypertension with preeclampsia. *Am. J. Obstet. Gynecol.* **2013**, *209*, 438.e1–438.e12. [CrossRef]
23. Tang, Y.; Zhang, J.; Dai, F.; Razali, N.S.; Tagore, S.; Chern, B.S.; Tan, K.H. Poor sleep is associated with higher blood pressure and uterine artery pulsatility index in pregnancy: A prospective cohort study. *BJOG Int. J. Obstet. Gynaecol.* **2021**, *128*, 1192–1199. [CrossRef] [PubMed]
24. Madigan, S.; Oatley, H.; Racine, N.; Fearon, R.P.; Schumacher, L.; Akbari, E.; Cooke, J.E.; Tarabulsy, G.M. A Meta-Analysis of Maternal Prenatal Depression and Anxiety on Child Socioemotional Development. *J. Am. Acad. Child Adolesc. Psychiatry* **2018**, *57*, 645–657.e8. [CrossRef] [PubMed]
25. Becker, M.; Weinberger, T.; Chandy, A.; Schmukler, S. Depression During Pregnancy and Postpartum. *Curr. Psychiatry Rep.* **2016**, *18*, 32. [CrossRef] [PubMed]
26. ACOG Committee on Practice Bulletins–Obstetrics. ACOG Practice Bulletin: Clinical management guidelines for obstetrician-gynecologists number 92, April 2008 (replaces practice bulletin number 87, November 2007). Use of psychiatric medications during pregnancy and lactation. *Obstet. Gynecol.* **2008**, *111*, 1001–1020. Available online: https://pubmed.ncbi.nlm.nih.gov/18378767/ (accessed on 6 October 2022). [CrossRef] [PubMed]
27. Woods, S.M.; Melville, J.L.; Guo, Y.; Fan, M.-Y.; Gavin, A. Psychosocial Stress during Pregnancy. *Am. J. Obstet. Gynecol.* **2009**, *202*, 61.e1–61.e7.
28. Dennis, C.L.; Falah-Hassani, K.; Shiri, R. Prevalence of antenatal and postnatal anxiety: Systematic review and meta-analysis. *Br. J. Psychiatry* **2017**, *210*, 315–323. [CrossRef] [PubMed]
29. Du, M.; Liu, J.; Han, N.; Zhao, Z.; Yang, J.; Xu, X.; Luo, S.; Wang, H. Maternal sleep quality during early pregnancy, risk factors and its impact on pregnancy outcomes: A prospective cohort study. *Sleep Med.* **2021**, *79*, 11–18. [CrossRef] [PubMed]
30. Sedov, I.D.; Cameron, E.E.; Madigan, S.; Tomfohr-Madsen, L.M. Sleep quality during pregnancy: A meta-analysis. *Sleep Med. Rev.* **2018**, *38*, 168–176. [CrossRef]
31. Míguez, M.C.; Vázquez, M.B. Risk factors for antenatal depression: A review. *World J. Psychiatry* **2021**, *11*, 325–336. [CrossRef]
32. Biaggi, A.; Conroy, S.; Pawlby, S.; Pariante, C.M. Identifying the women at risk of antenatal anxiety and depression: A systematic review. *J. Affect. Disord.* **2016**, *191*, 62–77. [CrossRef]
33. Lancaster, C.A.; Gold, K.J.; Flynn, H.A.; Yoo, H.; Marcus, S.M.; Davis, M.M. Risk factors for depressive symptoms during pregnancy: A systematic review. *Am. J. Obstet. Gynecol.* **2010**, *202*, 5–14. [CrossRef] [PubMed]
34. Yin, X.; Sun, N.; Jiang, N.; Xu, X.; Gan, Y.; Zhang, J.; Qiu, L.; Yang, C.; Shi, X.; Chang, J.; et al. Prevalence and associated factors of antenatal depression: Systematic reviews and meta-analyses. *Clin. Psychol. Rev.* **2021**, *83*, 101932. [CrossRef] [PubMed]
35. Cohen, S.; Kamarck, T.; Mermelstein, R. A Global Measure of Perceived Stress. *J. Health Soc. Behav.* **1983**, *24*, 385–396. [CrossRef]
36. Spielberger, C.; Gorsuch, R.; Lushene, R.; Vagg, P.R.; Jacobs, G. *Manual for the State-Trait Anxiety Inventory (Form Y1 − Y2)*; Consulting Psychologists Press: Palo Alto, CA, USA, 1983; Volume IV.

37. Topp, C.W.; Østergaard, S.D.; Søndergaard, S.; Bech, P. The WHO-5 well-being index: A systematic review of the literature. *Psychother. Psychosom.* **2015**, *84*, 167–176. [CrossRef] [PubMed]
38. Buysse, D.J.; Reynolds, C.F.; Monk, T.H.; Berman, S.R.; Kupfer, D.J. The Pittsburgh sleep quality index: A new instrument for psychiatric practice and research. *Psychiatry Res.* **1989**, *28*, 193–213. [CrossRef] [PubMed]
39. Remor, E. Psychometric properties of a European Spanish version of the Perceived Stress Scale (PSS). *Span. J. Psychol.* **2006**, *9*, 86–93. [CrossRef] [PubMed]
40. Guillén-Riquelme, A.; Buela-Casal, G. Metaanálisis de comparación degrupos y metaanálisis de generalización de lafiabilidad delcuestionario state-trait anxiety inventory (stai). *Rev. Esp. De Salud Publica* **2014**, *88*. [CrossRef]
41. Julian, L.J. Measures of Anxiety. *Arthritis Care* **2011**, *63*, 1–11. [CrossRef]
42. Bonnín, C.; Yatham, L.; Michalak, E.; Martínez-Arán, A.; Dhanoa, T.; Torres, I.; Santos-Pascual, C.; Valls, E.; Carvalho, A.; Sánchez-Moreno, J.; et al. Psychometric properties of the well-being index (WHO-5) spanish version in a sample of euthymic patients with bipolar disorder. *J. Affect. Disord.* **2018**, *228*, 153–159. [CrossRef]
43. Sutter-Dallay, A.L.; Cosnefroy, O.; Glatigny-Dallay, E.; Verdoux, H.; Rascle, N. Evolution of perinatal depressive symptoms from pregnancy to two years postpartum in a low-risk sample: The MATQUID cohort. *J. Affect. Disord.* **2012**, *139*, 23–29. [CrossRef]
44. Mora, P.A.; Bennett, I.M.; Elo, I.T.; Mathew, L.; Coyne, J.C.; Culhane, J.F. Distinct Trajectories of Perinatal Depressive Symptomatology: Evidence From Growth Mixture Modeling. *Am. J. Epidemiol.* **2009**, *169*, 24. [CrossRef] [PubMed]
45. Bayrampour, H.; Ali, E.; McNeil, D.A.; Benzies, K.; MacQueen, G.; Tough, S. Pregnancy-related anxiety: A concept analysis. *Int. J. Nurs. Stud.* **2016**, *55*, 115–130. [CrossRef]
46. Sattler, M.C.; Jelsma, J.G.M.; Bogaerts, A.; Simmons, D.; Desoye, G.; Corcoy, R.; Adelantado, J.M.; Kautzky-Willer, A.; Harreiter, J.; van Assche, F.A.; et al. Correlates of poor mental health in early pregnancy in obese European women. *BMC Pregnancy Childbirth* **2017**, *17*, 404. [CrossRef] [PubMed]
47. ACOG. ACOG Committee Opinion No. 757: Screening for Perinatal Depression. *Obstet. Gynecol.* **2018**, *132*, E208–E212. Available online: https://journals.lww.com/greenjournal/Fulltext/2018/11000/ACOG_Committee_Opinion_No__757__Screening_for.42.aspx (accessed on 13 October 2022).
48. Bjelland, I.; Krokstad, S.; Mykletun, A.; Dahl, A.A.; Tell, G.S.; Tambs, K. Does a higher educational level protect against anxiety and depression? The HUNT study. *Soc. Sci. Med.* **2008**, *66*, 1334–1345. [CrossRef] [PubMed]
49. Mirowsky, J.; Ross, C.E. Education, personal control, lifestyle and health: A human capital hypothesis. *Res. Aging* **1998**, *20*, 415–449. [CrossRef]
50. Grigoriadis, S.; Graves, L.; Peer, M.; Mamisashvili, L.; Tomlinson, G.; Vigod, S.N.; Dennis, C.L.; Steiner, M.; Brown, C.; Cheung, A.; et al. Maternal Anxiety during Pregnancy and the Association with Adverse Perinatal Outcomes: Systematic Review and Meta-Analysis. *J. Clin. Psychiatry* **2018**, *79*, 813. [CrossRef]
51. Couto, E.R.; Couto, E.; Vian, B.; Gregório, Z.; Nomura, M.L.; Zaccaria, R.; Passini Junior, R. Quality of life, depression and anxiety among pregnant women with previous adverse pregnancy outcomes Qualidade de vida, depressão e ansiedade em gestantes com má história gestacional. *Sao Paulo Med. J.* **2009**, *127*, 185. [CrossRef]
52. Pascal, R.; Crovetto, F.; Casas, I.; Youssef, L.; Trilla, C.; Larroya, M.; Cahuana, A.; Boada, D.; Foraster, M.; Llurba, E.; et al. Impact of the COVID-19 Pandemic on Maternal Well-Being during Pregnancy. *J. Clin. Med.* **2022**, *11*, 2212. [CrossRef]
53. Ceulemans, M.; Hompes, T.; Foulon, V. Mental health status of pregnant and breastfeeding women during the COVID-19 pandemic: A call for action. *Int. J. Gynecol. Obstet.* **2020**, *151*, 146–147. [CrossRef] [PubMed]
54. Berthelot, N.; Lemieux, R.; Garon-Bissonnette, J.; Drouin-Maziade, C.; Martel, É.; Maziade, M. Uptrend in distress and psychiatric symptomatology in pregnant women during the coronavirus disease 2019 pandemic. *Acta Obstet. Gynecol. Scand.* **2020**, *99*, 848–855. [CrossRef] [PubMed]
55. Ravaldi, C.; Ricca, V.; Wilson, A.; Homer, C.; Vannacci, A. Previous psychopathology predicted severe COVID-19 concern, anxiety and PTSD symptoms in pregnant women during lockdown in Italy. *medRxiv* **2020**. [CrossRef] [PubMed]
56. Christian, L.M.; Carroll, J.E.; Porter, K.; Hall, M.H. Sleep quality across pregnancy and postpartum: Effects of parity and race. *Sleep Health* **2019**, *5*, 327–334. [CrossRef]
57. Guinhouya, B.C.; Bisson, M.; Dubois, L.; Sériès, F.; Kimoff, J.R.; Fraser, W.D.; Marc, I. Body Weight Status and Sleep Disturbances During Pregnancy: Does Adherence to Gestational Weight Gain Guidelines Matter? *J. Women's Health* **2019**, *28*, 535–543. Available online: https://www.liebertpub.com/doi/10.1089/jwh.2017.6892 (accessed on 13 October 2022). [CrossRef]
58. Bjertrup, A.J.; Væver, M.S.; Miskowiak, K.W. Prediction of postpartum depression with an online neurocognitive risk screening tool for pregnant women. *Eur. Neuropsychopharmacol.* **2023**, *73*, 36–47. [CrossRef]
59. Fusar-Poli, P.; Santini, Z.I. Promoting good mental health in the whole population: The new frontier. *Eur. Neuropsychopharmacol.* **2022**, *55*, 8–10. [CrossRef]

Disclaimer/Publisher's Note: The statements, opinions and data contained in all publications are solely those of the individual author(s) and contributor(s) and not of MDPI and/or the editor(s). MDPI and/or the editor(s) disclaim responsibility for any injury to people or property resulting from any ideas, methods, instructions or products referred to in the content.

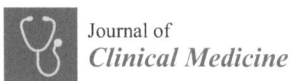

Brief Report

Gestational Weight Gain Is Associated with the Expression of Genes Involved in Inflammation in Maternal Visceral Adipose Tissue and Offspring Anthropometric Measures

Renata Saucedo [1], María Isabel Peña-Cano [2], Mary Flor Díaz-Velázquez [3], Aldo Ferreira-Hermosillo [1], Juan Mario Solis-Paredes [4], Ignacio Camacho-Arroyo [5] and Jorge Valencia-Ortega [5,*]

[1] Unidad de Investigación Médica en Enfermedades Endocrinas, Hospital de Especialidades, Centro Médico Nacional Siglo XXI, Instituto Mexicano del Seguro Social, Mexico City 06720, Mexico; sgrenata@yahoo.com (R.S.); aldo.nagisa@gmail.com (A.F.-H.)
[2] Hospital de Gineco Obstetricia 221, Instituto Mexicano del Seguro Social, Toluca 50000, Mexico; isabelpenacano@hotmail.com
[3] Hospital de Gineco Obstetricia 3, Centro Médico Nacional La Raza, Instituto Mexicano del Seguro Social, Mexico City 02990, Mexico; mary.diaz@imss.gob.mx
[4] Department of Reproductive and Perinatal Health Research, Instituto Nacional de Perinatología Isidro Espinosa de los Reyes, Mexico City 11000, Mexico; juan.solis@inper.gob.mx
[5] Unidad de Investigación en Reproducción Humana, Instituto Nacional de Perinatología-Facultad de Química, Universidad Nacional Autónoma de México, Mexico City 11000, Mexico; camachoarroyo@gmail.com
* Correspondence: j.valencia.o@hotmail.com; Tel.: +52-55-33564905

Abstract: Background: Adequate gestational weight gain (GWG) is essential for maternal and fetal health. GWG may be a sign of higher visceral adipose tissue (VAT) accretion. A higher proportion of VAT is associated with an inflammatory process that may play a role in the fetal programming of obesity. This study aimed to (1) compare the expression of genes involved in inflammatory responses (TLR2, TLR4, NFκB, IKKβ, IL-1RA, IL-1β, IL-6, IL-10, TNF-α) in the VAT of pregnant women according to GWG and (2) explore whether VAT inflammation and GWG are related to offspring anthropometric measures. Material and methods: 50 women scheduled for cesarean section who delivered term infants were included in the study. We collected maternal omental VAT, and the expression of genes was examined with RT-qPCR. Results: Women with excessive and with adequate GWG had significantly higher expressions of most inflammatory genes than women with insufficient GWG. Neonates from mothers with excessive GWG had greater birth weight and chest circumference than those from mothers with insufficient GWG. GWG was positively correlated with fetal birth weight. Conclusions: The VAT expression of most genes associated with inflammatory pathways was higher in excessive and adequate GWG than in pregnant women with insufficient GWG. Moreover, GWG was found to be positively associated with newborn weight.

Keywords: gestational weight gain; visceral adipose tissue; cytokines; birthweight; inflammation

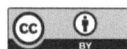

1. Introduction

Gestational weight gain (GWG) is a critical physiological process that supports adequate fetal growth and development. Insufficient or excessive GWG is associated with a higher risk of adverse pregnancy outcomes [1]. Insufficient GWG confers a higher risk for small-for-gestational-age infants and preterm birth [2]. In contrast, women with excessive GWG are at increased risk of adverse obstetric outcomes, including cesarean delivery, gestational diabetes mellitus, and preeclampsia [3]. Moreover, excessive GWG is associated with postpartum weight retention and pre-pregnancy adiposity in subsequent pregnancies [4]. The neonates also have adverse consequences, such as macrosomia and being large for their gestational age [5]. In addition, women with excessive GWG and their offspring have lifelong health disturbances, including obesity and a higher risk of type 2 diabetes and cardiovascular disease [6].

The Institute of Medicine (IOM) has recommended the ideal GWG to ensure the optimal health of the mother and the offspring [7]. The IOM proposes less GWG for women with overweight/obesity than for target-weight women. It has been estimated that only 28–32% of pregnant women have adequate GWG, almost 25% have insufficient weight gain, and half of the pregnancies gain in excess of the IOM recommendations [2]. In this context, women with overweight and women with obesity have the highest prevalence of excessive GWG, which is becoming increasingly prevalent among pregnancies worldwide [8,9].

GWG includes the fetus, placenta, uterus, amniotic fluid, maternal blood volume, breast tissue, and adipose tissue (AT). Maternal body fat accounts for about 30% of GWG and provides an energy source for the fetus and the mother [10]. Body fat distribution changes throughout pregnancy; there is a gradual decrease in subcutaneous fat accretion and an increase in visceral fat accumulation from early to late gestation [11]. Women with overweight and women with obesity have a higher proportion of visceral adipose tissue (VAT) than lean women, and this is associated with VAT inflammation, characterized by the increased release of pro-inflammatory signals (leptin, macrophage chemoattractant protein 1, IL-6, and IL-1β) and reduced production of anti-inflammatory molecules (adiponectin, IL-10) [12]. Adipose tissue inflammation has been related to the development of maternal metabolic disorders such as insulin resistance. Growing evidence supports that it also plays a relevant role in the fetal programming of obesity [13].

GWG may be a sign of higher VAT accretion during pregnancy [14]. Nevertheless, the relationship between GWG and VAT inflammation and offspring anthropometric measures at birth has not been tested. Therefore, the aim of this study was to (1) compare the expression of genes involved in inflammatory responses (TLR2, TLR4, NFκB, IKKβ, IL-1RA, IL1-β, IL-6, IL-10, TNF-α) in the VAT of pregnant women according to GWG and (2) explore whether VAT inflammation and GWG are associated with offspring anthropometric measures at birth.

2. Materials and Methods

Study population

This is a cross-sectional study conducted at the Hospital of Gynecology and Obstetrics 3, National Medical Center La Raza, and at the Hospital of Gynecology and Obstetrics 221, Instituto Mexicano del Seguro Social, and was approved by the Institutional Review Board (R-2018-785-026). All participants signed informed consent.

The study included 50 women aged 18 to 40 with singleton pregnancies and scheduled cesarean sections who delivered term infants. Indications for cesarean section were breech presentation and previous cesarean section. Exclusion criteria were smoking during pregnancy, pre-existing diabetes mellitus, major maternal comorbidities, and fetal malformations discovered at routine ultrasound examinations.

Maternal body mass index (BMI) was calculated from the weight measured at the first antenatal visit using a calibrated scale and the measured maternal height. BMI was categorized according to the WHO definitions: underweight < 18.5 kg/m^2, target weight 18.5–24.9 kg/m^2, overweight 25.0–29.9 kg/m^2, and obesity $\geq 30 \text{ kg/m}^2$. GWG was calculated as the difference between the weight measured at the first and last antenatal visit. GWG classification was determined using the IOM guidelines [7] and categorized as insufficient, adequate, or excessive GWG. Information on pregnancy was collected from hospital records.

Newborn anthropometric measurements (weight, length, foot length, head circumference, chest circumference, and abdominal circumference) were assessed at birth. The ponderal index was calculated as $100 \times [\text{birthweight (g)}/\text{length (cm}^3)]$.

Sample collection and biochemical analyses

Blood samples were collected in the morning on the day of the scheduled cesarean section after an overnight fast of 12 h. Glucose, total cholesterol, high-density lipoprotein

(HDL) cholesterol, and triglyceride serum levels were determined using an ARCHITECT Plus c4000 Clinical Chemistry Analyzer (Abbot Diagnostics, Abbott Park, IL, USA). Low-density lipoprotein (LDL) cholesterol levels were estimated with the Friedewald formula. According to manufacturer's guidelines, insulin levels were determined with a multiplex immunoassay using Magpix technology (Milliplex Map, Billerica, MA, USA). Homeostatic Model Assessment for Insulin Resistance (HOMA-IR) was estimated using the formula HOMA-IR = [fasting insulin concentration (μU/mL) × fasting glucose concentration (mmol/L)]/22.5 [15].

Gene expression analyses

Omental VAT fragments of about 5 cm^3 of volume were obtained from all participants within ten minutes of delivery, and they were dissected into small fragments, placed in TRIzol® Reagent (In-vitrogen™, Carlsbad, CA, USA), and stored at −70 °C until RNA extraction. A Direct-zolTM RNA MiniPrep kit (Zymo Research Corp, Irvine, CA, USA) was used for total RNA extraction in accordance with the manufacturer's protocol. RNA purity and quantity were measured using spectrophotometry (NanoDrop 2000, Thermo Fisher Scientific, Wilmington, DE, USA). cDNA was generated from RNA using a SuperScript®III First-Strand kit (Invitrogen™, Carlsbad, CA, USA) following the manufacturers' specifications. Subsequently, real-time PCR was performed using predesigned Taqman® Gene Expression Assays and Taqman® Universal PCR Master Mix (Applied Biosystems™, Foster City, CA, USA). The $2^{-\Delta Ct}$ relative method quantification was used to determine the fold change in the mRNA expressions with the GAPDH transcript as endogenous control. All the primers and probes were acquired from Applied BiosystemsTM: TLR2 (Hs02621280_s1), TLR4 (Hs00152939_m1), NFκB (Hs00765730_m1), IKKβ (Hs01559460_m1), IL-1RA (Hs00893626_m1), IL-1β (Hs01555410_m1), IL-6 (Hs00985639_m1), IL-10 (Hs00961622_m1), TNF-α (Hs01113624_g1), and GAPDH (PN 4326317E).

Statistical analysis

Statistical analyses were performed using IBM SPSS Statistics 23.0 (IBM SPSS Inc., Chicago, IL, USA). The normality was tested with Shapiro–Wilk tests. Data are presented as median (25th and 75th percentiles). Comparisons between groups were analyzed using Kruskal–Wallis test followed by a post hoc test for multiple group comparisons. The relationship of VAT gene expression and offspring anthropometric measures was analyzed using the Spearman test. Multiple linear regression was applied to analyze the correlations of GWG (independent variable) and birth weight (dependent variable) after adjusting for maternal age, gestational age at delivery, pregestational maternal weight, parity, maternal metabolic factors (glucose, insulin, and lipid profile), and sex of the newborn. A two-tailed p value < 0.05 was considered statistically significant.

3. Results

Participant characteristics

The maternal characteristics are presented in Table 1. Most women were in their second or subsequent pregnancy; 57.5% had overweight or obesity at the onset of pregnancy, and 56.8% had adequate GWG. Fasting plasma glucose and insulin resistance were in the normal healthy range; however, women had a dyslipidemic profile (total cholesterol > 5.2 mmol/L and triglycerides > 1.7 mmol/L). These biochemical measures were no different among the GWG groups (Table 2).

Women with overweight/obesity at the onset of pregnancy had a higher proportion of excessive GWG than women with a target weight (24.1% vs. 17.6%, p = 0.009). None of the underweight women had excessive GWG; 75% gained below the recommended level. Moreover, 29% of target-weight women and 17.4% of overweight women had GWG below the guidelines.

Table 1. Anthropometric and laboratory characteristics of the study group.

Characteristics	n = 50
Maternal age at delivery (years)	30.0 (22.0–33.3)
Previous pregnancies (%)	
None	31.9
At least one	68.1
Pre-pregnancy BMI n (%)	
<18 Underweight	4 (8.5)
18.0–24.9 Target weight	17 (34.0)
25.0–29.9 Overweight	23 (44.7)
>30 Obesity	6 (12.8)
Gestational weight gain n (%)	
Insufficient	12 (22.7)
Adequate	28 (56.8)
Excessive	10 (20.5)
Gestational age (weeks)	39.0 (38.0–40.0)
Fasting glucose (mmol/L)	4.2 (3.8–5.1)
Fasting insulin (pmol/L)	51.8 (30.1–73.4)
HOMA-IR	1.3 (0.82–2.0)
Total cholesterol (mmol/L)	6.1 (5.2–6.7)
HDL cholesterol (mmol/L)	2.7 (2.3–3.1)
LDL cholesterol (mmol/L)	1.9 (1.2–2.3)
Triglycerides (mmol/L)	3.0 (2.5–3.6)

Data are presented as counts and percentages as well as medians (interquartile range). BMI: body mass index, HOMA-IR: homeostasis model assessment-insulin resistance, HDL: high-density lipoprotein cholesterol; LDL low-density lipoprotein cholesterol.

Table 2. Biochemical parameters according to GWG.

	Insufficient GWG	Adequate GWG	Excessive GWG
Fasting glucose (mmol/L)	4.3 (3.6–6.2)	4.2 (3.8–4.5)	4.8 (3.7–5.4)
Fasting insulin (pmol/L)	55.9 (42.7–75.2)	51.1 (27.4–79.2)	50.3 (36.4–103.9)
HOMA-IR	1.3 (0.9–2.2)	1.3 (0.7–2.2)	1.4 (0.9–2.1)
Total cholesterol (mmol/L)	6.6 (5.6–7.5)	5.6 (5.0–6.5)	6.2 (5.4–6.8)
HDL cholesterol (mmol/L)	2.8 (2.4–3.4)	2.5 (2.3–3.2)	2.5 (2.2–3.0)
LDL cholesterol (mmol/L)	2.2 (1.3–3.7)	1.7 (1.1–2.1)	1.9 (1.0–3.1)
Triglycerides (mmol/L)	3.1 (2.6–3.7)	2.9 (2.4–3.6)	3.3 (2.8–4.0)

Data are presented as medians (interquartile range). HOMA-IR: homeostasis model assessment-insulin resistance, HDL: high-density lipoprotein cholesterol, LDL: low-density lipoprotein cholesterol.

Inflammatory gene expression and GWG

As shown in Figure 1, GWG was a relevant factor associated with the expression of genes involved in VAT inflammation. Women with excessive GWG had significantly higher TLR2, TLR4, IL-1RA, IL-6, IL-10, and NFκB expression than women with insufficient GWG. The GAPDH Ct values were not different among the groups [insufficient GWG: 23.8 (23.5–24.1); adequate GWG: 23.9 (23.3–24.3); excessive GWG: 23.6 (23.1–23.8); $p = 0.72$].

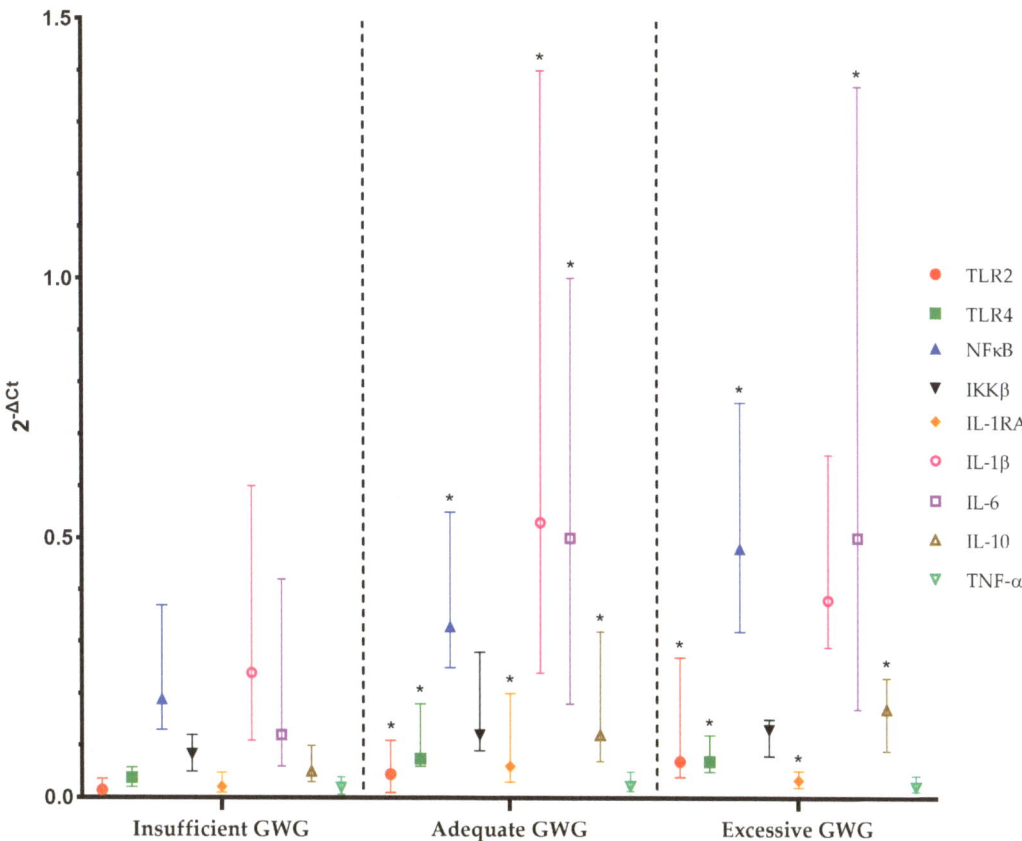

Figure 1. Inflammatory markers' mRNA expression (Q1, median, and Q3 of $2^{-\Delta Ct}$) in VAT according to GWG. GWG: gestational weight gain. * $p < 0.05$ vs. insufficient GWG.

Also, women with adequate GWG had higher TLR2, TLR4, IL-1β, IL-1RA, IL-6, IL-10, and NFκB expression than women with insufficient GWG. No differences in gene expression were observed between women with adequate GWG and those with excessive GWG. Concerning overweight/obesity at the onset of pregnancy, no association was observed between maternal pregestational BMI and gene expression in VAT.

GWG and offspring anthropometric measures

Neonates from mothers with excessive GWG had greater birth weights and chest circumferences than those from mothers with insufficient GWG, and newborns from mothers with adequate GWG had higher head circumferences than those from mothers with insufficient GWG (Table 3). No differences in offspring anthropometric measures were observed between women with adequate GWG and those with excessive GWG.

GWG was positively correlated with birth weight (r = 0.288, $p < 0.05$), and this correlation still existed after adjusting for maternal age, gestational age at delivery, pregestational maternal weight, parity, maternal metabolic factors, and sex of the newborn (β = 0.4, $p < 0.05$).

Gene expression related to VAT inflammation was not associated with offspring anthropometric measures.

Table 3. Offspring anthropometric measures according to GWG.

	Insufficient GWG	Adequate GWG	Excessive GWG
Gestational age (weeks)	39 (37.3–39.8)	38.9 (38.0–39.5)	39 (38.5–40.3)
Sex n (%) Female Male	 9 (75.0) 3 (25.0)	 9 (34.6) 17 (65.4)	 6 (66.7) 3 (33.3)
Birth weight (g)	2850 (2352.5–3100)	3025 (2787.5–3202.5)	3150 (3020–3395) *
Birth length (cm)	49 (48–50)	49 (47–50)	48 (47.25–51.25)
Ponderal index (g/cm^3)	2.47 (2.15–2.8)	2.63 (2.4–2.8)	2.67 (2.46–2.85)
Neonatal foot length (cm)	7.5 (7–8)	8 (7–8)	8 (7–8)
Neonatal head circumference (cm)	33 (32–34)	34 (33–35) *	34 (32.5–35.25)
Neonatal chest circumference (cm)	31 (29–32.75)	32 (31–33)	34.5 (32.0–35.0) *
Neonatal abdominal circumference (cm)	29 (28–30.75)	30.5 (29.5–32.25)	30.0 (29.0–33.5)

Data are presented as medians (interquartile range). * $p < 0.05$ vs. insufficient GWG.

4. Discussion

A meta-analysis of more than 1.3 million pregnancies worldwide reported that only 28–32% of pregnant women have adequate GWG [2]. In Mexico, the prevalence of excessive GWG ranges from 38% to 43%, and this frequency is higher in women with overweight and women with obesity [16,17]. Our results showed that 56.8% of the participants had adequate GWG, 22.7% had insufficient GWG, and 20.5% had excessive GWG. This frequency is lower than that in previous studies, probably due to the age and the pregestational BMI range in our study (BMI range: 15.24–32.81 kg/m^2). Additionally, we found that women with a higher pregestational BMI had higher GWG than those with a target weight. However, we did not observe significant differences in biochemical measures among the GWG groups. One explanation for this result could be the small sample size.

Maternal obesity is associated with impaired VAT function. We have previously reported that inflammatory genes in the VAT of women with obesity are upregulated compared with those in lean women late in pregnancy [18]. Inflammation during pregnancy has also been linked to GWG; recent studies have shown that the systemic inflammatory biomarkers C-reactive protein and interleukin 8 are positively correlated with GWG [19,20]. It has been suggested that inflammation stimulates the production of reactive oxidative species, which promote the expansion and terminal differentiation of adipocytes and sustained inflammation, leading to weight gain [21,22]. In the context of adipose tissue, TLR4 and TLR8 are involved in saturated fatty acid-mediated inflammation [23,24], IL-6 promotes macrophage infiltration [25], IL-1β is produced by activated macrophages [26], and NFκB is a transcription factor that triggers proinflammatory pathways in immune cells [27]. In turn, IL-10 is essential in resolving inflammation and subsequent tissue damage. IL-1RA inhibits the proinflammatory effects of IL-1, thus acting as an anti-inflammatory mediator [28]. We observed an up-regulation of most pro-inflammatory and of all anti-inflammatory genes in women with adequate or excessive GWG compared with the group with insufficient GWG. The down-regulation of these genes in insufficient GWG may reflect an energetic maladaptation of VAT that could partly explain the high risk of small-for-gestational-age infants [2,29]. Moreover, there may have been a difference in the pattern of adipose distribution between those women with insufficient GWG and those with adequate and excessive GWG; lean women gain more subcutaneous adipose tissue, and women with overweight and women with obesity have a greater proportion of VAT during pregnancy [30].

Interestingly, it has been suggested that maternal inflammation should contribute to the fetal programming of obesity through changes in organs that release pro-inflammatory cytokines as AT and the placenta [31]. Notably, in our study, the increased expression of the inflammatory cytokines in VAT was not associated with anthropometric neonatal measures. However, there is evidence that the placenta substantially contributes to maternal cytokine concentrations and nutrient transport to the fetus [32].

Several studies have shown that excessive GWG and pregestational BMI are associated with offspring birth weight and adiposity [2,13]. However, in our study, we did not observe an association between BMI and newborn weight. Only GWG was found to be independently and positively associated with newborn weight. Excessive GWG is accompanied by increased fat mass associated with birthweight because of the increased availability of plasma fatty acids for placental transport [33].

The present study is strengthened by the adjustment for several major elements that may confound the relationship between GWG and neonatal anthropometric measures. However, our study has some limitations. We had a modest sample size, which may limit the study's power to identify GWG-related metabolic profiles. Additionally, we were unable to obtain information regarding dietary patterns, lifestyle behaviors, and socioeconomic status during pregnancy. Newborn and maternal fat mass were not examined. At the same time, we investigated the overall GWG at the end of pregnancy instead of weight gain during each trimester. It has been suggested that GWG during the first and early second trimesters is related to somatic growth [34]. Finally, although our study demonstrates associations, we cannot determine causation.

5. Conclusions

The expression of most genes associated with inflammatory pathways was higher in excessive and adequate GWG than in pregnant women with insufficient GWG. However, VAT inflammation was not related to offspring anthropometric measures. Further longitudinal studies on bigger samples are required to evaluate the role of VAT inflammation on maternal and neonatal outcomes.

Additionally, GWG was found to be positively associated with newborn weight. This suggests that interventions, information, and counseling to optimize GWG should be evaluated for their ability to reduce excessive fetal growth.

Author Contributions: M.I.P.-C., J.V.-O., I.C.-A. and R.S. planned and designed the study. M.I.P.-C., J.M.S.-P. and J.V.-O. performed laboratory biomarker analysis. M.F.D.-V., A.F.-H., I.C.-A. and R.S. drafted the manuscript. M.I.P.-C., J.M.S.-P. and R.S. performed the data analysis. All authors provided significant intellectual contributions in interpreting data and critical review of the manuscript. All authors have read and agreed to the published version of the manuscript.

Funding: This work was supported by scientific grants from Instituto Mexicano del Seguro Social (FIS/IMSS/PROT/G18/1826). This source did not have a role in the preparation of data or the manuscript.

Institutional Review Board Statement: The research was conducted ethically in accordance with the World Medical Association Declaration of Helsinki. The protocol was reviewed and approved by the Institutional Ethics and Scientific Committees of the Instituto Mexicano del Seguro Social, approval number R-2018-785-026.

Informed Consent Statement: Informed consent was obtained from all subjects involved in the study.

Data Availability Statement: The data used to support the findings of this study are available from the corresponding author by request.

Acknowledgments: R.S., M.I.P.-C., A.F.-H., J.M.S.-P., I.C.-A. and J.V.-O. hold a fellowship from the National System of Investigators, Consejo Nacional de Ciencia y Tecnología. J.V.-O. receives a postdoctoral fellowship from the Dirección General de Asuntos del Personal Académico (DGAPA), Universidad Nacional Autónoma de México.

Conflicts of Interest: The authors declare no conflict of interest.

References

1. Voerman, E.; Santos, S.; Inskip, H.; Amiano, P.; Barros, H.; Charles, M.A.; Chatzi, L.; Chrousos, G.P.; Corpeleijn, E.; Crozier, S.; et al. Association of gestational weight gain with adverse maternal and infant outcomes. *JAMA* **2019**, *321*, 1702–1715. [CrossRef] [PubMed]
2. Goldstein, R.F.; Abell, S.K.; Ranasinha, S.; Misso, M.; Boyle, J.A.; Black, M.H.; Li, N.; Hu, G.; Corrado, F.; Rode, L.; et al. Association of gestational weight gain with maternal and infant outcomes: A systematic review and meta-analysis. *JAMA* **2017**, *317*, 2207–2225. [CrossRef] [PubMed]
3. Poston, L.; Caleyachetty, R.; Cnattingius, S.; Corvalán, C.; Uauy, R.; Herring, S.; Gillman, M.W. Preconceptional and maternal obesity: Epidemiology and health consequences. *Lancet Diabetes Endocrinol.* **2016**, *4*, 1025–1036. [CrossRef]
4. Catalano, P.M. Obesity, insulin resistance, and pregnancy outcome. *Reproduction* **2010**, *140*, 365–371. [CrossRef] [PubMed]
5. Marchi, J.; Berg, M.; Dencker, A.; Olander, E.K.; Begley, C. Risks associated with obesity in pregnancy, for the mother and baby: A systematic review of reviews. *Obes. Rev.* **2015**, *16*, 621–638. [CrossRef]
6. Catalano, P.M.; Shankar, K. Obesity and pregnancy: Mechanisms of short term and long term adverse consequences for mother and child. *BMJ* **2017**, *356*, j1. [CrossRef] [PubMed]
7. Institute of Medicine and National Research Council. *Weight Gain during Pregnancy: Reexamining the Guidelines*; The National Academies Press: Washington, DC, USA, 2009. [CrossRef]
8. Deputy, N.P.; Sharma, A.J.; Kim, S.Y. Gestational weight gain—United States, 2012 and 2013. *MMWR Morb. Mortal Wkly. Rep.* **2015**, *64*, 1215–1220. [CrossRef]
9. Devlieger, R.; Benhalima, K.; Damm, P.; Van Assche, A.; Mathieu, C.; Mahmood, T.; Dunne, F.; Bogaerts, A. Maternal obesity in Europe: Where do we stand and how to move forward?: A scientific paper commissioned by the European Board and College of Obstetrics and Gynaecology (EBCOG). *Eur. J. Obstet. Gynecol. Reprod. Biol.* **2016**, *201*, 203–208. [CrossRef]
10. Butte, N.F.; King, J.C. Energy requirements during pregnancy and lactation. *Public Health Nutr.* **2005**, *8*, 1010–1027. [CrossRef]
11. Sidebottom, A.C.; Brown, J.E.; Jacobs, D.R. Pregnancy-related changes in body fat. *Eur. J. Obstet. Gynecol. Reprod. Biol.* **2001**, *94*, 216–223. [CrossRef]
12. Trivett, C.; Lees, Z.J.; Freeman, D.J. Adipose tissue function in healthy pregnancy, gestational diabetes mellitus and pre-eclampsia. *Eur. J. Clin. Nutr.* **2021**, *75*, 1745–1756. [CrossRef] [PubMed]
13. Schmatz, M.; Madan, J.; Marino, T.; Davis, J. Maternal obesity: The interplay between inflammation, mother and fetus. *J. Perinatol.* **2010**, *30*, 441–446. [CrossRef] [PubMed]
14. Berggren, E.K.; Groh-Wargo, S.; Presley, L.; Hauguel-de Mouzon, S.; Catalano, P.M. Maternal fat, but not lean, mass is increased among overweight/obese women with excess gestational weight gain. *Am. J. Obstet. Gynecol.* **2016**, *214*, 745.e1–745.e5. [CrossRef] [PubMed]
15. Matthews, D.R.; Hosker, J.P.; Rudenski, A.S.; Naylor, B.A.; Treacher, D.F.; Turner, R.C. Homeostasis model assessment: Insulin resistance and beta-cell function from fasting plasma glucose and insulin concentrations in man. *Diabetologia* **1985**, *28*, 412–419. [CrossRef] [PubMed]
16. Jiménez-Cruz, A.; Bacardí Gascón, M.; Martínez-Nuñez, A.E.; Newell Morison, P.; Silva-Pérez, I.; Calzada-Tello, A.; Mora-Santillana, M.; Gastellum-Dagnino, M. Gestational Weight Gain Among Pregnant Women in the Mexico–US Border City of Tijuana, Mexico. *J. Negat. No Posit. Results* **2021**, *6*, 545–556. [CrossRef]
17. Zonana-Nacach, A.; Baldenebro-Preciado, R.; Ruiz-Dorado, M.A. The effect of gestational weight gain on maternal and neonatal outcomes. *Salud Publica Mex.* **2010**, *52*, 220–225. [CrossRef]
18. Peña-Cano, M.I.; Valencia-Ortega, J.; Morales-Ávila, E.; Díaz-Velázquez, M.F.; Gómez-Díaz, R.; Saucedo, R. Omentin-1 and its relationship with inflammatory factors in maternal plasma and visceral adipose tissue of women with gestational diabetes mellitus. *J. Endocrinol. Investig.* **2022**, *45*, 453–462. [CrossRef]
19. Perng, W.; Rifas-Shiman, S.L.; Rich-Edwards, J.W.; Stuebe, A.M.; Oken, E. Inflammation and weight gain in reproductive-aged women. *Ann. Hum. Biol.* **2016**, *43*, 91–95. [CrossRef]
20. Rugină, C.; Mărginean, C.O.; Meliţ, L.E.; Huţanu, A.; Ghiga, D.V.; Modi, V.; Mărginean, C. Systemic inflammatory status—A bridge between gestational weight gain and neonatal outcomes (STROBE-compliant article). *Medicine* **2021**, *100*, e24511. [CrossRef]
21. Lee, H.; Lee, Y.J.; Choi, H.; Ko, E.H.; Kim, J.W. Reactive oxygen species facilitate adipocyte differentiation by accelerating mitotic clonal expansion. *J. Biol. Chem.* **2009**, *284*, 10601–10609. [CrossRef]
22. Seals, D.R.; Bell, C. Chronic sympathetic activation: Consequence and cause of age-associated obesity? *Diabetes* **2004**, *53*, 276–284. [CrossRef]
23. Petrus, P.; Rosqvist, F.; Edholm, D.; Mejhert, N.; Arner, P.; Dahlman, I.; Rydén, M.; Sundbom, M.; Risérus, U. Saturated fatty acids in human visceral adipose tissue are associated with increased 11- β-hydroxysteroid-dehydrogenase type 1 expression. *Lipids Health Dis.* **2015**, *14*, 42. [CrossRef]
24. Hwang, D.H.; Kim, J.A.; Lee, J.Y. Mechanisms for the activation of Toll-like receptor 2/4 by saturated fatty acids and inhibition by docosahexaenoic acid. *Eur. J. Pharmacol.* **2016**, *785*, 24–35. [CrossRef]
25. Han, M.S.; White, A.; Perry, R.J.; Camporez, J.-P.; Hidalgo, J.; Shulman, G.I.; Davis, R.J. Regulation of adipose tissue inflammation by interleukin 6. *Proc. Natl. Acad. Sci. USA* **2020**, *117*, 2751–2760. [CrossRef]
26. Bing, C. Is interleukin-1β a culprit in macrophage-adipocyte crosstalk in obesity? *Adipocyte* **2015**, *4*, 149–152. [CrossRef] [PubMed]

27. Liu, T.; Zhang, L.; Joo, D.; Sun, S.C. NF-κB signaling in inflammation. *Signal. Transduct. Target. Ther.* **2017**, *2*, 17023. [CrossRef] [PubMed]
28. Mingomataj, E.Ç.; Bakiri, A.H. Regulator Versus Effector Paradigm: Interleukin-10 as Indicator of the Switching Response. *Clin. Rev. Allergy. Immunol.* **2016**, *50*, 97–113. [CrossRef] [PubMed]
29. Resi, V.; Basu, S.; Haghiac, M.; Presley, L.; Minium, J.; Kaufman, B.; Bernard, S.; Catalano, P.; Mouzon, S.H.-D. Molecular inflammation and adipose tissue matrix remodeling precede physiological adaptations to pregnancy. *Am. J. Physiol. Endocrinol. Metab.* **2012**, *303*, E832–E840. [CrossRef]
30. Ehrenberg, H.M.; Huston-Presley, L.; Catalano, P.M. The influence of obesity and gestational diabetes mellitus on accretion and the distribution of adipose tissue in pregnancy. *Am. J. Obstet. Gynecol.* **2003**, *189*, 944–948. [CrossRef]
31. Ingvorsen, C.; Brix, S.; Ozanne, S.E.; Hellgren, L.I. The effect of maternal Inflammation on foetal programming of metabolic disease. *Acta Physiol.* **2015**, *214*, 440–449. [CrossRef]
32. Aye, I.L.; Lager, S.; Ramirez, V.I.; Gaccioli, F.; Dudley, D.J.; Jansson, T.; Powell, T.L. Increasing maternal body mass index is associated with systemic inflammation in the mother and the activation of distinct placental inflammatory pathways. *Biol. Reprod.* **2014**, *90*, 129. [CrossRef] [PubMed]
33. Whitaker, R.C.; Dietz, W.H. Role of the prenatal environment in the development of obesity. *J. Pediatr.* **1998**, *132*, 768–776. [CrossRef] [PubMed]
34. Rifas-Shiman, S.L.; Fleisch, A.; Hivert, M.F.; Mantzoros, C.; Gillman, M.W.; Oken, E. First and second trimester gestational weight gains are most strongly associated with cord blood levels of hormones at delivery important for glycemic control and somatic growth. *Metabolism* **2017**, *69*, 112–119. [CrossRef] [PubMed]

Disclaimer/Publisher's Note: The statements, opinions and data contained in all publications are solely those of the individual author(s) and contributor(s) and not of MDPI and/or the editor(s). MDPI and/or the editor(s) disclaim responsibility for any injury to people or property resulting from any ideas, methods, instructions or products referred to in the content.

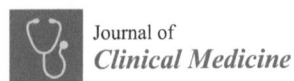

Article

Multifactorial Colonization of the Pregnant Woman's Reproductive Tract: Implications for Early Postnatal Adaptation in Full-Term Newborns

Piotr Gibała [1], Anna Jarosz-Lesz [2], Zuzanna Sołtysiak-Gibała [1], Jakub Staniczek [1,*] and Rafał Stojko [1]

[1] Chair and Department of Gynecology, Obstetrics and Gynecologic Oncology, Medical University of Silesia, 40-211 Katowice, Poland; piotr.gibala1@gmail.com (P.G.); zuzannasoltysiakk@gmail.com (Z.S.-G.); rsojko@sum.edu.pl (R.S.)

[2] Neonatology Unit, The Guardian Angels Hospital of the Brothers Hospitallers of St. John of God in Katowice, 40-211 Katowice, Poland; jaleszczan@gmail.com

* Correspondence: jstaniczek@sum.edu.pl; Tel.: +48-324-616-370

Abstract: This retrospective study aimed to investigate the impact of microorganisms identified in the reproductive tract on disorders during the early adaptation period in newborns. A cohort of 823 patients and cervical canal cultures were analyzed to identify the presence of microorganisms. Newborns included in the study were divided into two groups due to the number of pathogens identified in the swab from the cervical canal of the mother. The first group consisted of newborns whose mothers had one pathogen identified (N = 637), while the second group consisted of newborns whose mothers had two or more pathogens identified (N = 186). The analysis of disorders of the early adaptation period included the incidence of respiratory distress syndrome, the number of procedures performed with the use of CPAP, oxygen therapy, antibiotic therapy and parenteral nutrition. Respiratory distress syndrome was more common in group II than in group I (85 vs. 31, $p = 0.001$). In group II, CPAP (63 vs. 21, $p = 0.001$), oxygen therapy (15 vs. 8, $p = 0.02$) and antibiotics were used more frequently (13 vs. 8, $p = 0.01$). The findings of this study revealed that the number of pathogens colonizing the reproductive tract had a significant influence on the early adaptation period in newborns. Multifactorial colonization of the reproductive tract was associated with an increased incidence of infections in newborns and a higher prevalence of acid–base balance disorders. This study highlights the importance of monitoring and addressing the microbial composition of the reproductive tract during pregnancy.

Keywords: early postnatal adaptation; newborns; infection in pregnancy; vaginal infection; vaginal microbiome

1. Introduction

1.1. Background

The moment of birth is a rapid transition for the newborn from the intrauterine environment to the external environment. During fetal life, the ambient temperature is constant and optimal, oxygen and nutrients are supplied with the umbilical cord blood and the skin is covered with a protective layer of fetal fluid. Birth, the clamping of the umbilical cord together with thermal and tactile stimulation lead to the aeration of the lungs, the stabilization of regular breathing and gas exchange. An increase in systemic arterial pressure together with a decrease in pulmonary vascular resistance initiates changes in the circulatory system, adapting the heart to work with altered pulmonary circulation. In the following hours of life, the remaining organs of the newborn adapt to the changed conditions of functioning. Postnatal adaptation to extrauterine life is a physiological process and normally does not require medical intervention. However, there are situations that go beyond the limits of physiology, which may manifest themselves throughout the period of early adaptation to the 7th–10th day of a newborn's life. In Poland, newborns are usually discharged from the hospital after the age of 2 days; therefore, the assessment of a newborn rests with primary care physicians and community midwives, whose role is to notice the moment when the physiology of the neonatal period turns into pathology [1].

Cervico-vaginal infections are not without significance for both the fetus and the newborn. They are still the most common cause of morbidity and mortality in the postnatal period. It has been proven that bacteria commonly colonizing the mother's genital tract can be transferred to the child's body both intrauterine and during delivery [2]. The immaturity of the newborn's immune system increases its susceptibility to intrauterine or perinatal infections [3].

In clinical practice, smears are most often performed to identify group B streptococci (GBS—group B—streptococcal), bacteria that are an important cause of complications in the child in the perinatal period. Based on numerous meta-analyses carried out in the 1990s, the use of perinatal prophylaxis of GBS, which contributes to the reduction of infectious complications in newborns, has been demonstrated [4,5].

The factors contributing to neonatal infections and disorders of the early adaptation period in newborns are: [6,7]

1. Premature rupture of membranes (especially before 37 weeks of gestation),
2. Drainage of amniotic fluid for more than 18 h,
3. Maternal fever,
4. Chorioamnionitis,
5. Birth of a child with a history of GBS infection,
6. Colonization of GBS during pregnancy, especially urinary tract infection,
7. Maternal diabetes,
8. Prematurity,
9. Low birth weight.

The most common causative agents of early neonatal infections (occurring before 72 h of age) in industrialized countries include group *B streptococci*, *E. coli*, *Enterobacter*, *S. Aureus* and *S. Pneumoniae* [8]. In developing countries, infections caused by *E.coli*, *Klebsiellapneumoniae*, *Staphylococcus Aureus* and *Acinetobacter* predominate [9]. The most common form of early-onset infection is sepsis (EOS—Earlyonsetsepsis), beginning in the first hours of life and often progressing rapidly in newborns < 7 days of age. In addition to sepsis, pneumonia or meningitis may develop, being an isolated infection or complicating sepsis in about 25% of cases [6–10]. Recent studies indicate that bacterial vaginosis is a polymicrobial condition in which the processes occurring between the bacteria colonizing the vagina contribute to the formation of infection [11]. Disturbances of the microbiological balance consisting of a decrease in the physiological flora of *Lactobacilius* spp. and displacing it by pathological microbes, including *Streptococcus agalactie*, *Escherichia coli*, *Haemophilusinfluenze*, *Enterococcusfecalis* and *Peptoniphilus*, contribute to intra-amniotic infections and result in increased infectious complications in the newborn [12].

1.2. Objectives

The aim of this study was to analyze the microorganisms identified in the reproductive tract and their impact on disorders of the adaptation period in newborns. The neonatal assessment included the Apgar score, severity of jaundice, respiratory distress, the need for continuous positive airway pressure (CPAP) in the first 48 h of life and laboratory and microbiological tests.

The aim was to check the incidence of adjustment disorders among newborns, depending on the number of microorganisms detected in the reproductive tract of mothers.

2. Methods

2.1. Study Design and Data Sources

The study received consent from the Bioethics Committee of the Medical University of Silesia in Katowice, Poland, on 8 January 2019, number KNW/022/KB/307/18. Patient records were analyzed retrospectively for this study. The newborn's condition was based on the results of Apgar scores at 1, 3, 5 and 10 min of life, acid–base balance tests, complete blood count, urine and microbiological tests and inflammatory parameters, i.e., procalcitonin (PCT) and C-reactive protein (CRP) blood levels. We evaluated the need for respiratory support, parenteral nutrition, antibiotic treatment and the occurrence of severe or prolonged jaundice within the first 48 h after birth to assess adaptation issues to extrauterine life.

We analyzed the early adaptation of newborns in both groups to determine the incidence of respiratory disorders. No neonate required intubation or mechanical ventilation; frequency of use CPAP and oxygen therapy procedures were used to compare between groups. We also evaluated the rate of antibiotic therapy, parenteral nutrition and pathological jaundice in both groups.

2.2. Settings and Participants

Patients who gave birth between 1 January 2018 and 29 February 2020 were analyzed. The study included a group of 823 pregnant women who gave birth with positive cervical canal culture results from the Department of Gynecology, Obstetrics and Gynecologic Oncology, Medical University of Silesia, Katowice, Poland, and the Neonatology Department of the Hospital of the Order of Bonifraters in Katowice. On the day of admission to the hospital, before the gynecological examination, material for bacteriological examination was collected from the cervical canal in each patient by a gynecologist. Taking a vaginal swab upon admission to the hospital is a standard procedure for every pregnant woman.

The criteria for inclusion in this study were: uncomplicated single pregnancy, culture from the lower genital tract on the day of admission to the ward, natural delivery during the same hospitalization and complete medical documentation. The criteria for exclusion from the study were: cesarean section, multiple pregnancies, complicated pregnancies, pre-eclampsia, eclampsia, gestational diabetes, gestational hypertension, thrombophilia, cholestasis of pregnancy, uterine defects, fetal defects and incomplete medical records. Newborns delivered by cesarean section were excluded from this study to eliminate the possible overlapping of postnatal adaptation issues that may arise during childbirth by this method with disorders resulting from maternal colonization.

Newborns included in the study were divided into two groups due to the number of pathogens identified in the swab from the cervical canal of the mother. The first group consisted of newborns whose mothers had one pathogen identified (N = 637), while the second group consisted of newborns whose mothers had two or more pathogens identified (N = 186). Enrolment is presented in the CONSORT 2010 diagram—Figure 1.

2.3. Statistics Methods

The normality of the distributions was checked using the Shapiro–Wilk test. The analysis for normally distributed qualitative unrelated variables was performed using the Chi^2 test. The analysis for normally distributed unrelated quantitative variables was performed using the student's t-test. Quantitative variables not meeting the criteria of normal distribution were compared using the Mann–Whitney U test. All results were statistically processed in Statistica™ 12 PL software. The significance level of $p < 0.05$ was adopted as the criterion for statistical inference.

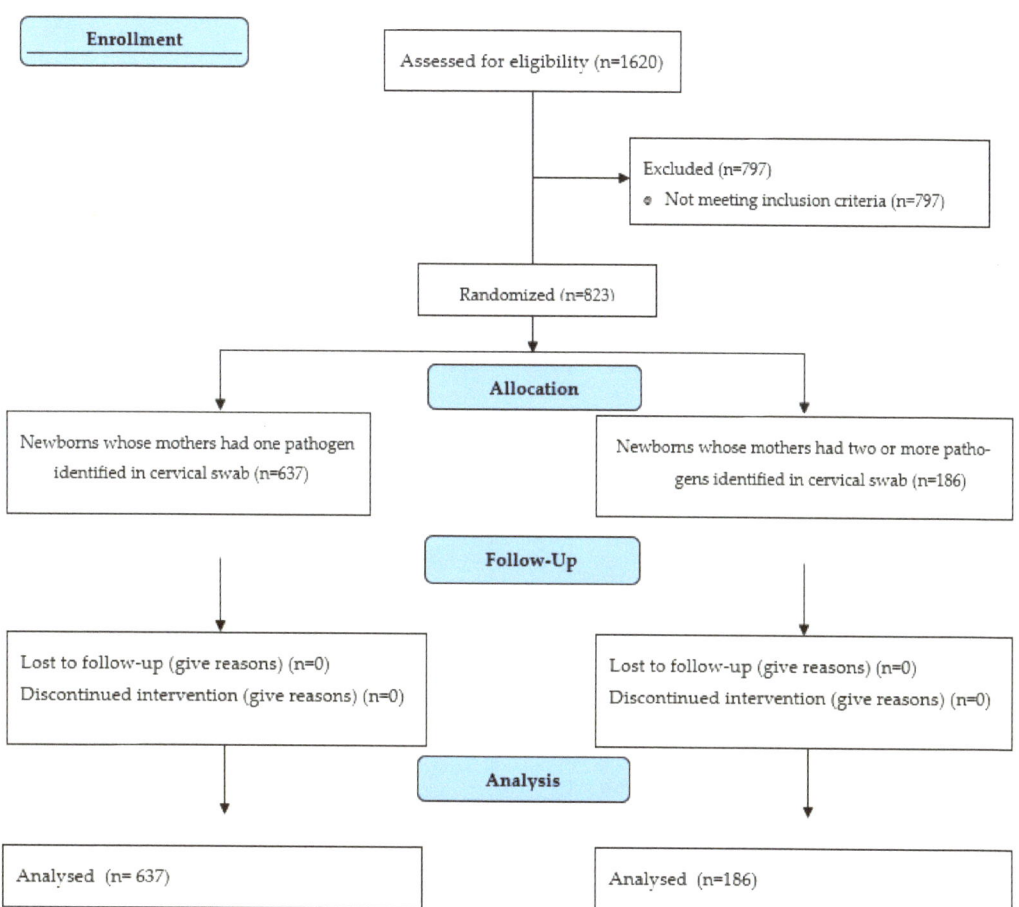

Figure 1. The CONSORT 2010 diagram—Enrolment of participants.

3. Results

The general characteristics of the study group and the control group are presented in Table 1. Both groups did not differ statistically significantly in terms of all parameters analyzed in Table 1.

The most frequently identified microorganisms in the genital tract in the presented groups were *Candida albicans* and *Streptococcus agalactiae*. All microorganisms identified in the endocervical swabs are listed in Table 2.

Table 1. General characteristics of the study and control groups—analysis with the T-student test of variables: mother's age, week of pregnancy, number of pregnancies, number of deliveries, BMI, birth weight and Apgar score. *p* value > 0.05—statistically non-significant result.

Variable	Group I (N = 637)	Group II (N = 186)	p	Effect Size
Mother's age	31.03 (SD ± 4.23)	32.1 (SD ± 4.52)	0.54	0.244
Gestational age (weeks)	39.4 (SD ± 1.94)	39.1 (SD ± 1.88)	0.32	0.157
Pregnancy	1.75 (SD ± 0.91)	1.83 (SD ± 0.89)	0.08	0.089
Parity	1.59 (SD ± 0.80)	1.45 (SD ± 0.68)	0.77	0.189
BMI (kg/m^2)	27.1 (SD ± 3.45)	26.7 (SD ± 2.88)	0.63	0.126
Birth weight (g)	3366 (SD ± 493)	3402 (SD ± 456)	0.37	0.076
Apgar score (1 min)	8.83 (SD ± 0.57)	8.33 (SD ± 1.03)	0.20	0.601
Apgar score (3 min)	9.78 (SD ± 0.77)	9.79 (SD ± 0.92)	0.83	0.012
Apgar score (5 min)	9.37 (SD ± 0.54)	9.23 (SD ± 0.72)	0.44	0.220
Apgar score (10 min)	9.63 (SD ± 0.80)	9.67 (SD ± 0.74)	0.94	0.052

Table 2. Types of microorganisms identified in swabs from the cervical canal and their frequency.

Lp	Pathogen	Group I (N = 637)	Group II (N = 186)
1	Candida albicans	302	156
2	Streptococcus agalactiae	247	148
3	Candida glabrata	42	35
4	Staphylococcus aureus MSSA	29	26
5	Candida tropicalis	10	14
6	Enterococcus faecalis	2	3
7	Trichomonas vaginalis	1	0
8	Klebsiella pneumoniae	1	1
9	Candida krusei	1	1
10	Escherichia coli	1	18
11	Staphylococcus aureus MRSA	1	2

Comparing the parameters of the acid–base balance, inflammatory markers and bilirubin, lower pH values were observed in group II than in group I (7.31 ± 0.07 vs. 7.39 ± 0.02). Saturation values were also lower in group II than in group I (78.91 ± 13.1 vs. 83.44 ± 6.91). The concentration of HCO3- was statistically significantly lower in group II than in group I (19.17 ± 3.23 vs. 23.22 ± 2.64). The results of the parameters of inflammation from the first day of life were higher in group II than in group I (8.52 ± 8.02 vs. 7.24 ± 6.12), while statistical significance was observed when comparing the concentration of procalcitonin (1.74 ± 1.11 vs. 0.67 ± 0.52), bilirubin (8.92 ± 4.05 vs. 7.92 ± 3.67) and leukocytes (19.57 ± 7.48 vs. 12.51 ± 4.35) in the complete blood count of newborns. The results are presented in Table 3.

Table 3. Comparison of blood gas, inflammatory markers and bilirubin test results in the analyzed groups of newborns—analysis using the student t-test. p-values > 0.05—statistically non-significant result.

Variable	Group I (N = 637)	Group II (N = 186)	p	Effect Size
pH	7.39 (SD ± 0.02)	7.31 (SD ± 0.07)	0.0001	1.554
BE (mEq/l)	−3.61 (SD ± 2.21)	−6.13 (SD ± 3.72)	0.06	0.824
pO$_2$ (mmHg)	46.21 (SD ± 11.01)	45.78 (SD ± 13.11)	0.67	0.036
pCO$_2$ (mmHg)	36.75 (SD ± 8.61)	36.66 (SD ± 7.11)	0.88	0.011
HCO$_3-$ (mmol/L)	23.22 (SD ± 2.64)	19.17 (SD ± 3.23)	0.0001	1.373
Saturation (%)	83.44 (SD ± 6.91)	78.91 (SD ± 13.1)	0.03	0.433
CRP (mg/L)	7.24 (SD ± 6.12)	8.52 (SD ± 8.02)	0.34	0.179
Procalcitonin (ng/mL)	0.67 (SD ± 0.52)	1.74 (SD ± 1.11)	0.01	1.235
Bilirubin (mg/dL)	7.92 (SD ± 3.67)	8.92 (SD ± 4.05)	0.03	0.259
WBC (tys/µL)	12.51 (SD ± 4.35)	19.57 (SD ± 7.48)	0.0001	1.154
Granulocytes (%)	54.67 (SD ± 11.39)	56.42 (SD ± 9.76)	0.15	0.165

The analysis of disorders of the early adaptation period included the incidence of respiratory distress syndrome and the number of procedures performed with the use of CPAP, oxygen therapy, antibiotic therapy and parenteral nutrition. In addition, the number of newborns diagnosed with pathological jaundice was examined. Respiratory distress syndrome was more common in group II than in group I (85 vs. 31, p = 0.001). In group II, CPAP (63 vs. 21, p = 0.001), oxygen therapy (15 vs. 8, p = 0.02) and antibiotics were used more frequent (13 vs. 8, p = 0.01). The results are presented in Table 4.

Table 4. Analysis of disorders of the early adaptation period and procedures performed in a group of newborns from the study group and the control group—analysis with the Chi^2-Pearson test. p-values > 0.05—statistically non-significant result.

Variable	Group I (N = 637)	Group II (N = 186)	p	Cramer's V
Respiratory disorder syndrome	31	85	0.001	0.491
CPAP	21	63	0.001	0.422
Oxygen therapy	8	15	0.02	0.173
Antibiotics	8	13	0.01	0.152
Parenteral nutrition	7	8	0.2	0.100
Jaundice	122	98	0.04	0.317

Infections occurred in 21 neonates and were statistically significantly more common in group II—13 (61.9%)—than in group I: 8 (38.1%), p = 0.01. We studied the correlation between premature amniotic fluid leakage in mothers and neonatal infections. However, the results showed no statistical significance (p > 0.05). There were no incidents of early sepsis in both groups of neonates. Most common in both groups were infections of undetermined origin: II—8 (61.5%) vs. I—4 (38.5%). This difference was statistically significant (p = 0.01). For other types of infections, the differences were not statistically significant.

The relationship between infections was also analyzed statistically using neonates and premature amniotic fluid leakage in the mother; however, the results were not statistically significant ($p > 0.05$).

A division was also made according to the type and number of infections. Infections were more frequently observed in group II than in group I. The most common infections were infections with an undetermined origin—8 (61.5%) vs. 4 (38.5%); this result was statistically significant ($p = 0.01$). No statistically significant differences were found for other types of infection. The results are presented in Table 5.

Table 5. Analysis of the type and frequency of infection in newborns in the study groups performed with the Chi^2–Pearson test. p-values > 0.05—statistically non-significant result.

Type of Infection	Group I (N= 8)	Group II (N = 13)	p	Cramer's V
Pneumonia	3	3	0.27	0.155
Urinary tract infection	1	2	0.14	0.040
Infection of undetermined origin	4	8	0.01	0.113

4. Discussion

There are data suggesting the possible intrauterine contact of the fetus with DNA and bacterial metabolites [13]. The results of studies on the importance of providing the child with the microbiota of the reproductive tract during childbirth clearly indicate the beneficial effect of such colonization on postnatal adaptation, the colonization of the newborn's gastrointestinal tract and the stimulation of its immune system. At the same time, however, colonization with the mother's bacterial flora may cause infection of the newborn [14].

Among the detected infections, the largest part were infections with an undetermined origin, followed by pneumonia and urinary tract infections. In the presented studies, no case of neonatal sepsis was found. According to the available worldwide data, the incidence of early-onset neonatal sepsis varies between 4 and 22 per 1000 newborns [8]. One of the aims of this study was to identify the relationship between the number of pathogens colonizing the cervical canal and the occurrence of infections in newborns. There were statistically significant differences between group II and group I: 13 (61.9%) vs. 8 (38.1%), $p = 0.01$. When dividing by the type of infection, a higher incidence of infections was also observed in group II. In a meta-analysis, Chan et al. confirmed the correlation between maternal infection and neonatal infection.

In the cited study, the authors analyzed the relationship between a positive smear result and the presence of infection in a newborn and showed a correlation. In the seven studies they reviewed, 5.0% (95% CI 1.9–8.2) of maternal colonization cases had clinical signs of neonatal infection. In this study's analyzed own material, the percentage of infections in newborns was 2.54%—21 cases of infection were recorded. These results confirm the legitimacy of using smears in women before childbirth, as the pathological bacterial flora of the mother's reproductive tract has an impact on the occurrence of infection in the newborn [8,15]. The presence of pathological flora in the cervix affects the occurrence of PROM in the mother, which may lead to the development of FIRS in the fetus. This can lead to birth asphyxia or the development of infection in the newborn. The colonization of the genital tract with a diverse pathological flora may also have an immunomodulatory effect on the fetus, as demonstrated by the studies of Gilbert et al. carried out on mice. The coexistence of different types of microorganisms, e.g., *Gardnerella vaginalis*, can stimulate the growth of other strains and cause infections, as evidenced by Gilbert's research. Antibiotic therapy used during pregnancy may also have an immunomodulatory effect on strains colonizing the reproductive tract. The development of resistance to antibiotics may be associated with an increased rate of infection with drug-resistant strains such as MRSA.

In recent years, an increase in the rate of infections in neonatal intensive care units with methicillin-resistant staphylococci has been observed [16,17].

The analysis of disorders of the early adaptation period in a newborn, carried out in our own study, indicates a more frequent occurrence of disorders in group II than in group I. Newborns exposed to many microorganisms present in the mother's cervical canal more often presented respiratory disorders in the first days of life. Respiratory disorders were present in 85 (10.3%) newborns in group II, while in group I there were 31 (3.7%) cases, $p = 0.001$. These results are confirmed by studies by Edwards et al., who indicate an infectious factor as one of the factors determining respiratory disorders in a newborn [18]. So far, it has been proven that breathing disorders in the early adaptation period affect about 7% of children. A higher percentage of respiratory disorders occurs in the group of newborns born before 37 weeks of gestation and amounts to 34%. Then, it gradually decreases until the 41st week of pregnancy, where it is about 0.5%. However, from year to year, the tendency of respiratory distress syndrome in neonates born at term is observed more and more often [16,17,19,20]. Breathing disorders in newborns from full-term pregnancies occur most often in the form of TTN (Transient Tachypnea of the newborn). This is confirmed by our own research where about 90% of breathing disorders observed in newborns covered by this study were transient breathing disorders. The analysis by Gizzi et al. comparing the use of oxygen therapy and CPAP respiratory support confirms the better effect and greater usefulness of CPAP in the group of newborns with TTN. In the collected research material, respiratory support with CPAP was more often used in group II than in group I, respectively, 63 vs. 21, $p = 0.001$. This is because more TTN cases were reported in the study group.

The acid–base balance parameters checked in the study show that in group I, newborns achieved higher results of saturation, pH and pO_2 compared to group II. This is also related to the parameters of inflammation examined in children in the first days of life. The levels of procalcitonin and WBC were statistically significantly higher in group II than in group I.

None of the infants observed developed sepsis and only three of the 63 infants requiring respiratory support in group II developed pneumonia. The results of our study suggest the possibility of the prolonged and complicated adaptation to the extrauterine life of full-term infants in the case of the multifactorial colonization of the mother's reproductive tract. However, in the observed group, prolonged and complicated early adaptation was not associated with the more frequent diagnosis of neonatal infection. The results of our study were similar to those of other centers [18,21]. Considering the widespread early use of antibiotics, the data obtained in our study suggest the vigilant observation of full-term newborns in the event of impaired early adaptation and the use of early-onset sepsis calculators to guide antibiotic management in Term Neonates, rather than the rapid initiation of antibacterial therapy.

This study was a retrospective analysis of the documentation of completed hospitalizations of mother–newborn couples. In the case of suspected infection in the neonate during the first 72 h of life, the scope of examinations depended on the clinical symptoms presented by the child. Not all children underwent the same diagnostic tests, which makes it difficult to compare the two groups of neonatal patients. This study included mother–child pairs in which the bacteriological examination of the genital tract at admission was positive in mothers. The goal was to compare differences in the adaptation of the newborns depending on the number of cultured microorganisms. The limitation of this study is the lack of comparison of the incidence of adaptation disorders and infections in newborns in the culture-positive group to the incidence of the same in newborns of mothers whose bacteriological tests were negative.

In addition, in the group of patients with multifactorial colonization regarding the reproductive tract, an attempt was made to divide into subgroups depending on the configuration of the cultured microorganisms. However, the population in each subgroup was too small to obtain statistical significance; therefore, the results were not credible and the reliable assessment of differences in the quality and severity of neonatal adaptation disorders depending on colonization was impossible.

5. Conclusions

1. The number of pathogens colonizing the reproductive tract affects the early adaptation period in newborns.
2. Polymicrobial colonization of the reproductive tract increases the incidence of acid–base balance disorders in newborns.
3. Multifactorial colonization of the reproductive tract increases the number of infections in newborns. However, it does not affect the incidence of early-onset sepsis or pneumonia in full-term newborns.

6. Implications

We understand the importance of conveying the practical implications of our findings. In the revised manuscript, we have expanded our discussion to include possible clinical implications based on our study results. Specifically, we have discussed the potential benefits and challenges of routine screening for cervicovaginal infections and the empirical use of antibiotic prophylaxis for these infections in pregnant women. We believe this will provide clearer guidance to the readers on the relevance of our study to clinical practice.

Author Contributions: Conceptualization, P.G., Z.S.-G., A.J.-L. and R.S.; methodology, P.G., Z.S.-G., A.J.-L. and R.S.; validation, P.G., A.J.-L. and J.S.; formal analysis, J.S. and R.S.; investigation, P.G., Z.S.-G. and A.J.-L.; resources, P.G., Z.S.-G., A.J.-L. and J.S.; data curation, P.G., Z.S.-G., A.J.-L. and J.S.; writing—original draft preparation P.G., Z.S.-G., A.J.-L. and R.S.; writing—review and editing, J.S.; visualization, P.G. and J.S.; supervision, J.S., A.J.-L. and R.S.; project administration, P.G. and R.S. All authors have read and agreed to the published version of the manuscript.

Funding: This research received no external funding.

Institutional Review Board Statement: The study received consent from the Bioethics Committee of the Medical University of Silesia in Katowice, Poland, on 8 January 2019, number KNW/022/KB/307/18.

Informed Consent Statement: Not applicable.

Data Availability Statement: The data presented in this study are available on request from the corresponding author.

Conflicts of Interest: The authors declare no conflict of interest.

References

1. Witkowska, K.; Głowacka, M.; Słodki, M.; Wierzba, W.; Piórkowska, K. Intensifying transition states in newborns depending on the gender and mode of delivery—A prospective, comparative analysis. *Med. Ogólna I Nauk. O Zdrowiu* **2020**, *26*, 134–138. [CrossRef]
2. Kumar, M.; Saadaoui, M.; Al Khodor, S. Infections and Pregnancy: Effects on Maternal and Child Health. *Front. Cell. Infect. Microbiol.* **2022**, *12*, 873253. [CrossRef] [PubMed]
3. Megli, C.J.; Coyne, C.B. Infections at the maternal–fetal interface: An overview of pathogenesis and defence. *Nat. Rev. Microbiol.* **2022**, *20*, 67–82. [CrossRef]
4. Yancey, M.K.; Duff, P.A. An analysis of cost-effectivenes of selected protocols for the prevention of neonatal group B streptococcal infection. *Obstet. Gynecol.* **1994**, *83*, 367–371. [PubMed]
5. Verani, J.R.; McGee, L.; Schrag, S.J. Prevention of perinatal group B streptococcal disease—Revised guidelines from CDC. *MMWR Recomm. Rep.* **2010**, *59*, 1–36.
6. O'Sullivan, C.P.; Lamagni, T.; Patel, D.; Efstratiou, A.; Cunney, R.; Meehan, M.; Ladhani, S.; Reynolds, A.J.; Campbell, R.; Doherty, L.; et al. Group B streptococcal disease in UK and Irish infants younger than 90 days, 2014–2015: A prospective surveillance study. *Lancet Infect Dis.* **2019**, *19*, 83–90. [CrossRef]
7. Esper, F. Postnatal bacterial infections. In *Fanaroff & Martin's Neonatal-Perinatal Medicine. Diseases of the Fetus and Infant*, 11th ed.; Martin, R.J., Fanaroff, A.A., Walsh, M., Eds.; Elsevier Saunders: Philadelphia, PA, USA, 2020.
8. Glaser, M.A.; Hughes, L.M.; Jnah, A.; Newberry, D. Neonatal Sepsis: A Review of Pathophysiology and Current Management Strategies. *Adv. Neonatal. Care* **2021**, *21*, 49–60. [CrossRef]

9. Birhane Fiseha, S.; Mulatu Jara, G.; Azerefegn Woldetsadik, E.; Belayneh Bekele, F.; Mohammed Ali, M. Colonization Rate of Potential Neonatal Disease-Causing Bacteria, Associated Factors, and Antimicrobial Susceptibility Profile Among Pregnant Women Attending Government Hospitals in Hawassa, Ethiopia. *Infect. Drug Resist.* **2021**, *14*, 3159–3168. [CrossRef]
10. Ohlsson, A.; Shah, V. Intrapartum antibiotics for known maternal Group B streptococcal colonization. *Cochrane Database Syst. Rev.* **2009**, *3*, CD007467.
11. Payne, M.S.; Bayatibojakhi, S. Exploring preterm birth as a polymicrobial dis-ease: An overview of the uterine microbiome. *Front. Immunol.* **2014**, *5*, 595. [CrossRef] [PubMed]
12. Brown, R.G.; Al-Memar, M.; Marchesi, J.R.; Lee, Y.S.; Smith, A.; Chan, D.; Lewis, H.; Kindinger, L.; Terzidou, V.; Bourne, T.; et al. Establishment of vaginal microbiota composition in early pregnancy and its association with subsequent preterm prelabor rupture of the fetal membranes. *Transl. Res.* **2018**, *207*, 30–43. [CrossRef] [PubMed]
13. Stinson, L.F.; Boyce, M.C.; Payne, M.S.; Keelan, J.A. The Not-so-Sterile Womb: Evidence That the Human Fetus Is Exposed to Bacteria Prior to Birth. *Front. Microbiol.* **2019**, *10*, 1124. [CrossRef] [PubMed]
14. Mueller, N.T.; Bakacs, E.; Combellick, J.; Grigoryan, Z.; Dominguez-Bello, M.G. The infant microbiome development: Mom matters. *Trends Mol. Med.* **2015**, *21*, 109–117. [CrossRef] [PubMed]
15. Chan, G.J.; Lee, A.C.; Baqui, A.H.; Tan, J.; Black, R.E. Prevalence of early-onset neonatal infection among newborns of mothers with bacterial infection or colonization: A systematic review and meta-analysis. *BMC Infect. Dis.* **2015**, *15*, 118. [CrossRef] [PubMed]
16. Qian, L.-L.; Liu, C.-Q.; Guo, Y.-X.; Jiang, Y.-J.; Ni, L.-M.; Xia, S.-W.; Liu, X.-H.; Zhuang, W.-Z.; Xiao, Z.-H.; Wang, S.-N.; et al. Chinese Collaborative Study Group for Neonatal Respiratory Diseases. Current status of neonatal acute respiratory disorders: A one-year prospective survey from a Chinese neonatal network. *Chin. Med. J.* **2010**, *123*, 2769–2775. [PubMed]
17. Gizzi, C.; Klifa, R.; Pattumelli, M.G.; Massenzi, L.; Taveira, M.; Shankar-Aguilera, S.; De Luca, D. Continuous Positive Airway Pressure and the Burden of Care for Transient Tachypnea of the Neonate: Retrospective Cohort Study. *Am. J. Perinatol.* **2015**, *32*, 939–943. [CrossRef] [PubMed]
18. Edwards, M.O.; Kotecha, S.J.; Kotecha, S. Respiratory distress of the term newborn infant. *Paediatr. Respir. Rev.* **2013**, *14*, 29–36. [CrossRef] [PubMed]
19. Alfarwati, T.W.; Alamri, A.A.; Alshahrani, M.A.; Al-Wassia, H. Incidence, Risk factors and Outcome of Respiratory Distress Syndrome in Term Infants at Academic Centre, Jeddah, Saudi Arabia. *Med. Arch.* **2019**, *73*, 183–186. [CrossRef] [PubMed]
20. Consortium on Safe Labor; Hibbard, J.U.; Wilkins, I.; Sun, L.; Gregory, K.; Haberman, S.; Hoffman, M.; Kominiarek, M.A.; Reddy, U.; Bailit, J.; et al. Respiratory morbidity in late preterm births. *JAMA* **2010**, *304*, 419–425. [CrossRef] [PubMed]
21. Frymoyer, A.; Joshi, N.S.; Allan, J.M.; Cohen, R.S.; Aby, J.L.; Kim, J.L.; Benitz, W.E.; Gupta, A. Sustainability of a Clinical Examination-Based Approach for Ascertainment of Early-Onset Sepsis in Late Preterm and Term Neonates. *J. Pediatr.* **2020**, *225*, 263–268. [CrossRef] [PubMed]

Disclaimer/Publisher's Note: The statements, opinions and data contained in all publications are solely those of the individual author(s) and contributor(s) and not of MDPI and/or the editor(s). MDPI and/or the editor(s) disclaim responsibility for any injury to people or property resulting from any ideas, methods, instructions or products referred to in the content.

MDPI AG
Grosspeteranlage 5
4052 Basel
Switzerland
Tel.: +41 61 683 77 34

Journal of Clinical Medicine Editorial Office
E-mail: jcm@mdpi.com
www.mdpi.com/journal/jcm

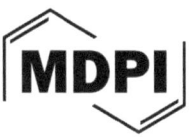

Disclaimer/Publisher's Note: The title and front matter of this reprint are at the discretion of the Guest Editors. The publisher is not responsible for their content or any associated concerns. The statements, opinions and data contained in all individual articles are solely those of the individual Editors and contributors and not of MDPI. MDPI disclaims responsibility for any injury to people or property resulting from any ideas, methods, instructions or products referred to in the content.

www.ingramcontent.com/pod-product-compliance
Lightning Source LLC
LaVergne TN
LVHW072325090526
838202LV00019B/2351